Health Education Evaluation and Measurement

A Practitioner's Perspective
Second Edition

Health Education Evaluation and Measurement

A Practitioner's Perspective
Second Edition

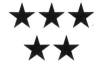

Robert J. McDermott
University of South Florida College of Public Health
Department of Community and Family Health

Paul D. Sarvela
Southern Illinois University
Center for Rural Health and Social Services Development
and
Department of Health Education and Recreation

WCB/McGraw-Hill

*A Division of The **McGraw-Hill** Companies*

HEALTH EDUCATION EVALUATION AND MEASUREMENT:
A PRACTITIONER'S PERSPECTIVE, SECOND EDITION

This book is printed on acid-free paper.

2 3 4 5 6 7 8 9 0 DOC/DOC 9 3 2 1 0 9

ISBN 0–697–22322–1

Vice president and editorial director: *Kevin T. Kane*
Publisher: *Edward E. Bartell*
Editorial assistant: *Kristine Fisher*
Senior marketing manager: *Pamela S. Cooper*
Senior project manager: *Kay J. Brimeyer*
Production supervisor: *Sandy Ludovissy*
Designer: *JoAnne Schopler*
Printer: *R. R. Donnelley & Sons Company/Crawfordsville, IN*

Library of Congress Catalog Card Number: 98–88621

In honor of our family members, those living,
as well as those who have passed on,
our other loved ones, our dearest friends,
our esteemed colleagues, and our students,
from whom we have learned so much,
we dedicate this book.

Table of Contents

11 Qualitative Evaluation: Methods and Designs 224

12 Survey Methods and Evaluation 243

13 Methods and Strategies for Sampling 264

From the Authors

Once an Olympic skier makes a downhill run, it is over. Once a concert artist performs a solo, it is done. For a sculptor who completes a piece of work, it becomes a finished monument to the effort that inspired it. For us, as authors, this second edition has given us the ability to "fine tune" our run, improve our cadenza, and better define our sculpture.

New features emanate from recommendations of students and colleagues. The two of us are more skilled and learned than we were when set out to compose the first edition. Where possible, we draw upon our experiences. We are purposely redundant on occasion, because experiences have taught us that certain things need to be said more than once.

As with the first edition, our goal is to present a "user friendly" book. We have retained, updated, and expanded the learning tools (chapter objectives, key terms, case studies, and chapter summaries). We have included recommended readings at the end of each chapter, and an expanded glossary for quick reference and study.

We have added sections on important areas such as gathering data from young children, working with persons of other languages or cultural traditions, and conducting surveys via the Internet. We have expanded our coverage of ethics in guiding evaluation decisions. We have added two new chapters: Chapter 2, which addresses the use of conceptual models that drive evaluation; and Chapter 12, prepared initially by Dr. Karen M. (Kay) Perrin, which addresses how to plan and conduct surveys.

We wish to give special thanks to our colleagues and friends at the University of South Florida and Southern Illinois University-Carbondale, for their help, support, and occasional inspiration in preparing the second edition. We also recognize the experiences provided by persons at the Florida and Illinois Departments of Health that have made us better program evaluators; and Dr. Klaus Klein, of the University of Cologne, who has given us some international opportunities and perspectives. We are deeply appreciative.

Evaluation can be an enjoyable and exciting challenge. This potential is especially realized if evaluators work in concert with other program stakeholders to develop a responsive and useful evaluation plan. To conduct evaluations under these circumstances is a pleasure, and the delivery of a timely report to the sponsoring agency is a rewarding achievement.

This satisfaction extends for us in the process of writing this book. We have enjoyed climbing the mountain for the second "run" at writing. We hope that you will enjoy the ride down the hill, and will, at the end, be both a better consumer of evaluation reports, and a person confident in initiating your own evaluation projects.

Robert J. McDermott, Ph.D.,
Tampa, FL

Paul D. Sarvela, Ph.D.,
Carbondale, IL

Chapter

1

Program Evaluation:
Who?Whom?What?Why?Where?When?How?

Chapter Objectives

After completing this chapter, you should be able to:

1. Define evaluation from several different viewpoints and philosophies.
2. Highlight the history of program evaluation with particular attention to health education evaluation.
3. Give an array of purposes for performing evaluation.
4. Distinguish among different types of evaluation.
5. Conduct an evaluability assessment of a program.
6. Identify the targets of program evaluation.
7. Establish a realistic scope of evaluation efforts.

Key Terms

continuous quality improvement
evaluability assessment
formative evaluation
impact evaluation
outcome evaluation
process evaluation

program evaluation
quality assurance
quality control
summative evaluation
total quality management

Introduction

Benjamin Franklin once wrote:

"In this world, nothing can be said to be certain except death and taxes."

Today, there should be a modification to this statement:

"In this world, nothing can be said to be certain except death, taxes, and being *evaluated*."

After all, from the moment we are born to the moment we die, we are evaluated. Just after birth, a baby is given a number of tests. The baby is measured and weighed, checked for birth defects, and given an Apgar test at one and five minutes that measures basic physiological functioning. The physician uses these data and others to determine a course of care for the newborn. These data also are reported on a birth certificate, which is sent to the local health department. Thus, not only is the baby being evaluated, but so is the general public health of the community. The birth certificate data are analyzed to determine prevalence of such things as premature births, low birth weight babies, birth defects, and demographic characteristics of the parents. Extending the discussion a step further, one may argue that today, babies are frequently evaluated even before they are born, using sophisticated procedures such as ultrasound, amniocentesis, and emerging biomedical tests that assess the health status of the baby.

The cycle of evaluation continues throughout life. We are tested (some would say *over*-tested) throughout our school years. Again, not only is the individual evaluated when taking an important test (e.g., when taking an ACT or SAT test), but so are the schools. Every year, newspapers report how local school districts compare to each other in terms of standardized test scores, and how the local schools compare to state and national averages. Legislative bodies take interest too, sometimes withholding appropriations to "underachieving schools" or threatening to scrutinize teachers' tenure.

One might finish university studies, fraught with evaluation throughout the course of study, and then be required to take a licensing or certification test (e.g., an exam to be a teacher, a registered nurse, or a certified health education specialist) just to work in the profession for which one was prepared. Persons who join the armed forces face a barrage of tests (e.g., medical physicals and fitness, aptitude, and qualification tests). Nursing programs, law schools, medical schools, and other professional schools are frequently evaluated, in part, by how many of their students pass professional examinations.

Even during the final stages of life, and thereafter, one is evaluated. The physician tests our brain to see if we are dead. Once we die, our age, cause of death, and other personal characteristics are reported on a death certificate. And of course, these data are reported to the health department, so, again, our community can be evaluated in terms of mortality rates as compared to the norms established by state and federal health agencies.

Clearly, evaluation is an important part of daily life, and customary in some form for all professions. In business and industry it is known as quality control; in health care, it might instead be called quality assurance. Many school systems employ evaluators in some capacity, as public expectations concerning accountability of educational programs increase. Like other professionals, health educators view evaluation as an important part of delivering quality programs to target populations.

Just as health education evaluators work in an array of settings, they also are charged with a variety of tasks. The achievement of each task can be evaluated in different ways. Through this text, we seek to introduce you to some of the basic elements of conducting effective and defensible evaluations of health education and promotion programs and materials.

A Historical Overview of Program Evaluation

Program evaluation is often viewed as a recent phenomenon, first achieving prominence in the 1960s. However, program evaluation has taken an active role in the educational process for thousands of years. Shortell and Richardson (1978) indicate that the evaluation of medical programs is centuries old. Today's evaluations are related to sanctions in Egypt around 3000 B.C., where if a patient lost his or her eye unnecessarily, the physician could lose a hand. Worthen and Sanders (1987) note that Chinese officials, as early as 2000 B.C., used civil service examinations to measure proficiency of public officials. They further indicate that Socrates and other early Greeks used verbal exams as an important component of teaching.

Madaus, Stufflebeam, and Scriven (1983) describe the evolution of evaluation in six stages:

- The Age of Reform (pre-1900)
- The Age of Efficiency & Testing (1900-1930)
- The Tylerian Age (1931-1945)
- The Age of Innocence (1946-1957)
- The Age of Expansion (1958-1972)
- The Age of Professionalization (1973-1983)

We would add that a seventh stage, an "age of accountability," has evolved in the past 15 years or so that places evaluation in the context of being more responsive to program stakeholders than ever before.

The Age of Reform took place before the 1900s. In 1870, the Royal Commission of Inquiry into Primary Education in Ireland, after conducting an evaluation based on testimony and examining evidence indicated:

> *"The progress of the children in the national schools of Ireland is very much less than it ought to be."*

Members of the Commission indicated that a "Payment by Results" strategy could be used to remedy the situation; a teacher's salary would be dependent on student performance. During this time period, school evaluations were frequent. They were conducted by an inspectorate charged with assessing school performance. In the U.S., the first recorded school-based evaluation took place in Boston in 1845, where test scores were used to evaluate the effectiveness of an instructional program.

Written exams, modeled after the ones used in Europe, were introduced by Horace Mann at this same time. The written exams replaced the *viva voce* or oral exams that had been in use. The historically interesting point is that there was a hidden agenda behind the move to use written exams. Written exams were used to enable administrators to compare schools, and to facilitate decisions concerning the annual appointments of headmasters. Obviously, it would have been difficult, if not impossible, to compare schools if only oral exams were used.

In the late 1800s Joseph Rice conducted the first formal educational program evaluation in the U.S., finding no significant learning gains between those school systems spending 200 minutes a week studying spelling and those spending as few as 10 minutes a week on this task. His investigation can be seen as one of the first "experimental" studies that compared different educational treatments (in this case, different time lengths spent on studying spelling) and achievement.

At this time, the North Central Association of Colleges and Secondary Schools was established. This association and similar accrediting organizations were responsible for setting certain minimum standards that schools had to meet to gain accreditation status. In addition, these associations assessed the degree to which minimum standards were met through systematic site reviews by teams of experts.

The Age of Efficiency & Testing (1900-1930) was a period of time when scientific management was seen as an important administrative tool. The emphasis was on systemization, standardization, and efficiency.

Experts conducted large-scale surveys that focused on school and teacher effectiveness. A report entitled "Methods for Measuring Teachers' Efficiency and the Standards for the Measurement and the Efficiency of Schools and School Systems" was published during this time. In addition, standardized testing, which was used on a large scale basis for selection purposes during World War I, also became popularized. Schools extensively used standardized tests to evaluate effectiveness and efficiency.

The Tylerian Age (1931-1945) is named after Ralph Tyler, who many evaluation specialists consider the "inventor" of educational evaluation. The Tyler Rationale for evaluation and curriculum building came from the now-famous "Eight-Year Study." Tyler examined the effectiveness of various types of schooling, comparing for example, "traditional" schools with "liberal" schools. Tyler (1949) emphasized that evaluation should focus on the *outcomes* of the program. He is given credit as the first person to institute objective-based testing programs, or what eventually became known as goal-oriented evaluations.

The Age of Innocence (1946-1957) was a time of great expansion in schools. Plenty of two key ingredients, optimism and money, were available for school program development. However, little work was done in the general area of evaluation, with the exception of test development and the use of experimental designs to assess educational programs, and little emphasis was given to how one improves schools.

The Age of Expansion (1958-1972) began as a response to the launching of the Russian Sputnik satellite. Sputnik had a tremendous impact on the American educational system because of the outcry that educational programs lagged far behind their Soviet counterparts. In the face of this criticism and the growing fear of the "Red menace" of communism, the American educational system made widespread policy and curriculum changes.

Major evaluations of important social programs also took place at this time. For example, evaluations of Title I programs designed for disadvantaged youth often were based on classical evaluation strategies, such as objective-based testing. These methods were unsuccessful in assessing needs and achievement gains of Title I populations. On the basis of these and other findings, educators argued that new methods of program evaluation must be developed and implemented.

In 1971, a commission founded by Phi Delta Kappa, an educational honorary society, indicated that "evaluation was seized with great illness." New ideas were needed for evaluation. Professionals recognized the tremendous need for the evaluation of the implementation *process*, instead of focusing strictly on program *outcomes*. New models and ideas were developed based on the notion that one must look at inputs, implementation, and intended and unintended outcomes, and not just whether the program met its stated objectives.

The Age of Professionalization (1973-1983) is identified by two simple events: (1) the recognized existence of a body of literature specific to program evaluation; and (2) the development of professional organizations devoted to the practice and improvement of program evaluation. The American Evaluation Association is an important professional organization, and the results of program evaluations are an important part of most meetings about health services, health education, or general public health. Evaluation methods are now emphasized, and new ways of evaluating programs are proposed continuously.

The Age of Accountability (1984-present) is where we now find ourselves. As early as 1971, Stufflebeam (1971) talked about accountability in education through better program evaluation. House (1990) indicates that between 1965 and 1990, there were changes in methodology, philosophy, and politics of evaluation. Evaluation changed from a quantitative process restricted to quasi-experimental designs, to one that includes qualitative and mixed qualitative-quantitative approaches. Today, skilled evaluators recognize that many tools are available to them. A primary task in evaluation, as with any task, is in the selection of the right tool for the right job. Moreover, at virtually every level and function, accountability to CEOs, stockholders, rank and file workers, taxpayers, the electorate, and legislative bodies rules the day and necessitates sound, precise, and valid evaluations performed by skilled individuals.

History of Health Education Evaluation

Health education evaluation has a more recent history. Pigg (1976) suggests that there was little evaluation activity in school health education in the nineteenth century because before that time, there was no organized school health education. Although Pigg (1976) describes a number of different "demonstration" projects that took place in the early 1900s, he argues that the most influential evaluation study that focused on school health instruction did not occur until the "School Health Education Study" (SHES) was conducted in the 1960s (Sliepcevich, 1964). This monumental study involved the collection of student health practices data and information concerning health education programs from teachers and administrators in thirty-eight states. Historically, the SHES can be seen as an "overture" to the health education evaluation work that began in earnest during the 1970s. In the 1970s, most state and federal grant programs required rigorous evaluations as integrated features of almost all projects. To be approved for grant monies, evaluation components typically had to be included in proposals. Many administrators viewed evaluation as an excellent decision-making tool. In the 1980s, results of the School Health Education Evaluation (1985) demonstrated that certain conditions could maximize the effects of comprehensive school health education. In the 1990s, ongoing data acquired through the Centers for Disease Control and Prevention's (1994) Youth Risk Behavior Surveillance System (YRBSS) provides health educators with a plethora of information for program needs assessment and evaluation.

In addition, the Society for Public Health Education (SOPHE) indicated that evaluation was a critical skills area for health educators (Green & Lewis, 1986). Evaluation was now considered an important element in the professional preparation of all health educators. This point is reinforced by the fact that most collegiate health education programs offer such courses. Moreover the National Commission on Health Education Credentialing, Inc. (NCHEC), incorporates "evaluation" as one of the seven areas of responsibility, and this subject matter is part of the national test given to persons seeking to earn the certified health education specialist (CHES) credential (NCHEC, 1996).

The Purposes of Evaluation

Why should health education specialists be concerned with evaluating programs they deliver? Green and Lewis (1986) argue that health educators should demonstrate the effectiveness of their programs through evaluation to improve the credibility of their specific program and of health education in general. In addition, they indicate that because major health organizations (e.g., The American Cancer Society, the National Institute on Drug Abuse, Robert Wood Johnson Foundation) invest large sums of money for health education and human services program development and implementation, administrators from these organizations want evidence that indicates that programs are "good." Historically, health and human services programs have received financial support on the basis of their presumed or "intrinsic good" (Burchard & Schaefer, 1992) rather than on their actual effectiveness and true cost (Gore & Brown, 1993). As Nelson (1993) writes: "It has become a well-worn observation that success in human services is too often measured by persons served or services provided and too rarely by results achieved" (p.4). Unfortunately, the question of "whether to evaluate" when resources are so scarce is a persistent one that funders, policymakers, and program leaders all face (Peck, 1996). Wouldn't one do more good just investing the resources in program delivery?

What does the term *evaluation* mean? Verduin and Clark (1991) indicate that the root word of evaluation is "value," which comes from the Latin *valere* meaning "to be strong" or "to have worth." This origin reflects the notion that values are an important element in evaluation. Program evaluation uses various qualitative and quantitative procedures to determine if a program has been implemented as planned. It also determines the degree to which the program has met its goals and objectives.

Grotelueschen (1982) and House (1983) argue that how people define evaluation is dependent on their philosophy of education, evaluation methods, and audiences. Their definition is also based on how the evaluation results are to be used. A few of the more prominent evaluation theorists and their unique perspectives on evaluation as described by Grotelueschen and House are identified below.

Tyler (1949) argues that evaluation is the process of examining the match between learner outcomes and program objectives (see Chapter 2). He recommends the use of achievement tests in evaluating programs. A typical evaluation question from the Tylerian perspective is: *Are the students attaining the program objectives and are the teachers producing?* Major audiences of Tylerian evaluations include managers and psychologists.

Other theorists believe that evaluation is the process of examining the differences between actual performance and commonly accepted standards. While methods recommended by Tyler are used frequently, there is interest by some program managers and evaluators to use systems analysis to determine whether programs are being implemented in an efficient, cost-effective manner. Both managers and economists frequently use systems analysis.

Evaluation sometimes is comprised of procedures that specify, obtain, and provide data for judging decision alternatives. The evaluator might use surveys, questionnaires, and interviews to determine whether or not a program is effective or which specific aspects of a program are more useful than others. These decision-facilitative approaches are used especially by administrators.

Another perspective has been proposed by Scriven (1972). He indicates that evaluation is the process of comparing the actual effects of a program with demonstrated target population needs. By using various logical analyses, *all* the effects of a program, *intended* or *unintended*, are examined. Major audiences of this form of evaluation are the consumers of different programs.

Judging a program's merit against the values of stakeholders is yet another approach to evaluation (Stake, 1975). Particularly important is the ability to understand what the program looks like to different people through case studies, interviews, and observations. Both clients and practitioners are major audiences of this evaluation model.

Eisner (1979) feels that evaluation is the process of examining a program critically using expert knowledge. The bottom-line question here is "would a critic approve of this program?" Consumers as well as "connoisseurs" find this approach appealing when designing evaluations.

It is clear that the definition of evaluation will strongly influence the type of evaluation conducted, as well as the way the evaluation data will be used. For example, if one designed a program evaluation based on the ideas of Scriven (1972), one would examine all the effects of the program (both intended and unintended)) to see if the program is meeting the needs of the target population. This approach would differ from

Tyler's perspective, where the evaluator would carefully measure the degree to which the program obtained prespecified goals and objectives.

We believe it is best to synthesize the many different ideas concerning **program evaluation** when conducting your own evaluations. Usually, no one definition will best fit your needs. Using the example above, evaluators are almost always interested in finding out if a program has met prespecified objectives (the Tylerian perspective). However, unintended effects (both positive and negative) in health education are especially important. For instance, as a result of a cigarette smoking cessation program, an evaluator could look at not only how many people quit or reduced their smoking (the intended effect) but also how many began an exercise program (not specifically an intended effect, but certainly related to overall health promotion). House (1990) argues that because evaluators frequently serve many different interest groups, often times, multiple methods, measures, criteria, perspectives, audiences, and interests must be considered when evaluating a single program.

The fact that evaluators frequently deal with an array of interest groups is responsible for there being many perspectives to consider, when examining the purpose of evaluation. Shortell and Richardson (1978) present the viewpoints from five different groups concerning evaluation: the organization; the program administrator; the funding agency; the public; and the program evaluator. These perspectives are summarized in Figure 1.1.

Windsor, Baranowski, Clark, and Cutter (1984) describe a similar set of purposes for program evaluation. They indicate that evaluation can be used to:

- Determine the rate and level of attainment of program objectives.
- Assess the strengths and weaknesses of a program.
- Help make decisions.
- Monitor standards of performance.
- Establish quality assurance and control mechanisms.
- Determine the generalizability of an overall program or program elements to other populations.
- Contribute to scientific knowledge.
- Identify hypotheses for future study.
- Meet the demand for public or fiscal accountability.
- Improve the professional staff's skill in program planning, implementation, and evaluation activities.
- Promote positive public relations and community awareness.
- Fulfill grant or contract requirements.

Stufflebeam (1971) indicates that the purposes of evaluations are to *improve* rather than to *prove*, while Guba and Lincoln (1989) argue that evaluation is the process of sharing accountability, not assigning accountability. These are important ideas when attempting to help people understand the benefits of evaluation. In addition, one must note

Organization's Perspective

    to demonstrate program effectiveness to other groups
    to justify program costs
    to determine program costs
    to gain support for program facilities, equipment, or activities
    to satisfy funding agency demands for accountability
    to determine future program plans

Program Administrator's Perspective

    to bring favorable attention to the program
    to increase one's status in the organization
    to increase the probability of promotion
    to be fashionable (i.e., evaluation is a popular activity at this time for some organizations)
    to gain greater control of the program
    to provide evidence for more program support

Funding Agency's Perspective

    to ensure efficiency
    to determine program effects
    to demonstrate program effects for political purposes

Public's Perspective

    to ensure that tax dollars are spent efficiently
    to learn about the benefits/disadvantages of the program
    to learn about the value of planned change
    to increase the public's participation in social/health/education programs

Program Evaluator's Perspective

    to contribute to disciplinary and applied knowledge
    to advance professionally
    to help support the program's goals
    to ensure that evaluation is used to help make the program meet program and societal goals

---

Figure 1.1 Reasons for Program Evaluation

From Shortell, S.M., & Richardson, W.C. (1978). *Health Program Evaluation.* St. Louis: C.V. Mosby, Copyright S.M. Shortell, Reprinted by permission.

that evaluation is a sociopolitical process (Guba & Lincoln, 1989). Social, cultural, and political considerations must be considered when designing the evaluation study. For these reasons, the stakeholders of the evaluation must be considered when designing an evaluation study. Stakeholders are those individuals who are affected by the evaluation. Political issues of evaluation are discussed in more detail later in this textbook.

Formative and Summative Evaluation

Although there are many different types of evaluation models, most evaluators organize the models into two general areas: formative and summative.

Formative evaluation refers to the ongoing process of evaluation while the program is being developed and implemented. You also will hear of it called **process evaluation**. The primary goal is to improve the program. Quality assurance and control are important elements of formative evaluation.

Quality control refers to a set of procedures used to assess the quality of a program and its materials. It is also used throughout the design and development phases. **Quality assurance** refers to the application of quality control procedures as well as examinations of critical processes, programs, projects, standards, materials, and outcomes as they relate to the program's overall goals and objectives. More recently, two other terms have emerged: **total quality management** (TQM) and **continuous quality improvement** (CQI). TQM is unlike earlier views of assuring quality in that it sees product (or service) improvement as a phenomenon that is not incompatible with cost control (Fottler, Hernandez & Joiner, 1994). With TQM, improvement is linked closely to both outcome and process. Moreover, TQM requires that the foundation of change consists of the actual needs expressed by customers and workers, as opposed to earlier bureaucratic, top-down approaches to management and quality control. The potential relevance to health promotion and reform of health care in general is enormous. The one common denominator in all CQI programs is the available of data. According to Fottler, et al., (1994): "...*data are critical* for understanding the variables in a process, a prerequisite to improvement" (p.502). Output quality is a cornerstone of CQI as illustrated by its two significant questions: (1) Are we doing the right things? and (2) Are we doing things right?

Typical formative evaluation questions include whether or not the program's content and materials were developed in a manner so that they match the program's objectives, or, whether or not the program is being implemented as planned. Pilot studies are also methods of conducting formative evaluation. In pilot studies, programs that have just been developed are tested with a small group of people to detect and correct any errors before the program is released on a large-scale basis. Sometimes formative evaluations are referred to as process evaluations because they are designed to examine the processes that are taking place while the program is being developed and implemented.

Formative evaluations are often qualitative in nature, meaning that the data collection techniques used include observation, interviews, and open-ended questions in surveys. Often with formative evaluations, only a small number of staff or program participants are solicited for feedback. Also, formative evaluations are often conducted by staff employed by the program being developed. These people are called *internal evaluators*.

Table 1.1 Comparing Formative and Summative Evaluation Methods

Issue	Formative Evaluation	Summative Evaluation
Purpose	Program improvement	Program achievement
Stakeholders	Managers and staff	Consumers, funders, management
Evaluator	Internal staff member	External consultant
Measures	Qualitative	Quantitative
Sample size	Small	Large
Key queries	What is working? What should be improved? How should it be changed?	What has happened? Who was affected? What was the most effective treatment? Was it cost-effective?

From: Grotelueschen, A.D. (1982). Program evaluation. In A.B. Knox and Associates (Eds.) *Developing, Administering and Evaluating Adult Education.* Copyright Jossey-Bass: San Francisco. Reprinted by permission.

Summative evaluation is that form of evaluation which we most frequently associate with program evaluation. With summative evaluation, one usually is interested in assessing the degree to which the program has met some prespecified objectives, or the degree to which the program has been of use to the target population.

Summative evaluations frequently use quantitative approaches. Quantitative procedures include experimental designs and the use of standardized achievement tests or other "objective" measures. The procedures are usually conducted using large groups of people. For purposes of objectivity, summative evaluations are often conducted by outside evaluators, known as *external evaluators*.

Evaluators may speak of two different forms of summative evaluation: impact and outcome evaluation (Green & Kreuter, 1991). In an **impact evaluation**, the evaluator assesses the immediate effects of a program (e.g., gains in knowledge as a result of enrolling in a prenatal education program of self-care and infant care). **Outcome evaluations** are designed to examine the long-term effects of the program, in terms of morbidity and mortality rates (e.g., did program participants have lower rates of stroke than those who did not participate in the program?). A comparison of formative and summative evaluation is made in Table 1.1.

The Evaluability of Programs

No introduction to the study of evaluation would be complete without at least a cursory examination of what it means for a program to be evaluated, and what state of development a program should be in before assessment of any possible outcomes proceeds. Experienced evaluators conduct what is known as an **evaluability assessment**. According to Smith (1989):

Evaluability assessment is a diagnostic and prescriptive tool for improving programs and making evaluations more useful. It is a systematic process for describing the structure of a program (i.e., the objectives, logic, activities, and indicators of successful performance); and for analyzing the plausibility and feasibility for achieving objectives, their suitability for indepth evaluation, and their acceptability to program managers, policymakers, and program operators (p.1).

It is possible for an evaluation to be conducted prematurely, especially one of the summative variety. How does one know when a program is "ready" to be evaluated? Before undertaking an evaluation, one should be able to answer some key questions that relate to what might be called the program's "descriptive elements." One relevant question relates to what the *scope* and *size* of the program is. For example, does the program serve individuals? groups? persons in a certain firm, community, or geographic setting? What issues are covered in this program? What is the target group and how many people are eligible? If one doesn't know who the participants are or what the program is supposed to achieve, an evaluation of outcomes is not of much value.

A second question has to do with the *duration* of the program. What is the time frame for the program -- is it six prenatal education classes held one week apart, or is it an ongoing employee wellness program in a major company that has been in existence for 15 years? Over what period of time is the evaluation to take place? Will the entire program be evaluated or merely a segment of it? Has the program been in existence for a sufficient amount of time for it to have attained the intended change? Defining the scope of the evaluation will to a large extent be dependent on one's understanding of this particular element.

A third area of interest in determining a program's evaluability is related to the *clarity and specificity* of the program. What is the program supposed to accomplish? What are its reasons for existing? What does the program look like to the different "actors" who must interface with it? Is there common agreement about program objectives? A CEO's view of an employee wellness program may be that it exists to reduce health care costs, and that may be the only reason he or she sees for having the program. On the other hand, a junior executive with the firm may see the program as a way to motivate employees, produce more "widgets" during the year, and earn a big bonus from the CEO. The employees themselves may see the program of screening, stress reduction, counseling, and personal fitness as more trouble than fun, and may sabotage it from the start. The question of clarity/specificity may be as simple a one as "who's in charge?" If a program's mission, objectives, and hierarchy of responsibility are vague, one will be hard pressed to draw worthwhile conclusions about its operational value.

At the very least, one should also have a notion of the *complexity and time frame* of the program's objectives. Usually programs have short term objectives (get medically underserved women into prenatal care) that relate to long term objectives (fewer low birthweight babies) or a long term goal (healthier and higher achieving children and youth). Similarly, some objectives are fairly general (increase knowledge of tobacco's health risks among fifth-graders) to specific (delay experimentation with tobacco and other gateway drugs until at least high school) to even more specific (reduce the number of high school seniors who are regular cigarette smokers). The role of the evaluator is to take these different types of objectives and translate them to variables that are measurable.

The evaluator, in conjunction with program managers, policymakers, and other stakeholders, has the task of deciding whether evaluation is warranted. If the questions above are not answerable, or if they lack consensus, program evaluation may be a waste of time.

There are some circumstances under which program evaluation probably should *not* be undertaken. First, if there are no questions to be answered -- because the effect of the program is obvious, because the task of evaluation is merely an information gathering exercise with no focus, or because evaluation is not likely to result in any change. One might argue that there is an enormous need to evaluate the efficacy of the federally-subsidized, school-based meal program -- the so-called "hot lunch" program -- since it is so criticized for its dubious nutrition value and for the taste of the products that are presented to children and youth to eat. An evaluation could delineate the program's shortcomings quite specifically, and even suggest ways to improve both its nutritious and its gastronomical appeal. However, if the resources are not available to make warranted improvements, the evaluation may have little value outside of its value as an academic exercise.

Evaluation is of limited value if a program has no clear objectives, when they are ill-defined, or when the program boundaries are obscured. Moreover, if staff, administrators, and clients have vast discrepancies as to how they view the program, it may be wiser to perform some type of formative exercise to see if some common points of agreement related to what the program is to accomplish can be generated.

Lastly, program evaluation cannot be performed without resources -- both monetary and human. A "rule of thumb" about program budgets is that a minimum of 15 percent of the total resources should be dedicated to the evaluative component. In reality, the figure is probably too low, and it must include the array of staff, computer, paper, telecommunication, and other supplies and expenses, just as with any modern program operation. If there are no resources to allow for at least a minimal evaluation, and there is a clear commitment to the program, then the resources may just as well be pumped into the program or service itself, with "hope" that activities are effective and efficient.

An evaluability assessment is an important pre-evaluation activity. If successful, it can identify parts of a program lacking the elements described above, and help focus what is to be accomplished. Thus, according to Smith (1989), evaluability assessment can be a *summative tool* to determine which parts of a program are evaluable and which parts are of the greatest stakeholder interest. Moreover, it can be a *formative tool* to help decide what needs changing about a program in its current form to make it more effective, more efficient, or at the very least, more evaluable. Finally, it can be a *planning tool* to help define program objectives and the resources necessary to achieve quality.

The Targets of Evaluation: Another Aspect of Evaluability Assessment

As seen from the above discussion, program evaluation is a broad term that can be applied to many different fields. Despite these variations in philosophy, application, and expected outcomes, there are several common issues and questions that an evaluator must consider when planning an evaluation. In other words, the processes and principles used by an evaluator at the National Aeronautics and Space Administration will share similarities with the processes used by an evaluator from the National Institutes of Health, which in turn will be similar to the processes used by a health educator at a rural health department in this or any other country. When planning an evaluation, the evaluator must answer the following basic questions concerning the targets or foci of evaluation:

- Why will you evaluate?
- Whom will you evaluate?
- What will you evaluate?
- Where will you evaluate?
- When will you evaluate?
- How will you evaluate?
- Who will do the evaluating?

Why will you evaluate sets the evaluation design in motion. What are the particular questions the stakeholders are trying to address? For example, if one is only interested in knowledge and behavior change of the students (which would be an evaluation project with limited objectives) a survey of the students might suffice. However, if one is interested in the broad-based impact of the substance abuse prevention project on the community, multiple methods will need to be used to address the evaluation questions.

Whom will you evaluate refers to the individuals who will be evaluated. For example, in a school-based drug education program, students, parents, teachers, administrators, and community leaders all might be evaluated.

What will you evaluate is related to the targets of evaluation. For instance, in the drug education program, evaluators might appraise knowledge, attitudes, and behaviors of the students, while they would ask teachers if the materials were "easy to use." Administrators could be questioned in terms of their teachers' willingness to implement the program as well as their own perceptions of the program's success. In addition, program costs could be the target of the evaluation. Evaluators might survey parents and community leaders about where the program has helped the students and community, as well as areas that are in need of improvement.

Where will you evaluate means considering the many sites of evaluation. For example, students could be given questionnaires in school, but could also be observed at their local "hangouts." Evaluators could also collect data in homes, at PTA meetings, or at hospitals or police departments.

When will you evaluate refers to the important issue of timing the evaluation. Should students be tested concerning their knowledge of drug use immediately after the program has been completed or two months later? When should they be questioned about their drug use behaviors? One month, one year, or even two or three years later?

How will you evaluate considers the evaluation designs that will be used, such as experimental research or surveys, and the data collection methods, such as self-completion questionnaires, urinalyses of drug use, or observations.

Who will do the evaluating is also no trivial issue. Will certain people elicit certain kinds of reactions (positive or negative) from subjects if they perform face-to-face interviews, or even by being present in an evaluation setting when subjects are completing a questionnaire? What influence might the "who" have on the data that are reported by subjects?

The answers to these questions constitute the evaluation plan. The purpose of this text is to provide you with a variety of strategies and techniques to be a better consumer of evaluation studies, to answer questions like those above, and finally, to teach you how to conduct actual evaluations.

Summary

This chapter began with a historical overview of the process of evaluation. People often think that evaluation is a rather new and innovative idea. To the contrary, evaluation has been an evolving process covering many thousands of years. Health education program evaluation has a more recent history, primarily because health education is a rather new form of education. The purposes of evaluation were discussed next, along with the two major forms of evaluation: formative and summative. The definition of evaluability assessment and the context in which it is performed was discussed. The chapter concluded with a discussion of the various foci of evaluation to be considered when planning an evaluation study. Overall, in this, and other chapters of the textbook, we attempt to make you a better consumer of evaluation studies, whether you are a program developer, program manager, or actually, the program evaluator.

Case Study

Paperny, D.M.N. (1997). Computerized health assessment and education for adolescent HIV and STD prevention in health care settings and schools. *Health Education & Behavior, 24*(1), 54-70.

In this paper, Paperny assessed a decade's worth of computer applications, computerized health assessments for adolescents, and automated health education in a wide array of health care settings (HMOs, detention settings, military facilities, clinics) and schools. As a result of this study, many recommendations concerning future applications were made, especially related to HIV and other STD prevention in adolescents. What barriers and facilitating factors would you anticipate in achieving widespread implementation of computer-based education in schools on these topics? What descriptive elements would need to be in place before evaluation of such a computer-based learning program would be feasible? Describe how an evaluability assessment in such a study could be (1) a summative tool; (2) a formative tool; and (3) a planning tool.

Student Questions/Activities

1. Consider the scenarios described below. Decide how you would conduct the evaluation by answering the questions listed below:

    a. Why will you evaluate?
    b. Whom will you evaluate?
    c. What will you evaluate?
    d. Where will you evaluate?
    e. When will you evaluate?
    f. How will you evaluate?
    g. Who will do the evaluating?

Compare and contrast the methods and ideas you generated for each scenario.

Scenario 1
You have been hired as a consultant by the State of Missouri Department of Health to evaluate the quality of its health education network program to update the knowledge and skills of health educators in the region through in-service education workshops.
Scenario 2
You have been hired by a small rural public health clinic to evaluate the effectiveness of its teenage pregnancy prevention program.
Scenario 3
You have been hired by a large metropolitan hospital to evaluate the quality of its diabetes patient education program.

2. Consider each of the evaluation perspectives described by Grotelueschen. Describe how you would evaluate a high school sex education program using each evaluation definition. Compare and contrast the descriptions.
3. Identify in the local newspapers several evaluation activities that are taking place in your community. Are these activities formative or summative in nature? What do you think are the purposes of these evaluations?

Recommended Readings

Wills, T.A., & Cleary, S.D. (1997). The validity of self-reports of smoking: Analyses by race/ethnicity in a school sample of urban adolescents. *American Journal of Public Health*, *87*(1), 56-61.

This research compared variation in the validity of self-reported cigarette smoking in African-American, Hispanic, and White adolescent respondents, and concluded that the validity of reporting was comparable across groups. It is an excellent paper to read and think through the formative processes for conducting such a study, and for identifying the targets (foci) of evaluation.

Swain, R.C., Beauvais, F., Chavez, E.L., & Oetting, E.R. (1997). The effect of school dropout rates on estimates of adolescent substance use among three racial/ethnic groups. *American Journal of Public Health*, *87*(1), 51-55.

The study examined substance use among Mexican-American, White non-Hispanic, and Native American adolescents. It demonstrates the extent to which the *what* and *where* and *whom* measures could impact the later design of responsive health education programs. In this case, should programs target special groups who have dropped out, or should they emphasize the reformation of schools to reduce the level of dropping out?

Apel, M., Klein, K., McDermott, R.J., & Westhoff, W.W. (1997). Restricting smoking at the University of Köln, Germany: A case study. *Journal of American College Health*, *45*(5), 219-223.

This study examined the effects of a policy change to limit the areas where smoking could occur at a German university, where the point prevalence of smoking is approximately 1.5 times what it is in the United States. It illustrates the potential value of performing an evaluability assessment. What might have been concluded from a thorough evaluability assessment before undertaking the study? In addition, consider all the targets of evaluation, and speculate on what other targets of evaluation might have been. Given the cultural differences between the United States and Germany regarding smoking, might there be different standards in evaluating a program such as this one as whether or not it could be called successful?

References

Burchard, J.D., & Schaefer, M. (1992). Improving accountability in a service delivery system in children's mental health. *Clinical Psychology Review*, *12*, 867-882.

Centers for Disease Control and Prevention. (1994). Health risk behaviors among adolescents who do and do not attend school - United States, 1992. *Morbidity & Mortality Weekly Report*, 43, 129-132.

Eisner, E. (1979). *The Educational Imagination*. New York: MacMillan.

Fottler, M.D., Hernandez, S.R., & Joiner, C.L. (1994). *Strategic Management of Human Resources in Health Services Organizations*. (2nd ed.). Albany, NY: Delmar Publishers, Inc.

Gore A., & Brown, R. (1993). *The National Information Infrastructure: Agenda for Action*. Washington, DC: White House.

Green, L.W., & Kreuter, M.W. (1991). *Health Promotion Planning: An Educational and Environmental Approach*. (2nd ed.). Mountain View: Mayfield.

Green, L.W., & Lewis, F.M. (1986). *Measurement and Evaluation in Health Education and Health Promotion*. Palo Alto: Mayfield.

Grotelueschen, A.D. (1982). Program evaluation. In A.B. Knox and Associates (Eds.). *Developing, Administering, and Evaluating Adult Education*. San Francisco: Jossey-Bass.

Guba, E.G., & Lincoln, Y.S. (1989). *Fourth Generation Evaluation*. Newbury Park: Sage.

House, E.R. (1990). Trends in evaluation. *Educational Researcher 19*(3), 24-28.

House, E.R. (1983). Assumptions underlying evaluation models. In G.F. Madaus, M.S. Scriven, & D.L. Stufflebeam (Eds.). *Evaluation Models: Viewpoints on Educational and Human Services Evaluation*. Boston: Kluwer-Nijhoff.

Madaus, G.F., Stufflebeam, D.L., & Scriven, M.S. (1983). *Evaluation Models: Viewpoints on Educational and Human Services Evaluation*. Boston: Kluwer-Nijhoff.

National Commission for Health Education Credentialing, Inc. (1996). *A Competency-Based Framework for Professional Development of Certified Health Education Specialists*. New York: NCHEC.

Nelson, D.W. (1993). Introduction. In Anne E. Casey Foundation and Center for the Study of Social Policy, *Kids Count Data Book*. Washington, DC: Center for the Study of Social Policy.

Peck, M. (1996). Reinventing evaluation. *City Lights*, 5(4), 1.

Pigg, R.M. (1976). A history of school health program evaluation in the United States. *Journal of School Health, 46*, 583-589.

Results of the School Health Education Evaluation. (1985). Special issue: Journal of School Health. *Journal of School Health*, 55, 295-355.

Scriven, M.S. (1972). Pros and cons about goal-free evaluation. *Evaluation Comment, 1*, 1-7.

Shortell, S.M., & Richardson, W.C. (1978). *Health Program Evaluation*. St. Louis: C.V. Mosby.

Sliepcevich, E.M. (1964). *School Health Education Study: A Summary Report*. Washington, DC: School Health Education Study.

Smith, M.F. (1989). *Evaluability Assessment: A Practical Approach*. Boston: Kluwer Academic Publishers.

Stake, R.E. (1975). *Evaluating the Arts in Education: A Responsive Approach*. Columbus, OH: Charles E. Merrill.

Stufflebeam, D.L. (1971). The relevance of the CIPP evaluation model for educational accountability. *Journal of Research and Development in Education, 5,* 19-25.

Tyler, R.W. (1949). *Basic Principles of Curriculum and Instruction.* Chicago: University of Chicago Press.

Verduin, J.R., Jr., & Clark, T.A. (1991). *Distance Education: The Foundation for Effective Practice.* San Francisco: Jossey-Bass.

Windsor, R.A., Baranowski, T., Clark, N., & Cutter, G. (1984). *Evaluation of Health Promotion and Education Programs.* Palo Alto: Mayfield.

Worthen, B.R., Sanders, J.R. (1987). *Educational Evaluation: Alternative Approaches and Practical Guidelines.* New York: Longman.

Models for Conducting Program Evaluation

Chapter Objectives

After completing this chapter, you should be able to:

1. List and describe the salient or defining features of eight different approaches to, or models of, program evaluation.
2. Formulate appropriate and measurable program objectives.
3. Describe the characteristics of a well-written behavioral objective.
4. Demonstrate the successful construction of specific behavioral objectives for a given scenario.
5. Analyze a completed evaluation and examine how alternative approaches could have been used to replace, supplement, or enhance the approach that was actually used.

Key Terms

accreditation/professional review approach
adversarial/quasi-legal approach
art criticism/connoisseurship approach
CIPP model
cost-benefit evaluation

discrepancy evaluation
goal-free approach
goal-/objectives-oriented approach
systems analysis
transactional evaluation

Introduction

In the text below we discuss some evaluation models that demonstrate the wide array of approaches that can be applied in evaluation settings. It is often argued (and practiced) that programs are set up, goals and objectives are established, and then it becomes the evaluator's task in consultation with program stakeholders to figure out if the program is achieving its objectives. If it is, the program is declared a success. If it isn't, and the reason is not explained by a lack of good and faithful implementation, the program is declared a failure and is either revamped or scrapped entirely. While "objective-oriented" evaluations are indeed the most common, especially in health education and other education programs, they are by no means the only methods available. We would like to acquaint you in this chapter with a series of other models, and be a little provocative in looking at their possible applications in examining and assessing health programs. Patton (1990) suggests that these alternative models be viewed not as "recipes," but as "frameworks."

Evaluation Models in Review

Evaluation can be complex. Because of this reality, the evaluator must have a wide array of approaches available, and not be restricted to just one model, or only "traditional" strategies. The evaluation of health education and promotion programs in the future might benefit from the application of creative techniques. The remainder of this chapter presents different models for measuring and comparing programs.

Goal-oriented Evaluations

Ralph Tyler's evaluation of curricula in the 1940s revolutionized educational assessment (Tyler, 1949). Evaluators employing a **goal-oriented** (also called **objectives-oriented**) **approach** take the stated goals of a program, and collect evidence using appropriate means to see whether the goals have been met. The confluence of the program goals and actual program effects is the measure of program success. This strategy for program evaluation got its origin in the education arena, and became popularized in the 1940s and 1950s through the work of such persons as Ralph Tyler and Benjamin Bloom (House, 1980). In subsequent decades, Suchman (1967) showed its value in public health and human service programs. According to Suchman (1967): "The most identifying feature of evaluative research is the presence of some goal or objective whose measure of attainment constitutes the main focus of the research problem" (p.37). More recently, Guild (1990) has demonstrated how goal-oriented evaluations can be used to determine progress toward both short-term and long-term goal attainment. This approach to evaluation is particularly well suited for the evaluator when program goals are stated as behavioral objectives. "Given a list of 50 different food items, the learner will be able to divide them into high, medium, and low saturated fat items within 10 minutes making no more than five errors" is an example of such a behavioral objective. According to Green and Kreuter (1991), well written behavioral objectives should answer: *Who?* (the person or persons expected to change), *What?* (the action or change in knowledge, attitude, or behavior to be attained), *How much?* (the extent of the condition to be attained or the degree of accuracy that is acceptable), and *When?* (the time span over which the change is to occur).

Other evaluators have developed models that are outgrowths of Tyler's philosophy of evaluation being measurement of the extent to which specific objectives are attained. Provus (1971) for example coined the term **discrepancy evaluation** because of its emphasis on examining discrepancies between program objectives and actual achievement, and subsequently, the analysis of those discrepancies to guide management decisions. Levin (1971) presented **cost-benefit evaluation** as another example of an objectives-based model. Evaluators employing Levin's approach can compare program costs versus objectives met, and in turn, look at how one program compares to another to promote selection of the program that yields the lowest cost per unit. The need for models that diversify approaches to evaluation continues.

Transactional Approach

According to Rippey (1973), Stake (1978), and Patton (1990), evaluation needs to be more *responsive* to the needs of the people who are part of programs. Thus, evaluation has to be more "personal" and "humanizing" than just a simple assessment of to what extent particular sets of objectives were met. The transactional approach concentrates on program processes and how various people associated with the program actually view it. The major question asked, according to House (1980), is *What does the program look like to various people who are familiar with it?* The customary strategy for conducting **transactional evaluation** is to conduct interviews with as many people as possible who can offer views about the program's operation. The evaluator organizes these interviews and presents the program information as a sort of case study. A most appropriate application of the transactional model is when the purpose of the inquiry is *understanding* rather than *explanation and propositional knowledge* (House, 1980).

Suppose one was interested in evaluating the patient-provider relationship and the overall delivery of health care in a clinic setting. One could view patient visits to physicians as a series of "transactions," not altogether different in principle from the types of transactions a consumer might have with a merchant from whom he or she made a purchase. By interviewing patients, receptionists, nurses, technicians, physicians, pharmacists, patient services coordinators, and other key individuals, the evaluator could gain a great deal of understanding about how health care is perceived by various people. The value of such understanding might be especially valuable in the event that patient compliance to scheduled visits or medication-taking was low. Poor compliance might be traced to discrepant expectations or miscommunication on the part of the patient and the physician, waiting times that were too long, lack of courtesy on the telephone by reception staff, or other reasons that would emerge only through such in-depth qualitative evaluation.

CIPP Approach

The **CIPP model** was developed by Daniel L. Stufflebeam and his colleagues (1971) in response to the need of managers to have data that can assist in key decision making. Its utility is found especially in educational settings. *CIPP* is an acronym that stands for the four types of evaluation that are considered by the model: context, input, process, and product.

    Context evaluation is the identification of the problems and needs of a specific educational setting. *Input evaluation* is the assessment of resources and strategies for achieving desired program outcomes. This stage in the CIPP approach may deal with the feasibility of obtaining or employing certain resources, and consequently, with acceptable compromises between what is desired versus what is feasible. *Process evaluation* allows one to examine a program's operation in its formative stages. It may include monitoring students' attendance, teachers' fidelity to a plan when delivering a curriculum, adherence to the program's specific operational procedures, and other features. Feedback gives program managers a chance to "fine tune" the program before it goes out of control, or may give some clues later on if the program yields less than what was expected, so that subsequent programs can perform better. *Product evaluation* is the extent to which program objectives were achieved, and to that extent somewhat follows from Tylerian philosophy. According to Borg and Gall (1989) the CIPP approach can be separated from a pure goal-oriented evaluation in that: "The CIPP model is distinguished by its comprehensiveness, by the fact that it is an ongoing process, and by its purpose, which is to guide in the decision-making in program management" (p.768).

Systems Analysis

This approach to evaluation goes beyond examining the effectiveness of a program (or the relative levels of goal attainment of two or more programs), by assessing program efficiency as well. That is, **systems analysis** is like the approach attributed above to Levin (1971) in that it seeks better operating procedures so as to achieve the most effect for the least amount of resources expended. If a program is effective, managers want to know if the same level of effectiveness can be achieved more economically. Thus, cost-benefit measures are some of the critical defining aspects of systems analysis. As you might guess, the systems analysis technique is of great interest to economists, program fiscal officers, and other persons whose interest is unit cost. Since the interests and concerns of program participants (i.e., the human and social contexts in which the program operates) take a back seat to simple economics, the systems analysis approach is readily criticized on the grounds that it lacks "warmth."

Art Criticism or Connoisseurship Approach

An old saying in the art world goes something like: "I may not know art, but I do know what I like." Whether one is speaking of examining art, critiquing movies, eating good food, or tasting fine wine, if one partakes often enough in any of these activities, there is some expertise that develops. The label attached to this technique is **art criticism** or **connoisseurship**. Eisner (1979) believes that through the development of personal standards and criteria, a certain connoisseurship also can be developed where the evaluation of programs is concerned. If you are having a difficult time imagining this model put into practice, simply consider the popular televised reviews of new movies offered for years by Chicago writers Gene Siskel and Roger Ebert. Incorporating elements of casting, acting, writing, directing, and editing, these reviewers give a critique of a movie that provides a professional judgment to consumers.

Using criteria related to program structure (scope and size), duration, management, clarity, and other standards, evaluators of health education and promotion programs also can make judgments that are oriented toward the consumer. Program weaknesses, strengths, and key or unique features can be identified by benefit of expert review. The drawbacks of this model include an absence of universal standards, standards for identifying skilled evaluators, and the reluctance of program personnel to accept criticisms. One of the best applications of this approach may be to corroborate other evidence, when used in conjunction with more widely accepted evaluative standards and practices.

Adversarial or Quasi-legal Approach

In a courtroom, it is common practice for two opposing attorneys to argue the facts of a case, each presenting a body of evidence for a judge or jury to consider. Upon hearing all of the evidence, the judge (or panel of jurists if it is a jury trial) weighs the evidence and renders a decision for one side or the other. Wolf (1975) and House (1980) were some of the first professional evaluators to describe the use of this approach for program evaluation.

The **adversarial evaluation** or **quasi-legal approach** has four distinct phases. In the first phase a broad range of issues is generated. These issues may be established through interviews with key stakeholders using evaluative questions such as: *Should this program be expanded? funded again but with close scrutiny? curtailed? eliminated altogether? To what extent is the program meeting (or not meeting) its objectives?* In the second phase, a lengthy list of issues is trimmed to one of manageable size by having key informants rank-order the issues and discuss them until a consensus is reached. The third phase is to form two teams that will take adversarial positions on the issues decided upon in phase two. Teams can interview "witnesses" to obtain "testimony" supporting their point of view, or actually perform other investigations that may turn up new evidence or data. The fourth phase is to conduct the sessions in which the teams present their opposing arguments.

We can imagine how it might be applied to a health education setting. Suppose a company's worksite health promotion program has been in place for several years, but because of budgetary and other considerations, its performance and value to the company is now "under the gun." One way to determine its future survival may be for managers (acting as judges or jurists) to have two factions (acting as "defense" and "prosecuting" attorneys) argue the pros and cons of the program. The side in support of the program offers evidence concerning the program's contributions (e.g., attendance at work, morale, etc.) while the side in favor of eliminating the program offers evidence to the contrary. Upon weighing the evidence from both sides, management personnel can examine where the program fits into the company's long range plans. This approach is not always used to assess whether a program is to be eliminated or further supported. It can be used to examine needed modifications or to weigh the comparative benefits of two programs competing against one another. Like the art criticism approach, its best application may be in conjunction with other evaluative techniques. The adversarial approach may suffer from discrepant abilities of the two sides to collect and present available evidence. The personal qualities, dynamics, and charisma of the presenter may interfere with objective interpretation of the evidence.

Accreditation or Professional Review Approach

Professional associations conduct evaluations of professional preparation programs to set and maintain standards, stimulate an upward spiral in program performance, and be responsive to public accountability. Several examples of accreditation bodies exist. Among the more familiar to institutions of higher education where health educators are prepared include the Council for Education in Public Health (CEPH), the National Council on Accreditation of Teacher Education (NCATE), the American Association for Health Education (AAHE), and the Society for Public Health Education (SOPHE).

While some variation occurs, a typical **accreditation** or **professional review** process involves a self-study by the institution, followed by on-site visits by expert panelists (professional peers) appointed by the accrediting body. Interviews, checklists, and other tools are used to assess an institution's performance. In the case of colleges and universities, standards that are applied relate to quality of instruction, quality of research, quality of service to the institution, community, and profession, unique features of the program, and potential for high performance in the future. Review teams that make site visits examine an institution's curriculum. A curriculum also can be assessed and revised more easily when clearly established standards exist. One example is the Standards for the Preparation of Graduate Level Health Educators (Dennison, 1997). By comparing course content with standards, faculty can fine tune an entire program so that professional responsibilities and competencies are linked to the curriculum. Moreover, students are able to assess their own strengths and weaknesses better when they compare expected standards of knowledge and performance to their own perceived competencies.

The accreditation approach is sometimes criticized as being political. Evaluations may be uneven if some peer reviewers are substantially less skilled than others, or apply evaluative criteria with vastly different levels of specificity. Overall, the model enjoys widespread adoption, and is generally praised for its emphasis on self-study, peer review, ongoing evaluation, inclusion of multiple stakeholders, and responsiveness to identified weaknesses.

Goal-free Approach

While the strength of the goal-oriented approach is that it provides the evaluator with a framework for conducting his or her work, its glaring weakness is that it may distract one from finding (or even looking for) effects other than the ones than were planned for and desired. Moreover, the same characteristics that provide the evaluator with direction also enhance the possibility of introducing biases to the evaluation. Because of these dangers, Scriven (1973) has proposed an alternative to this model called the **goal-free approach**. According to House (1980):

The goal-free approach reduces the bias of searching for only the program developer's prespecified intents by not informing the evaluator of them. Hence, the evaluator must search for all outcomes. Many of these outcomes are unintended side effects, which may be positive or negative (p.30).

House (1980) points out that the goal-free evaluation is perhaps the least often employed approach, "even to the point where some people would question it as a major model" (p.40). Evaluators do have some difficulty envisioning the occasion where a program manager would not insist on sharing program goals. Other evaluation aficionados argue that even in the case where program goals are unknown, wouldn't evaluators simply guess or make up their own? On many occasions wouldn't the likely program goals be obvious to the evaluation team? It is the lack of answers to these types of questions that causes skepticism about goal-free evaluation. Furthermore, advocates of the approach have been unsuccessful in clearly delineating methods for evaluators to follow. Nevertheless, it is an important strategy to be alert to since it forces the evaluator to be sensitive to measuring side effects occurring from programs. In smoking cessation programs, the possibility of many unintended side effects is possible. These side effects might be positive (increased awareness of proper nutrition, higher activity level, better attention to stress management, improved self-esteem) or negative (increased anxiety and nervousness, weight gain from higher level of food consumption, grief and depression, avoidance or social isolation by friends who do smoke). Without attention to program side effects, an evaluator might find an intervention to perform worse (or better) than it really does.

Patton (1987) lists the following reasons why one might consider the goal-free evaluation: (1) to reduce the risk of studying program objectives too narrowly, and therefore, missing unanticipated outcomes; (2) to reduce the "negative connotations" often attached to finding side-effects; (3) to use these unanticipated effects to one's advantage in terms of establishing new or future priorities; and (4) to reduce the bias introduced to the evaluation setting when the program goals are known, and thus, promote evaluator objectivity.

The array of models explored briefly in this chapter is not exhaustive. We hope that the discussion of alternative approaches has been provocative enough to get you to think "outside the box" as you begin to contemplate evaluation tasks. Some of the key elements of these models are summarized in Table 2.1.

Table 2.1 Key Elements of Different Evaluation Models

Model	Audience	Major Strength	Major Weakness
Goal-oriented	managers educators	links program with outcomes	value-laden
Transactional	clients practitioners	links client and practitioner points of view	value-laden; susceptible to evaluator bias
Decision-oriented (e.g., CIPP)	administrators	links method with decision need	vulnerable to bias
Systems analysis	economists fiscal staff	links causes with effects	may exclude participants' views, thereby lacking "warmth"
Art criticism	consumers connoisseurs	links "feelings" of participants with other evaluative data	lacks clear criteria and definition of "connoisseur"
Adversarial	managers acting as "jurists"	all positive and negative aspects of one or more programs can be "aired"	requires good "jurists;" susceptible to "charisma" bias
Accreditation	CEOs general public	self-evaluative; on-going study sets professional criteria	vulnerable to evaluator bias; can promote disharmony
Goal-free	consumers	not biased by pre-specified goals and objectives	lack of clear methodology

Summary

We began this chapter by examining goal-oriented (objectives-oriented) evaluation strategies, and came full-circle until we finished with a discussion of goal-free evaluation. In this chapter we gave numerous examples of alternative strategies that may have utility for increasing one's view of the evaluation process and its aims. Some approaches will work better for certain evaluation situations than for others. Sometimes, it may be valuable to combine approaches to increase perspective about the program under concern. The most important point to take away from this chapter is that evaluation approaches are diverse and continue to be developed in an effort to be responsive to the numerous stakeholders affected both by programs and their evaluation.

Case Study

Lowe, J.B., Windsor, R., Balanda, K.P., & Woodby, L. (1997). Smoking relapse prevention methods for pregnant women: A formative evaluation. *American Journal of Health Promotion, 11*(4), 244-246.

In this paper, Lowe and his colleagues perform a formative evaluation on a program designed to prevent smoking relapse in pregnant women. Specifically, they determine how faithfully the program was delivered. Suppose you were going to replicate this study in another setting. Given what you learned in this chapter about other evaluation models, tell how you might approach this evaluation differently than these investigators did. Be sure to consider at least three different approaches to evaluation that are described in this chapter.

Student Questions/Activities

1. One controversial aspect of professional preparation in health education is the development of a uniform set of standards for entry-level and graduate-level preparation across all institutions of higher learning. Select teams of people in your class and evaluate the relative pros and cons of "standardizing" professional preparation using the adversarial evaluation approach described in this chapter.
2. In this chapter we cite Patton as saying that models ought to be used as "frameworks" rather than as "recipes" for conducting evaluation. What do you think he means by that? Explain.
3. Examine an existing health education or health promotion program with which you are familiar. Are the "behavioral objectives" for that program as concrete as the one illustrated in this chapter? Create a hypothetical program and write at least three specific behavioral objectives for it.
4. Try to locate and interview some teachers who have used two or more of the widely disseminated comprehensive school health education curricula, or curricula specific to a particular topic (e.g., drug education, sex education). Take

an art criticism approach to probe for how they view and compare these curricula. How could this information be useful in lieu of, or in addition to, data you might have on student achievement related to being exposed to these curricula?

Recommended Readings

Guild, P.A. (1990). Goal-oriented evaluation as a program management tool. *American Journal of Health Promotion, 4*(4), 296-301.

> This article illustrates how to quantify the extent to which program goals are achieved using concepts such as a "short-term achievement index" and a "long-term achievement index." The author also explains how use of these indices can help one plan a subsequent year's program.

Raynal, M.E., & Chen, W.W. (1996-97). Evaluation of a drug prevention program for young high risk students. *International Quarterly of Community Health Education, 16*(2), 187-195.

> This article reports the effectiveness of a multifaceted drug use prevention program for high risk elementary and junior high school students. Results were determined by paper-and-pencil tests on students and subjective evaluations performed by teachers, and specific instrumentation is described by the authors. When you read this paper consider the possibilities brought about by using multidimensional evaluation approaches to assess a multicomponent prevention program.

Tappe, M.K., Galer-Unti, R.A., & Bailey, K.C. (1997). Evaluation of trained teachers' implementation of a sex education curriculum. *Journal of Health Education, 28*(2), 103-108.

> This study evaluated the long-term implementation of the *Understanding Sexuality* curriculum by teachers who had been trained to use the curriculum. This article successfully demonstrates the importance of the concept of "fidelity of implementation" in program evaluation, and identifies barriers to more successful implementation, such as the limitations imposed by the sparseness of resources (e.g., time, adequate support personnel). When you read this article consider the procedures in the CIPP approach described in this chapter, and how their utilization might be able to make teacher training, curriculum implementation, and program monitoring more successful.

References

Borg, W.R. & Gall, M.D. (1989). *Educational Research*. (5th ed.). New York: Longman.

Dennison, D. (1997). Health education graduate standards: Expansion of the framework. *Journal of Health Education, 28*(2), 68-73.

Eisner, E. (1979). *The Educational Imagination*. New York: MacMillan.

Green, L.W., & Kreuter, M.W. (1991). *Health Promotion Planning: An Educational and Environmental Approach*. (2nd ed.). Mountain View, CA: Mayfield.

Guild, P.A. (1990). Goal-oriented evaluation as a program management tool. *American Journal of Health Promotion, 4*(4), 296-301.

House, E.R. (1980). *Evaluating with Validity*. Beverly Hills, CA: Sage.

Levin, H.M. (1971). *Cost-Effectiveness: A Primer*. Beverly Hills, CA: Sage.

Patton, M.Q. (1987). *How to Use Qualitative Methods in Evaluation*. Newbury Park, CA: Sage.

Patton, M.Q. (1990). *Qualitative Evaluation and Research Methods*. (2nd ed.). Newbury Park, CA: Sage.

Provus, M. (1971). *Discrepancy Evaluation*. Berkeley: McCutchan.

Rippey, R.M. (ed.) (1973). *Studies in Transactional Evaluation*. Berkeley, CA: McCutchan.

Scriven, M.S. (1973). Goal-free evaluation. In E.R. House (ed.). *School Evaluation: The Politics and Process*. Berkeley: McCutchan.

Stake, R.E. (1978). The case study method in social inquiry. *Educational Researcher, 7*, 5-8.

Stufflebeam, D.L., Foley, W.J., Gephart, W.J., Guba, E.G., Hammond, R.L., Merriman, H.O., & Provus, M.M. (1971). *Educational Evaluation and Decision Making*. Itasca, IL: F.E. Peacock.

Suchman, E.A. (1967). *Evaluative Research: Principles and Practice in Public Service and Social Action Programs*. New York: Russell Sage Foundation.

Tyler, R.W. (1949). *Basic Principles of Curriculum and Instruction*. Chicago: University of Chicago Press.

Wolf, R.L. (1975). Trial by jury: a new evaluation method. *Phi Delta Kappan, 57*, 185-187.

Chapter

3

Politics, Ethics, and Program Evaluation

Chapter Objectives

After completing this chapter, you should be able to:

1. Compare and contrast the advantages and disadvantages of external and internal evaluators.
2. Identify traits and skills in an evaluator-for-hire.
3. Analyze how to determine one's evaluation needs.
4. Examine contractual needs of program managers and evaluators.
5. Identify the program interests of various stakeholders.
6. Describe the political context in which program evaluation occurs.
7. Evaluate the ethical dilemmas faced in program evaluation.
8. Identify the steps taken to assure protection of human subjects' rights.

Key Terms

academic evaluation
anonymity
beneficence
compliance/regulatory evaluation
confidentiality
deception
ethics
external evaluator
fidelity
hatchet evaluation
information gathering evaluation

informed consent
ingratiating evaluation
institutional review board (IRB)
justice
least publishable unit
nonmalficence
respect/autonomy
right of privacy
stakeholders
untreated control group
whistle-blower

Introduction

Just as program interventions do not occur in a vacuum, neither do the evaluations of those interventions. Program evaluation may involve a network of organizations and groups, and many complex individual personalities. In this chapter we will examine some of the political ramifications of health education program evaluation. We will consider how to select an evaluator for your program, and how to participate effectively as an evaluator of your own or someone else's program. Furthermore, we will explore some of the ethical dilemmas with which the evaluator of health education and promotion programs may be confronted.

Evaluation: Who Should Do the Job?

According to Johnson (1981): "All of us evaluate. We judge whether the bread in our sandwich is fresh, whether the baseball manager should have substituted another pitcher at a particular point in the game..." (p.vi), and so on. While everyone has some evaluative abilities, there is no single model or method for performing evaluations, no universally recognized set of skills or qualities for evaluators to possess, no particular professional preparation programs for evaluators, and no uniform role for evaluators to play. Consequently, there are no "rules" carved in granite about when to conduct your own evaluations, and when to seek outside help. In some respects, though, the person who evaluates his or her own program is like the lawyer who defends himself, or the physician who treats himself. Just as the self-defending lawyer may have a fool for an attorney, the program manager who is his own evaluator may have an incompetent alter ego with which to contend. Objectivity may be lost completely when evaluation is performed strictly as an "inside job." If evaluation is done from the inside, the evaluator needs to play certain roles and possess unique skills (Clifford & Sherman, 1983). These features are highlighted in Table 3.1.

Having an **external evaluator** may not be the perfect solution, either. Worthen and Sanders (1987) identify several advantages and disadvantages in using external evaluators. These points are summarized in Table 3.2.

The motivations underlying an evaluation impact upon which aspects of a program are evaluated, how the results get used, the level of involvement of various program **stakeholders**, and the selection of an evaluator. Evaluators, as a rule, may come from three sources: *the funding agency*, *the program itself*, or *an organization that specializes in evaluation*, and which has no particular ties to either the program or the funding source. The choice of who performs the evaluation may rest with the funding agency or the program manager.

If you have a funded project and are seeking to hire an evaluator, the following considerations may be helpful in thinking through your specific evaluative needs. First, you might examine the issue of whether or not the project really needs to be evaluated. The reasons for carrying out evaluations are numerous, and are discussed at some length in Chapter 1. Certainly if one can define the purpose, scope, target audience, and objectives of a program clearly, evaluation is of great value in fine tuning implementation and delivery, as well as providing feedback concerning early achievements. However, one also should consider when evaluation might be premature or unwarranted. For example, evaluation may just represent wasted effort if there are no questions to be answered, if the effect of a program has been established previously or is obvious, when evaluation findings are not going to be used, or when findings are not going to result in change.

Table 3.1 Traits of the Effective Internal Evaluator

Able to be a management decision-support specialist
- planner
- operations researcher
- manager
- organizational development consultant
- management trainer

Able to process data and be a management information specialist

Able to analyze and interpret data

Able to communicate using interpersonal skills

Able to adopt a manager's perspective

Able to raise management's consciousness about evaluation

Able to project the costs of evaluation

Able to negotiate evaluation and management needs

Able to organize and lead an internal evaluation team

Adapted from: Clifford, D.L., & Sherman, P. (1983). Internal evaluation: Integrating program evaluation and management. In Arnold J. Love, (Ed.). *Developing Effective Internal Evaluation*. San Francisco, CA: Jossey-Bass, Inc., pp.26-36.

Assuming you decide that evaluation *is* a critical need, what traits do you look for in an evaluator? Evaluation is a "young" discipline, but already has developed into a number of areas of specialization. Johnson (1981) points out several competencies that evaluators may possess, the relevance of which may be worthwhile considering before making your choice of an evaluator: (1) *knowledge/skill base*. How familiar is the evaluator with programs of similar scope and aims? Does the person have the survey development, statistical, interviewing, or other technical competencies that may be needed? (2) *authority*. Does the person have the professional credentials, eminence, track record, and interpersonal abilities to work effectively with a wide range of people? (3) *communication skills*. Can the evaluator write a report that can be interpreted and used by an intended audience of stakeholders? Does the person have strong oral communication ability? (4) *interactive style*. What posture does the evaluator take toward the client - one of supportive teamwork? one of aloofness? Will program manager and evaluator be able to "get along?" (5) *logistics*. To which other projects is the evaluator committed? Will the evaluator be able to commit adequate time to tasks I need done? and (6) *links*. Does the evaluator have particular biases or ideologies that will interfere with carrying out the needed tasks? Is the person familiar with the values of the various groups of people involved, and able to demonstrate respect for individual and cultural diversity?

Table 3.2 Advantages and Disadvantages of Using External Evaluators

---

Advantages

      Greater opportunity for impartiality
      Enhanced credibility, especially in controversial programs
      Taps expertise beyond that possessed by program staff
      Increases chance for fresh perspective
      May put staff at ease to disclose sensitive concerns

Disadvantages

      Evaluator competence may be a question mark
      Evaluator may not be familiar with program dynamics
      Negotiations may delay evaluation process
      Likely to be more costly than internal evaluations

Adapted from: Worthen, B.R., & Sanders, J.R. (1987). *Educational Evaluation*. New York: Longman, pp.173-174.

It is difficult, if not impossible, to say with absolute authority how one should prioritize evaluator qualities. Technical expertise is important, but if the evaluator's personality and style are impediments to communication and staff cooperation, all the technical wizardry in the world won't help. Popham (1988) puts this issue in appropriate perspective as he targets evaluators themselves:

Educational evaluators must realize that their expertise is no substitue for actual interactions with those around them. Evaluators who walk into an educational setting and expect deferential treatment, merely because they know that a *t* test is not a process used by the Lipton Company, are in for a surprise (p. 323).

The Evaluator-Client Contract

French, Fisher, and Costa (1983) identify seven "potentially troublesome issues" that should be ironed out between program managers and program evaluators prior to the initiation of the evaluation process. While these issues are important, to say the least, they do not necessarily have to be addressed in the form of a binding, legally implemented contract between the parties. Nevertheless, agreements are best if put in writing, because they can be referred to from time to time, and modified as needed. Among the issues of concern are: (1) *Division of labor*. Who is responsible for data collection? Who will duplicate and disseminate forms, surveys, questionnaires, and other documents? This pragmatic concern may seem trivial, but it should be resolved in advance. (2) *Division of resources*. Who provides resources such as computer access, typing, paper, postage, and other services and consumable resources? (3) *Timetable*. What steps need to be taken, in what order do they need to be taken, and when does each step need to be completed? Such forethought permits budgeting of time and other resources, and prevents reports from being submitted after it is too late for them to provide any insight about decision making needs. (4) *Deliverables*. What is/are the end product(s) for which the evaluator is responsible? Will there be only a final report, or will there be preliminary or ongoing reports prepared at specific intervals? In addition to a written document, will there be an oral presentation of data? Moreover, how long after project completion will the evaluator need to be available for interpretation of data? (5) *Distribution of results*. Although it may seem obvious, it should be made clear who has access to program reports, and when this access will occur. Typically, the evaluator will be asked to provide the report for the program manager directly, and control of access will be the purview of the manager. In some instances, evaluative data have been shared with the media first, a situation that can prove to be embarrassing to the program manager, and bad for the program evaluator's career. (6) *Right of preview*. To quote French, et al. (1983):

> Related to the issue of control of the report's distribution is control of its content. Without invoking debate about the integrity of the data, the issue here involves interpretation and emphasis. Managers will usually wish to see a preliminary or draft report and have the opportunity to recommend changes, make corrections, and discuss interpretation. The self-protective stance behind this wish is obvious enough; at the same time, an evaluator hoping to make a contribution to a program beyond the simple analysis of data will recognize the risk of Pyrrhic victories inherent in surprise attacks (p.51).

(7) *Authority to renegotiate*. Invariably, at least some minor changes in operating agreements will be necessary. Things do not always go according to plan. Unforeseen delays occur, subjects or clients become unavailable or uncooperative, staff workloads become unexpectedly heavy, and personnel come and go. Above all other aspects of the contract between the evaluator and the program manager is the need for flexibility with both parties.

Another issue that may be "sticky" is the ownership of data for publication purposes. On the one hand, a program manager may view *all* aspects of the program, including evaluative data, as being owned exclusively *by the program*. Its publication beyond that of a technical report (which might not even get disseminated beyond the manager) could be viewed with suspicion and hostility. The more negative the findings, the more likely it is that there will be reluctance to disseminate the report. Evaluators, while they get paid for their efforts, nevertheless can feel ownership of the information they produce and interpret. For the sake of their reputation as evaluators, as well as for other personal and professional reasons, they may want to publish it in the professional literature that can be shared with, and read by their colleagues. Shouldn't the field of evaluation have the opportunity to grow as a result of someone's efforts (failures as well as successes)? Does the evaluator's access to, and use of the data cease when payment is made? If publications *do* result, how will authorship be determined? These points can be quite substantive ones from the point of view of both the program manager and the program evaluator. They should be resolved prior to formalizing any contractual arrangement.

House (1980) provides an additional descriptive example of the components of an evaluation agreement that includes: (1) the evaluator's charge; (2) a listing of the audiences for the evaluation report presented in priority order; (3) stipulations about responsibility for report writing and editing; (4) release and dissemination of reports; (5) format of the evaluation report; (6) questions to be addressed by the report; (7) budgetary resources to support the evaluation effort; (8) report delivery schedule; (9) evaluators' access to relevant program data; and, (10) evaluative procedures to be employed. These lists of contract recommendations are not intended to be exhaustive. They should, however, provide some guidance to program evaluators and program managers who have not developed such contracts previously.

The Basic Needs of Stakeholders

According to Smith (1989) stakeholders are "those persons or groups who impact a program in very significant ways or who are similarly affected by the actions of a program" (p.82). Stated somewhat differently by Mitroff (1983), stakeholders are "...those interest groups, parties, actors, claimants, and institutions -- both internal and external to the corporation -- that exert a hold on it" (p.4). A stakeholder is more than just anyone in an organization with informational requirements, or someone who might take advantage of the availability of evaluation data. Rather, stakeholders are persons with a vested interest in the program, and are in a position to make decisions that affect the future of the program. Rossi and Freeman (1989) provide a list of stakeholders and explain the context in which their respective "stakes" occur. These people and organizations are identified in Table 3.3. More often than not, stakeholders of health education and promotion programs are decision makers within funding organizations, legislative committees, boards of directors, companies, or any of the administrative bodies of the numerous agencies, facilities, and organizations that carry out health education and promotion activities.

Preparation of a program for evaluation necessitates a focus on *technical*, as well as *context* issues. Technical concerns include examination of the current stage of program development and assessment of information (i.e., data) needs. For example, a program still in a developmental phase may have a greater need for formative data that can help refine it or put it on a corrective course, whereas a more established program may benefit from

Table 3.3 Potential Stakeholders of Program Evaluations

Policymakers and other decision makers	persons ultimately responsible for whether a program is started, maintained, expanded, curtailed, or eliminated
Program sponsors	individuals and organizations that fund the program
Evaluation sponsors	individuals and organizations that fund the evaluation of a program (often the same as the program sponsors)
Target participants	any of the participating units (individuals, groups, etc.) who are the recipients of the intervention being evaluated
Program management	individuals, groups, or organizations that oversee or coordinate the program being evaluated
Program staff	personnel who carry out implementation of the program
Evaluation staff	personnel who design and conduct the program evaluation
Program competitors	individuals, groups, or organizations that compete for finite available resources
Contextual stakeholders	individuals, groups, and organizations that reside in proximity of a program (e.g., agencies, government officials, or other persons with political influence)
Evaluation community	evaluators who read evaluation reports and make judgments about their technical adequacy

Adapted from: Rossi, P.H., & Freeman, H.E. (1989). *Evaluation: A Systematic Approach*, 4th edition. Newbury Park, CA: Sage Publications.

data that are summative in nature. Context concerns address the psychological and political "readiness" of the program, including attitudes, beliefs, and relationships of managers, staff, service recipients and clients, and advisory/governing boards.

A frequently voiced criticism of evaluations is that their results either are not used, or are not used effectively. Results of evaluations are more likely to be used if they address issues of importance to specific audiences. Thus, the primary groups of stakeholders, along with their information needs, should be identified at the time that the evaluation is planned. An evaluator who is apprised of the decision making requirements of the stakeholders will be in a better position to direct the evaluation, and to measure those indicators most critical to the decisions that ultimately have to be made. As Raizen and Rossi (1981) point out:

Such initial identification will help define the type of evaluation to be undertaken, the issues to be addressed, the sort of information to be collected, and the form of reporting and communication that is likely to be most effective (p.6).

The Political Nature of Evaluation

Evaluation of almost any variety is likely to be perceived by program staff as threatening. Anybody who has ever taken an examination, has had an important job interview or job performance review, or who has been "assessed" or "judged" in some other way, is familiar with the feeling of being placed "under a microscope." At best, program evaluations can cause some disruption of people's lives, often resulting in their having to perform more interviews, enter more records, or fill out more forms. At worst, evaluation can cast doubt on the value of programs, point fingers at the competence of certain staff members or managers, place a question mark on job security, and call into question the probability of a program's long term survival.

People being served by a program can be affected directly by the evaluation process, too. They may have to complete surveys, participate in in-depth interviews conducted by strangers, answer questions of a highly personal nature, and sign consent forms that surrender some of their rights. In summary, evaluations may affect people on a continuum ranging from mild irritation to distinct threat and suspicion.

In an ideal world, the evaluation of health education and promotion programs would be governed by powerful designs, objective measures, appropriate statistical applications, unbiased interpretation, and dissemination to stakeholders whose interest would be in program improvement. It is perhaps, not surprising to you that such ideal conditions rarely, if ever, present themselves to the professional evaluator. To understand why the real world is different from an "ideal" world, we must examine the motivations that underlie many evaluations.

Funding agencies typically require the submission of a sound evaluation plan before any money is passed to the grantee. This evaluation plan is likely to include a combination of process and outcome measures, perhaps with an emphasis on program effects. However, there can be a problem with using outcome evaluations of program effects to improve program management. If negative findings occur, there is the fear that a program will be curtailed or eliminated. This fear is heightened in today's environment of austerity and fiscal accountability. Consequently, program managers and other personnel are not likely to be warmly receptive to, nor cooperative with, evaluations that they perceive to have the potential of damaging the reputation of their programs (Raizen & Rossi, 1981).

For people who operate programs whose budgets are contingent on performance, highly positive evaluations are a survival necessity. Consequently, evaluators may be encouraged to emphasize program successes (possibly reporting *only* the achievements), while downplaying any program weaknesses or deficiencies. Under such circumstances, persons in a position to make policy decisions concerning widespread dissemination of a program to other sites, or to make recommendations about renewal of an existing program, will be presented with less than adequate information. This type of **ingratiating evaluation** in which the evaluator is asked to take on the role of "program advocate" may be the approach used when a modestly productive, but highly visible or popular program is being scrutinized. One would find it difficult to defend some drug education programs or driver education programs aimed at adolescents on the basis of results achieved. Yet, elimination of these highly institutionalized programs would be nothing short of blasphemy in the eyes of some health and safety education policymakers. Another strategy that takes the evaluator out of the role of "objective scientist" and gets employed for defending monetary allocations and promoting program survival, especially when program effects are unspectacular, is concentrating the evaluation report on program activities alone. In the early, formative stages of an intervention, the reporting of effort is appropriate and necessary, and may be the only evaluative information available. Moreover, monitoring an intervention in its beginning stages is critical in being able to articulate process with later outcome. However, when a program has existed for a period of time that is "long enough" to show effects, limiting an evaluation report to a discussion of effort and activity may be a ruse to avoid confronting the relevant issues.

Even for programs that do appear to have positive social value, and that can be defended with respect to their cost-effectiveness and other measures, evaluators must be cautious about the "trap" of becoming a program advocate. Some authors (House, 1988; Mathison, 1991) view this type of advocacy disapprovingly as substituting values for evaluation, thus removing the evaluator's independence as well as the credibility of the evaluation process. On the other hand, Braskamp (1994) argues that if the evaluator discloses this advocacy position, the consequences for the program and the evaluation can be positive, since the evaluator uses this caring position to show that the program's context is understood in the evaluation, and the evaluation's purpose is for real program improvement and not merely for the sake of accountability.

It is possible for program managers and evaluators to be at "odds" with each other about evaluation intent. According to French, et al. (1983):

......managers generally preferred evaluations focusing on process and development (to guide future program development) whereas evaluators preferred those emphasizing outcome and effectiveness to facilitate judgment of programs. When evaluations conformed more to the wishes and and beliefs of evaluators, managers tended to lose interest in the evaluations and to withdraw support (p.48).

Weiss (1977) suggests that a basic mistrust of motive and point of view can exist between evaluators and program managers. Evaluators may be seen as "fighting for the integrity of their data," while managers attempt to impose positive interpretations of the same data. Evaluators can see program managers as impediments to evaluation "often out of ignorance." Thus, a relationship of true animosity, or at least one with a significant conflict of interest can arise. Weiss (1972) stresses that personality and role conflict between managers and evaluators can be major impediments to the evaluation process. As French, et al. (1983) surmise:

Trying to compare managers and evaluators along a good-bad or positive-negative dimension is inappropriate. Far more productive is viewing each party as possessing integrity, ability, and devotion to certain kinds of truth. Both are dedicated to doing the best possible job, but they have different jobs with different success criteria. ......Evaluators develop [successful] careers by conducting methodologically competent evaluations useful in guiding social or program policy and contributing to general knowledge through publication. Whether the programs evaluated are successful is not their primary concern. For program managers in human service programs, success is usually defined in terms of longevity, growth, size of staff and budget, and number of people served. Because many human service programs are never adequately evaluated, and because evaluation reports are filed and forgotten more often than not, the actual effectiveness of a program may have little impact on a manager's career and reputation. ......Attending to some of these differences and similarities should help managers and evaluators see themselves not as antagonists, but as complementary and even synergistic partners in the enterprise of program evaluation (p.49).

According to Weiss (1972): "A characteristic of evaluation research that differentiates it from most other kinds of research is that it takes place in an action setting. Something else besides research is going on; there is a program serving people. In fact, the service program is the more important element on the scene" (p.92). Even a whole team of evaluators will not shift the priority from service delivery to evaluation. An evaluator who adjusts to this reality will enjoy his or her work more.

We have just examined what can happen when positive feedback about a program is of great concern to program managers, and who therefore, may attempt to orchestrate positive results. It is possible though that control of the evaluation is not in the hands of those individuals who would benefit most from a positive program review. To the contrary, control may lie with persons whose interests are in the *extinction* of the program. Under these circumstances, evaluation may be the process of gathering any information whatsoever that would reflect poorly on the program, its clients, or its managers. This **"hatchet" evaluation** becomes the mechanism for curtailing or eliminating a program that is perceived by high level managers or politicians as unnecessary. For instance, it is quite plausible that a hospital-based wellness program existing in a large health care facility could be effectively carrying out such activities as patient education and counseling, rehabilitation, and community outreach. The program may be meeting its objectives and be a good patient-provider bridge. However, if the evaluative criterion employed is the program's ability to generate revenue for the health care facility, its extinction may be justified in good conscience by policymakers whose primary motive is fiscal accountability to a board of directors or to stockholders.

The evaluation of a program does not have to be skewed intentionally for it to become a political "hot potato" though. Suppose that an objective, but strongly negative evaluation of a state health department program to reduce drug use among economically poor, pregnant minority women had just been completed. If the evaluator's principal recommendation concerning the program to the health department decision makers is "extinction," what consequences might arise? If this program represents a highly visible health department endeavor for disadvantaged minority women, what will its extinction mean in terms of political fallout? If, in addition, the program supports a staff of health educators, social workers, and other human service providers who are themselves members of ethnic or racial minorities, what will their dismissal mean in terms of morale, racial harmony, and trust in this governmental agency? Any evaluator who expects decision makers to accept a recommendation for program extinction without examining a broader range of issues is being presumptuous, if not altogther unrealistic.

Not all evaluations are used primarily to justify program survival or promote extinction. However, there may be motives surrounding an evaluation that are still highly political. For example, the **compliance** or **regulatory evaluation** is carried out when the principal objective is to protect the program or the organization in which it resides from violations of government regulations or standards of performance set forth by a professional review organization or an accrediting body. Such violations may have consequences such as fines, closer scrutiny in the future, reduced funding, lost prestige, or other "penalties." The compliance evaluator is likely to be a person from inside the organization whose role is one of watchdog. The activity involves information gathering of whatever kind that facilitates the monitoring of performance against a standard of practice or official operating code. The evaluator's main objective is to "keep the heat" from a regulatory agency off the program.

As we hinted previously, evaluators may wish to publish their findings in a forum beyond that of the obligatory technical report. If program evaluation is to grow as a discipline, it can do so only if methods and results are shared beyond just a closed circle of individuals. The driving force for publishing, therefore, may be the desire to make a contribution to the field of evaluation. We take the position that that motivation should be nurtured and encouraged.

Other factors may drive the desire to publish, however. The evaluator's professional survival, if he or she also is a member of a college or university faculty, may hinge on publish or perish criteria. If such is the case, it becomes extremely important to this person to attempt to publish any and all material that can be derived from a large scale effort. At least two factors seem to affect the subsequent course of the publication process: (1) the writer's desire to write as little as possible and still get published; and (2) the writer's desire to please the journal editor or board of reviewers. In regard to the former issue, the writer may partition the evaluation report into what are known as the **least publishable units** or LPUs. Bits and pieces of the original evaluation get written, and if the writer is fortunate enough to have them published, may get them spread diffusely among several journals. A reader who does not have access to all of the relevant journals, or who does not even know of the existence of companion articles, gets a most incomplete view of the evaluation as it actually occurred. Since becoming published means pleasing peer reviewers, a writer may include only selected findings, concentrate only on statistically significant relationships, or provide other abbreviated results. It should be obvious that such **academic evaluations,** driven by the need to publish, place academic integrity and completeness in peril.

In general, evaluations are used for one or more of three broad purposes: (1) To assist people in making value judgments about programs; (2) To serve the decision making needs of program managers; or (3) To collect information that might be tapped at some future point in time. An evaluation that is continuous or ongoing can be described as an **information gathering evaluation**. The data may be used for making a judgment or decision in the future, but until that point in time, all information is "neutral." An information gathering evaluation simply may report things such as: *The childbirth education classes were attended by 187 women. At the STD counseling program, 86 condoms were distributed. The education phase of cardiac rehabilitation costs $125 per patient. A little over 83% of the women in the cocaine addiction recovery program were* *drug-free after six months of the intervention.* Of the five varieties of evaluations discussed (ingratiating, hatchet, compliance, academic, and informational) it is probably the one least mired in politics -- at least until the data are used for a specific purpose.

As an illustration of how "idle information" can become explosive, Jones (1985) offers the following example:

......in 1981 the nation's air traffic controllers went out on strike for more pay......[several studies] ......purported to demonstrate how stressful the job was......Air traffic controllers were said to experience disorders such as ulcers and depression much more frequently than did members of the general population. The reason, or so the research seemed to indicate, was the nature of their high-pressure jobs, jobs that required constant alertness and in which a mistake could cost hundreds of lives. Those studies had been in the literature for years, and were generally considered noncontroversial. At the time of the strike, however, they were dug out and held up to ridicule. Their results were called into question. It was claimed by those who wanted to end the strike that the studies had been poorly conducted and sloppily done. Now, it appeared that air traffic controllers had one of the poshest jobs around -- short hours, high pay, and only a two-year training period. You did not even have to go to college to qualify. The point, of course, is when the stakes are high -- as they usually are in evaluation research -- different and more powerful motives come into play (pp.263-264).

At least one other issue that can have political ramifications, and which has not yet been touched on, should be addressed. Programs have a way of changing as they progress. This "drift" may be true especially of new programs. Weiss (1972) writes:

If the program has altered course, what does the evaluator do? If he goes ahead as if he were studying the same program, he will never know what it was that led to the observed effects or the lack of them -- the old program, the new one, the transition, or some combination of everything going on. If he drops the original evaluation and tries to start over again under the changed circumstances, he may lack appropriate baseline data (p.93).

As you can well imagine, programs with interventions that are forever changing (or seem to be) are nightmarish for an evaluation team. Some suggestions for handling this undesirable, but highly probable situation are provided by Weiss (1972): (1) Take frequent measures of program effect, rather than postponing data collection to one point in time; (2) If the intervention changes, try to define each successive intervention for the period of time it operates, along with the assumptions and procedures that characterize each phase, and make the transitions between interventions clear; (3) Note which clients, patients, or students participated at each phase of the program, and avoid any temptation to lump them all together; (4) Identify aspects of the program that are expected to remain stable, and focus at least part of the evaluation on these elements; and (5) If the program is truly amorphous, consider abandoning the thought of examining outcomes, and focus on an evaluation of the "what, how, and why of events."

The Ethics Continuum in Evaluation

The term **ethics** is one that is confused by many persons in virtually all fields of endeavor. The confusion may arise from expectations that ethical principles or guidelines have to be prescriptive to be useful, and must tell us what to do (or what *not* to do) in all conceivable situations. The definition of ethics may also be confused with religious dogma or simplified to a "do unto others" kind of philosophy. Ethical practice may also get presented as something we would do in an "ideal world," thus implying that what is practical, but "acceptable," is more likely to be the net outcome, and that what is "ethical" is something that cannot ever quite be achieved. Practice that is "ethical" gets characterized, therefore, as only an "ideal" rather than something actually attainable. Newman and Brown (1996) summarize three definitions of ethics:

...as the principles of morality, particularly those dealing with the right or wrong of an action; as the rules of conduct for members of a particular profession; and as the science of the study of ideal human behavior, the concepts of good behavior (p.20).

Though each of these definitions has merit, not any one of them is sufficiently comprehensive. Evaluators of health education and promotion programs are professionally prepared to devise poignant research questions and develop the strategies for answering them. But what if the most objective strategies for data gathering violate a person's privacy, such as occurs when hidden observers are used? What if procedures employed in an intervention or its evaluation could compromise a person's physical or psychological health? Under what circumstance should (1) potentially injurious activities be employed? (2) illegal activities be disclosed? (3) highly personal information (e.g., sexual behavior) be asked for? or (4) stress arousing situations be created? "The first responsibility of the evaluator, as it is with the basic researcher, is to protect people from harm" (Posavac & Carey, 1989, p.71).

The development of formal education and training in ethics among health education and promotion specialists is a recent innovation. Even with its occurrence, few individuals have had extensive experience with ethical decision making models, and even less opportunity in conducting evaluations. Concern about ethics in health education has inspired groups like the Society for Public Health Education (1993) and the Association for the Advancement of Health Education [now the American Association for Health Education] (1994) to develop codes of ethics. While such ethical codes may be necessary and valuable, they may not be sufficient for optimal practice. According to Newman and Brown (1996):

Codes, unfortunately, are too often designed to protect professionals from outside regulation and are often conservative. They are more likely to focus on what should not be done and on the minimal behavior rather than on what should be done and on ideal behavior......Another reason why ethical codes and rules for professionals may lack comprehensiveness is that they usually represent a consensus of opinions......Despite these limitations, statements of ethical codes and rules are a hallmark of maturity for a profession, serving as useful guidelines for both experienced and new professionals. They are insufficient, however, unless the practitioner also has the experience in relating these codes and rules to broader ethical theories and principles when thinking through ethical dilemmas (p.19).

Until the end of World War II, individual investigators were expected and presumed to safeguard the rights and personal well-being of their human subjects (Neale & Liebert, 1986). Fears of inappropriate research schemes had emerged as a result of the medical and social experiments carried out in Nazi concentration camps. Still, adequate protection of human subjects was not legislated in the United States for many years after the war. Concern over abuses in research led to the creation by the United States Congress in 1981 of the *National Commission for Protection of Human Subjects of Biomedical and*

Behavioral Research. As a result of this development, most colleges and universities, hospitals, and many school boards established **institutional review boards (IRBs)** that require a prior review of any research that uses human subjects in virtually any manner whatsoever (Ary, Jacobs & Razavieh, 1990).

According to Marshall and Rossman (1989), the researcher/evaluator is obliged to ask a series of questions concerning the proposed design. Will the study violate the participants' privacy or unduly disrupt their everyday lives? Are the participants placing themselves in danger or at risk by being in the study? Will any of the procedures violate their human rights, or in some way compromise their dignity?

Any research or evaluation involving human subjects must maintain certain basic standards of practice, including making participation voluntary and making it clear that subjects are free to withdraw from the study. At the minimum, study designs also must ensure that human subjects give their consent to any procedure that places them at any physical or psychological risk. Moreover, this consent must be **informed consent**, and all reasonable steps need to be taken to guarantee that clients, patients, and students (or their legal proxies) understand the risks of participation completely. In most instances where risk is possible, informed consent is obtained in writing. Yet, written consent may not necessarily meet the spirit of being "informed," if the written document is prepared at a reading level beyond the literacy level of the audience, or uses technical terms and jargon that subjects cannot be expected to know. Writes Kimmel (1988):

When studying minority group members, children, and non-English-speaking groups, certain difficulties arise from their differential status, including limited possibilities of articulation and understanding to judge adequately the purpose, risks, and other aspects of the investigation. These limitations further threaten the adequacy of the informed consent process, and increase the danger of subtly, perhaps unintentionally, coercing relatively powerless individuals into social research (p.70).

Nachmias and Nachmias (1987) report the six federal guidelines to be transmitted regarding matters of informed consent. The spirit of these six points is summarized in Table 3.4.

Ethical standards also entitle human subjects to their **right of privacy**. As Best and Kahn (1989) write:

Ordinarily, it is justifiable to observe and record behavior that is essentially public, behavior that others normally would be in a position to observe. It is an invasion of privacy to observe and record intimate behavior that the subject has reason to believe is private. Concealed observers, cameras, microphones, or the use of private correspondence without the subject's knowledge and permission are invasions of privacy. If these practices are to be employed, the researcher should explain the reasons and secure permission (p.43).

Moreover, **confidentiality** should be maintained with respect to any data about which the client might be sensitive. Generally speaking, confidentiality should apply to any information, since one can never be certain about which information clients would approve disclosure. Confidentiality is different than **anonymity**. The latter term means more than the fact that information about a particular individual will not be shared. It means that the identities of respondents to surveys or questionnaires, or of participants in experiments are unknown to the investigators. That is, information that is provided cannot be traced to a particular respondent. Anonymity is difficult to protect in small groups with which the investigator has close or regular contact. The confidentiality of records or responses is easier to guarantee than anonymity. Ethics extend beyond these points, however. Evaluation ethics extend to some other fundamental principles: **beneficence**, **nonmaleficence**, **respect/autonomy**, **justice**, and **fidelity**.

Table 3.4 Federal Guidelines for Conveyance of Informed Consent

---

Fair explanation of procedures to be followed, as well as their purposes

Description of any and all expected discomforts and risks

Description of benefits to be derived

Disclosure of any alternative procedures that might be advantageous to the person

Offer to respond to any inquiries concerning the procedures

Clear instruction that the person is free to withdraw consent and/or to discontinue participation in the study at any time without fear of prejudice or reprisal

---

Adapted from: Nachmias, D., & Nachmias C. (1987). *Research Methods in the Social Sciences*, 3rd edition. New York: St. Martin's Press, p.86

Beneficence asks what "good" can come to clients and participants as a result of the evaluation, whether maximum "good" is being achieved, and what "good" can be attained beyond just the expectations of professional codes of practice. Beneficence also seeks the avoidance of unnecessary harm and the promotion of optimal positive outcomes. Nonmaleficence queries as to what harm is likely to occur resulting from decisions and actions emanating from the evaluation. In this instance, the interpretation of "harm" must not only consider physical harm, but psychological harm as well. As we have explained previously, the evaluation process always invokes some level of stress among stakeholders. Thus, one must ask whether program staff (e.g., health care workers) will be exposed to excessive amounts of stress, or program participants (e.g., health care recipients) will have their privacy violated as a side effect of the evaluation. A critical examination of nonmaleficence versus beneficence is the weighing of the "good" that may be derived from a particular procedure or activity against the "bad" that may occur from it. Such an examination is a most suitable activity for evaluators and program managers to undertake in the evaluation planning process.

According to Sieber (1980), "respect refers to respect for autonomy or freedom of persons and for the well-being of nonautonomous persons (children, the mentally incompetent, prisoners)......justice refers to equitable treatment and equitable representation of subgroups within society" (p.54). A breach in the protection of individual rights is a serious malpractice issue for the investigator. House (1993) is emphatic in his remarks that direct evaluators to be advocates for the disadvantaged and the powerless, i.e., to bring "social justice" to bear on the standards against which evaluations are judged.

The issue of fidelity seeks to determine if evaluator and client are both being faithful to the contractual arrangements that have been made. Are they being honest with each other and with program participants? Are promises that were written or implied during negotiations for the evaluation being kept? Promises generally should be viewed as obligations. An evaluator who promises to conduct a certain type of evaluation, to provide a particular kind of analysis, or who asserts that he or she will devote a specified amount of time and effort to report preparation, needs to fulfill that expectation. The prospect of a competing evaluation contract that comes along and is more lucrative or more prestigious cannot be allowed to interfere with a previous contractual promise. On the other hand, Newman and Brown (1996) remind us that [fidelity] "is not an absolute principle" and that [promises] "to do something wrong are not binding" (p.50). Though contracts for evaluators ordinarily are binding, contracts can come into conflict with other duties or principles, and the fidelity or allegiance that one has to *all* of the stakeholders (e.g., program participants, taxpayers, other evaluation professionals, the society-at-large), and not just to the client who hires them, must be considered too.

Another issue of ethics concerns the deliberate use of **deception**. Deception is the purposeful or intentional withholding of, or misinforming about, details related to an investigation. The practice of deception in evaluation research probably grew out of a need that investigators have of protecting themselves against the reactive tendencies of their subjects. Stating it succinctly, when subjects know what is being evaluated, how it is being evaluated, and why it is being evaluated, they tend to act "differently" or "unnaturally." They may acquiesce, and tell the investigator exactly what they perceive he or she wants to hear (regardless of its factual nature). If they do not like the investigator or the process itself, they might engage in deliberate lying and deception themselves. Consequently, deception is a facet of investigations that may be critical in obtaining valid information. Writes Kimmel (1988):

[deception]...is seen as permissible as long as certain conditions are met (such as when no alternative means of investigation are available, risks are minimal, and adequate debriefing is provided)...Deception represents a potential violation of participants' rights, but without its use certain questions could not be investigated through valid research. However, the mere fact that a practice flourishes should not be taken as evidence that it is morally acceptable. That people lie, cheat, and steal are not moral defenses for those practices. That social researchers often deceive their subjects is not a defense of that practice (pp.34-35).

According to Nunnally (1983): "In many programs of evaluation research......the people who operate the program are highly committed to their evaluations even before the research evidence is in" (p.234). A consequence of this fact is that program managers (and evaluators, too) may be tempted to "fake" data, or at least manipulate it to their advantage (it's sometimes called "data massaging"). Motives may be good, but the end may not justify the means. Suppose you are funded to perform a statewide evaluation of need in which you will examine the gaps in the delivery of school health services. The political motive behind the study may be "to prove" that school boards and county health departments need to provide money to hire more nurses to work with children. In essence, the conclusion has been drawn before the study has even been started. The direction taken in the study, the data to be collected, and many other relevant issues will be focused on making the point. The possible benefit of having more nurses to perform more services for kids is a point that is hard to argue with philosophically, but it may not be one that can be demonstrated objectively through evaluation research. The issue of carrying out a "loaded" study is an ethical question with which an evaluator must wrestle.

The use of treatment and control groups in evaluation research will be discussed in detail later in this text (Chapter 10). However, a relevant ethical issue for the investigator is the assignment of subjects to one or the other of these groups. How will it be decided which subjects become part of the intervention, and which ones will be "control" group subjects? If the intervention is a favorable one, those persons in the control group will be deprived. If the intervention actually proves to cause harm, then the treatment group could be at a significant disadvantage. Does the investigator who provides a beneficial intervention to a treatment group have any kind of moral obligation to the untreated group? This dilemma is not resolved easily, but fortunately, it has little practical significance in most social or educational program evaluation. The use of an **untreated control group** often can be justified in at least two ways: (1) the assumption that resource limitations prohibit the dissemination of an intervention to all groups simultaneously; and/or (2) the promise that the untreated control or comparison group can be offered the intervention at the end of the experiment if it proves to be beneficial.

Newman and Brown (1996) believe that evaluators rely on four cues to guide their ethical thinking: *intuition*, *past experience*, *observations of conventional behavior among colleagues*, and *ethical rules as presented in ethical codes*. With respect to intuition, an evaluator may begin to suspect the existence of a problem if a client asks or demands to review such things as handwritten responses to open-ended questions, tapes of focus group interviews, a transcript or notes of an interview just completed with a member of the staff, or other original data sources that may allow the client to link individuals to particular responses, or to edit or actually "lose" some of the data. Evaluators may be confronted by situations that ask them to "react" on the spur of the moment, and must feel comfortable in deflecting a request from a client that "feels wrong at a gut level." Newman and Brown (1996) believe that an experienced evaluator can develop an "educated intuition" much like the wine connoisseur develops an educated palate. If a client request feels wrong, it may be wise to defer a response until adequate time to consider the request is available. If an immediate response is required, the educated intuitive response that comes from past experience must result in satisfying the client while also maintaining the goal of being ethical.

A bad past experience may be the reason that an evaluator insists to a client that their contract specifically deny the client the privilege of extracting portions of the evaluation report without the evaluator's permission. As discussed earlier in this chapter, negotiation of the evaluator-client is a critical stepping off point for the whole evaluation.

Not infrequently, a client is dissatisfied with the wording of what we as the evaluators expected to be the "final" submitted report of the evaluation. Naturally, we try to accommodate requests for modest changes, especially if they are in the interest of providing clarity for stakeholders. However, requests for content changes that significantly alter the interpretation of findings is quite another matter. Realizing that some evaluation reports are going to affect the interests of some stakeholders in a negative fashion, evaluators must always convey results in such a way as to preserve stakeholders' dignity and self-worth (American Educational Research Association, 1992). Expressing findings, even negative ones, in an objective manner is possible without offending individuals associated with the program or denigrating all aspects of the program. For the novice evaluator, seeking the counsel of more experienced peers may guide the resolution of matters that relate to controversial results. French, et al. (1983) and House (1980) emphasize that issues about final editing authority be determined prior to the onset of the formal evaluation, if possible, and we concur with that advice.

Professional evaluators may be confronted by special circumstances that require a particular type of role and ethical response. Perrin (1992) describes a clinical drug trial in which the effectiveness of a drug administered to high-risk pregnant women to improve fetal lung development was being evaluated. Evaluation required the use of multiple amniocentesis procedures, each one of which placed both the mother and the fetus at some physical harm. Patients were asked to sign a multiple-page consent form written in typical medical and legal jargon that might challenge even the most educated and literate of patients. In this particular case, the patients were all women for whom English was a second language or whose formal education was so low that reason to expect clear understanding of the implications of the procedure was dubious. A nurse who was not directly part of the evaluation, but who was involved in the care of these patients, was concerned that whatever "consent" was being given was not "informed," and attempted to have the clinical trial halted on ethical grounds. In this case there was an effort made to have the evaluator act as "**whistle-blower**." An evaluator *is* obliged to report to appropriate authorities whenever potential harm is feared (Kimmel, 1988). Similarly, Newman and Brown (1996) conclude that whenever information, especially negative information is being withheld from audiences, the evaluator's role as whistle-blower is an important one. For the internal evaluator a major conflict arises over the ethical role of whistle-blower versus that of the organizational "gatekeeper" role as the person who may determine which data get reported to decision makers and which data do not. Being loyal to the organization, the internal evaluator may withhold certain information which is counterproductive to the role of "non-biased scientist" and member of the society-at-large. As Newman and Brown write (1996): "For internal evaluators, the principle of fidelity may conflict with those of justice and beneficence" (p.142).

Evaluators, both novice and experienced, have at least four prominent resources to guide their ethical thinking and practice. These come from the American Educational Research Association (1992), the American Psychological Association (1992), the Joint Committee on Standards (1994), and the American Evaluation Association (1995).

The Responsibility of IRBs

Institutional review boards (IRBs) were created to assure the protection and welfare of human subjects. The Department of Health and Human Services (DHHS), as well as some other federal agencies, require that any grant, contract, cooperative agreement, or fellowship for research involving human subjects provide for an IRB to assure subject protection (Kimmel, 1988). The specific points covered under DHHS guidelines are presented in Table 3.5.

Table 3.5 Primary Functions of Institutional Review Boards (IRBs)

Obtaining voluntary informed consent and debriefing study participants

Protecting participants' privacy

Ensuring confidentiality

Reviewing protocols where deception is used

Weighing the relative risks of participants and benefits derived from the study

---

Adapted from: Newman, D.L., & Brown, R.D. (1996). *Applied Ethics for Program Evaluation.* Thousand Oaks. CA: Sage Publications.

Unfunded studies conducted within research-oriented institutions such as universities and some hospitals are not required to undergo IRB review as a matter of regulation. However, it is likely that most institutions of stature will require a review of the projects conducted by faculty and student researchers.

Investigators and IRBs alike will never be in a position to categorize all procedures, designs, methods, activities, and events as being 100% *ethical*, or 100% *unethical*. IRB committees are not perfect in their recommendations. Just because IRB approval has been sought and secured for an investigation does not guarantee that all ethical aspects of research and evaluation have been considered, or that the presumed context of the study will turn out to be the actual context, or that protocols will be conducted precisely in the manner in which they were proposed. The case study of the drug clinical trial involving pregnant women described above by Perrin (1992) was IRB-approved at its home institution, but still had several points of contention where ethical matters were concerned. Thus, while codes of ethics and professional practice standards may seem to imply that the ethics construct is dichotomous, it clearly is not. What is ethical is likely to be determined by precedent, particular circumstances, the values of the time in which one lives, and other matters. Ethics, like morality, cannot be legislated in a value-free manner.

Ethno-Cultural Issues and Evaluation

It has become increasingly common for evaluations not to be limited to the boundaries of the U.S., and subsequently, have procedures and protocols become confounded by divergent cultures, languages, and values. Even within the U.S., racial, ethnic, and social class differences can be so great in virtually any of the nation's large cities that evaluators may find themselves confronted with significant diversity issues that magnify already complex measurement concerns even within a single school district or zip code area.

Matsumoto (1994) points out that cross-cultural or cross-lingual investigations infringe on one's measurement ability. Cultures vary in the value they assign to such matters as authority, privacy, individuality, compliance, loyalty, trust, cooperation, independence, conflict, and other issues. According to Newman and Brown (1996): "Participants in more authoritarian cultures may be accustomed to acquiescing to requests for information coming from supposed official representatives. They may fear recriminations if they do not participate" (p.149). Ethical issues of little or no concern in the mainstream culture may abound when the study venue or the group of participants is altered.

Kirkhart (1995) points out that culturally unsophisticated or arrogant evaluators may reduce the accessibility of a population whose participation in a study is desired. Moreover, even if accessibility is obtained, evaluator behavior may be of a nature that compromises or invalidates study results.

Another potential confounder is the literacy of study participants. Variation in reading and comprehension skills may influence respondent bias and other forms of reporting error. Even if the written or spoken words used in translation are the same, such similarity is no guarantee that the words have identical meanings and idiomatic interpretation across languages or cultures. Some investigators now advocate for a careful "cultural tailoring" (Pasick, D'Onofrio & Otero-Sabogal, 1996) of questions or use of an extension of back-translation known as "decentering" to assure item equivalence as much as possible (Pasick, Sabogal, Bird, et al., 1996).

Direct involvement of community members (*critical stakeholders*) in the planning and delivery of an evaluation is especially important when the evaluation focus is on persons not part of the mainstream culture. Such direct involvement can provide credibility for the evaluation as well as to identify potential problems of cultural bias in data collection, definition of terms, social justice, and other issues that could later prove to invalidate findings (Madison, 1992; Travers, 1997). Negative social descriptors (e.g., *economically disadvantaged, culturally deprived, at-risk population*, and *hardcore unemployable*) can find their way into studies and carry a certain prejudicial status with them that is counterproductive to an evaluator's aims. Careful and planned involvement of critical stakeholders can minimize inappropriate bias that often accompanies studies.

Summary

Any program evaluation will arouse the attention and interests of the program's stakeholders. No evaluation, regardless of the program, occurs in an environment that is free of bias and values. Skills and competencies possessed by evaluators will determine, in part, the scope and content of evaluations. Evaluators will be confronted by ethical decisions regarding the integrity of their procedures, and pressure to conform to outcomes pleasing to program managers and evaluation sponsors. For many matters of decision making there are no clearly "right" or "wrong" answers. The evaluation process works best when evaluators and managers work cooperatively in attempting to understand their respective professional needs. Through whatever format an investigation is performed, persons responsible for conducting it must take into serious account, the rights of the human subjects to be involved. The benefits of conducting a research or evaluation study must be weighed against the potential threats, risks, or dangers faced by the people being studied. Investigators need to be able to make certain guarantees to subjects, or risk acting in an inappropriate sphere of ethics.

Case Study

Dickersin, K. (1997). How important is publication bias? A synthesis of available data. *AIDS Education and Prevention*, *9*(Supplement A), 15-21.

This paper elaborates on an issue that is raised in the chapter just completed -- reporting some but not all of the findings from a particular piece of research. If study participants consent to be studied based on the belief that they are "making a contribution" to science, but the results of the study are not reported or reported only selectively, has deception or another form of scientific misconduct occurred? Explain. What is the impact on the scientific community if results are reported (and published) on a highly selective basis? To what extent might publication bias be influencing choices related to HIV/AIDS education policy and practice? What are some ways that publication bias can be minimized, and under what circumstances are these mechanisms likely to be effective?

Student Questions/Activities

1.   Rank order each of the following "violations" of ethical practice from "1" (most serious) to "10" (least serious). Be prepared to defend your rankings. Compare your rankings to those of a peer or to the other members of your class.

- The evaluator changes the evaluation questions to match the data analysis.
- The evaluation plan necessitates major disruptions and significant changes in staff activities.
- The evaluator conducts an evaluation when he or she lacks sufficient skills or experience.
- The evaluation report is written so that partisan interest groups can delete embarrassing weaknesses.

- The evaluation report is available only to the hiring client with no provision for other audiences.
- The evaluator loses interest in the evaluation once the final report is written.
- The evaluator promises confidentiality when it cannot be guaranteed.
- The evaluator makes decisions without consulting with the client when consultation has been agreed to.
- The evaluator fails to note the limitations of the evaluation in the final report.
- The evaluator lacks adequate content knowledge of the program being evaluated.

2.   Elaborate on the ethical questions that may arise if subjects were recruited for participation in a research study under the following circumstances:

- Undergraduate students at a university are required to participate in instructor or graduate student research, or else their grade for the course suffers.
- Prisoners volunteer for participation in a study because they have been led to believe that a parole board will look more favorably upon their early release.
- Patients under care are encouraged to volunteer for a study because they believe that doing so will allow them to receive preferential treatment by physicians, nurses, and other health care workers.

3.   Investigate the IRB process at your particular institution. How is the membership of the IRB comprised? What effort is made to evaluate IRB effectiveness? Which projects have the IRB refused to approve? Have any IRB-approved projects that subsequently encountered complications resulted in queries about the thoroughness of the review that was conducted, or the qualifications of the persons who comprised the review?

4.   As an evaluator discuss how you would handle each of the following situations:

- You are pressured by a program manager to downplay negative results, and emphasize positive results.
- You receive reinforcement only for the nonthreatening or low obtrusive activities you employ in the design and conduct of the evaluation.
- You receive pressure from the program manager to make the evaluation activities appear visible even though management does not support the use of information that is being collected.
- You are told "in so many words" that your access to the power brokers of the organization for whom you are conducting the evaluation will be cut off if you fail to meet the expectations identified above.

Recommended Readings

Association for the Advancement of Health Education. (1994). Code of ethics for health educators. *Journal of Health Education, 25,* 196-200.

The AAHE code of ethics for health education practice, including research and evaluation endeavors, is presented. Professional and pre-professional health educators will find this published set of principles helpful in guiding discussions among colleagues for the refinement and evolution of the profession.

Newman, D.L., & Brown, R.D. (1996). *Applied Ethics for Program Evaluation.* Thousand Oaks, CA: Sage Publications.

Viewpoints of multiple stakeholders with varying perspectives on ethical practice in evaluation are considered. The book is particularly strong in its explanation and examples of the roles played by evaluators (e.g., objective scientist, reporter, administrator/manager, member of a profession, member of society) and the conflicts that can arise as one explores these various roles. The book has numerous useful vignettes that illustrate the application of ethical principles for decision making, and the utility of rules and codes of practice in arriving at decisions.

Perrin, K.M. (1992). Informed consent: a challenge for patient advocacy. In G.B. White (Ed.), *Ethical Dilemmas in Contemporary Nursing Practice.* Washington, D.C.: American Nurses Publishing, pp. 105-116.

Although this book chapter is designed primarily to be read by nurses, it is an excellent example of the role conflicts that can occur among various stakeholders (e.g., evaluator, program administrator, care provider, patient advocate, and so on).

References

American Educational Research Association. (1992). Ethical standards of the American Educational Research Association. *Educational Researcher, 21*(7), 23-26.

American Evaluation Association. (1995). *Guiding Principles for Evaluators.* Greensboro, NC: Author.

American Pyschological Association. (1992). Ethical principles of psychologists and code of conduct. *American Psychologist, 47,* 1597-1611.

Ary, D., Jacobs, L.C., & Razavieh, A. (1990). *Introduction to Research in Education,* 4th edition. Fort Worth, TX: Holt, Rinehart and Winston.

Association for the Advancement of Health Education. (1994). Code of ethics for health educators. *Journal of Health Education, 25*, 196-200.

Best, J.W., & Kahn, J.V. (1989). *Research in Education*, 6th edition. Englewood Cliffs, NJ: Prentice-Hall.

Braskamp, L.A. (1994, September). *The role of the advocate*. A panel presentation at the College of Education's 75th Anniversary Symposium. University of Illinois-Urbana.

Clifford, D.L., & Sherman, P. (1983). Internal evaluation: Integrating program evaluation and management. In A.J. Love, (Ed.), *Developing Effective Internal Evaluation*. San Francisco, CA: Jossey-Bass, Inc., pp.23-45.

French, J.F., Fisher, C.C., & Costa, S.J., Jr., (Eds.), (1983). *Working with Evaluators*. Rockville, MD: National Institute on Drug Abuse, DHHS Publication No. (ADM) 83-1233.

House, E.R. (1980). *Evaluating with Validity*. Beverly Hills, CA: Sage Publications.

House, E.R. (1988). *Jesse Jackson and the Politics of Charisma: The Rise and Fall of the PUSH/Excel Program*. Boulder, CO: Westview.

House, E.R. (1993). *Professional Evaluation: Social Impact and Political Consequences*. Newbury Park, CA: Sage Publications.

Johnson, R.R. (1981). *Directory of Evaluation Consultants*. New York: The Foundation Center.

Joint Committee on Standards. (1994). *Program Evaluation Standards*, 2nd edition. Thousand Oaks, CA: Sage Publications.

Jones, R.A. (1985). *Research Methods in the Social and Behavioral Sciences*. Sunderland, MA: Sinauer Associates, Inc.

Kimmel, A.J. (1988). *Ethics and Values in Applied Social Research*. Newbury Park, CA: Sage Publications.

Kirkhart, K.E. (1995). Seeking multicultural validity: A postcard from the road. *Evaluation Practice, 16*, 1-12.

Madison, A. (1992). Primary inclusion of culturally diverse minority program participants in the evaluation process. In A. Madison (Ed.), *Minority Issues in Program Evaluation* (New Directions for Program Evaluation No. 53, pp. 35-43). San Francisco: Jossey-Bass.

Marshall, C., & Rossman, G.B. (1989). *Designing Qualitative Research*. Newbury Park, CA: Sage Publications.

Mathison, S. (1991). Role conflicts for internal evaluators. *Evaluation and Program Planning, 14*, 173-179.

Matsumoto, D. (1994). *Cultural Influences on Research Methods and Statistics*. Pacific Grove, CA: Brooks/Cole.

Mitroff, I.I. (1983). *Stakeholders of the Organizational Mind*. San Francisco: Jossey-Bass.

Nachmias, D., & Nachmias, C. (1987). *Research Methods in the Social Sciences*. 3rd edition. New York: St. Martin's Press.

Neale, J.M., & Liebert, R.M. (1986). *Science and Behavior*, 3rd edition. Englewood Cliffs, NJ: Prentice-Hall.

Newman, D.L., & Brown, R.D. (1996). *Applied Ethics for Program Evaluation*. Thousand Oaks, CA: Sage Publications.

Nunnally, J.C. (1983). The study of change in evaluation research: Principles concerning measurement, experimental design, and analysis. In E.L. Struening & M.B. Brewer (Eds.), *Handbook of Evaluation Research*. Beverly Hills, CA: Sage Publications, pp.231-272.

Pasick R.J., Sabogal, F., Bird, J.A., D'Onofrio, C.N., Jenkins, C.N.H., Lee, M., Engelstad, L., & Hiatt, R.A. (1996). Problems and progress in translation of health survey questions: The *Pathways* experience. *Health Education Quarterly*, *23*(Supplement), S28-S40.

Pasick, R.J., D'Onofrio, C.N., & Otero-Sabogal, R. (1996). Similarities and differences across cultures: Questions to inform a third generation of health promotion research. *Health Education Quarterly*, *23*(Supplement), S142-S161.

Perrin, K.M. (1992). Informed consent: a challenge for patient advocacy. In G.B. White (Ed.), *Ethical Dilemmas in Contemporary Nursing Practice*. Washington, D.C.: American Nurses Publishing, pp. 105-116.

Popham, W.J. (1988). *Educational Evaluation*, 2nd edition. Englewood Cliffs, NJ: Prentice-Hall.

Posavac, E.J., & Carey, R.G. (1989). *Program Evaluation*, 3rd edition. Englewood Cliffs, NJ: Prentice-Hall.

Raizen, S.A., & Rossi, P.H., (Eds.), (1981). *Program Evaluation in Education: When? How? To What Ends?* Washington, D.C.: National Academy Press.

Rossi, P.H., & Freeman, H.E. (1989). *Evaluation: A Systematic Approach*, 4th edition. Newbury Park, CA: Sage.

Sieber, J.E. (1980). Being ethical: Professional and personal decisions in program evaluation. In R. Perloff & E. Perloff (Eds.), *Values, Ethics and Standards in Evaluation*. New Directions for Program Evaluation, No. 7. San Francisco: Jossey-Bass.

Smith, M.F. (1989). *Evaluability Assessment*. Boston: Kluwer Academic Publishers.

Society for Public Health Education. (1993). *Summary Code of Ethics*. Berkeley, CA: The Society.

Travers, K.D. (1997). Reducing inequities through participatory research and community empowerment. *Health Education & Behavior*, *24*, 344-356.

Weiss, C.H. (1972). *Evaluation Research*. Englewood Cliffs, NJ: Prentice-Hall.

Weiss, C.H. (1977). Between the cup and the lip. In: E.L. Struening, & M. Guttentag (Eds.), *Handbook of Evaluation Research*, Vol. I. Beverly Hills, CA: Sage Publications.

Worthen, B.R., & Sanders, J.R. (1987). *Educational Evaluation*. New York: Longman.

Chapter

4

Logistical Issues in Conducting Evaluations

Chapter Objectives

After completing this chapter, you should be able to:

1. Identify the relevance of numerous administrative tasks to the successful completion of an evaluation project.
2. Articulate the points that should be addressed in a contract or professional agreement to conduct an evaluation, and the rationale for the inclusion of each point.
3. Outline the key elements of a budget for conducting a program evaluation.
4. Compare the logistical strengths and weaknesses of employing selected data collection strategies in a program evaluation.
5. Use and compare various aides for planning and scheduling activities to be assigned and carried out in a program evaluation.
6. Discuss the uses of computer technology in conducting evaluations.

Key Terms

budget justification
codebook
cost reimbursement contract
critical path method
direct costs
fixed price contract
Gantt chart

GOAMs
indirect costs
key activity chart
overhead costs
PERT
request for proposal (RFP)

Introduction

A program evaluator preparing to initiate his or her project might be compared to a military general about to outfit his troops for battle. Both people need to be concerned about having a plan of action with clear objectives for management of the tasks at hand, having the array of quality personnel available who possess the necessary technical training and skills, and having other support personnel, finances, and hardware within reach to get the job done effectively and efficiently. In this chapter, we will look at a broad array of logistical issues that, if addressed wisely, can launch a project in a successful direction. In particular, we will focus on planning and managing an evaluation project, negotiating an evaluation contract agreement that is fair to all concerned parties, estimating expenses and preparing a budget, collecting data, scheduling key events and activities, and using available technology resourcefully.

Planning and Managing the Evaluation

One's ability to coordinate the activities that are integral to an investigation is crucial in determining the extent to which evaluation data are relevant and useful to stakeholders. A novice evaluator is benefitted by the presence of carefully prepared procedural guidelines for project operation. It is indeed wise even for experienced evaluators to be reminded of procedural steps from time to time. Fink and Kosecoff (1978) identify four principal activities whose coordination is of the utmost importance: (1) the establishment of schedules and deadlines; (2) the assignment and monitoring of staff; (3) the identification of activities to be carried out by staff; and (4) the preparation and ongoing review of budgetary matters.

Stufflebeam (1978) also provides six administrative guidelines for implementing and managing a program evaluation project. These guidelines for the chief or principal evaluator are indicated below:

- *Staff* - Provide the evaluation team with qualified personnel.
- *Orientation and training* - Acquaint all personnel who will be part of the evaluation team with their responsibilities; prepare them carefully (i.e., using a plan) to assume and carry out their responsibilities.
- *Planning* - Take care in developing the evaluation plan carefully, systematically, and collaboratively.
- *Scheduling* - Develop and maintain up-to-date projections of all relevant evaluation activities, when they are to occur, and the responsible parties for carrying them out.
- *Control* - Plan, monitor, and maintain control of all evaluation activities such that the evaluation is implemented according to a set, pre-established protocol. Careful monitoring will keep the evaluator abreast should changes in protocol become warranted.

- *Economy* - Time and resources need to be monitored to ensure that all factors related to the evaluation operate as smoothly and efficiently as possible.

According to Schaefer (1987) the successful achievement of evaluation tasks is assisted by having defined and stable relationships among the participating people, units, and agencies. Definition of these relationships requires, at a minimum, the following products: (1) a proposal on project organization, including the chain of command or line of authority; (2) approvals and agreements of the proposal, showing that all participating groups are familiar with, and are understanding of the evaluation plan; and (3) the actual making and acceptance of responsibility assignments.

Schaefer (1987) further explains that project execution may be compromised unless the conditions met by the following five actions are met. Consequently, the evaluator, working in conjunction with the program manager from the agency, needs to:

- Define the array of responsibilities for action (work) and coordination to be assigned.
- Clarify authority relationships to ensure the execution of work and coordination responsibilities.
- Specify and document the authority and responsibility assignments by position, in accordance with an overall pattern of relationships for direction, reporting, and ongoing decision making.
- Fix and establish overall (or "ultimate") responsibility for the project as a whole, specifying the project evaluator's relationship to the agency program manager, or other pertinent higher official or body.
- Ensure that the assigned responsibilities are realistic with regard to available time, authority status (intrinsic to the position or clearly delegated to it), and personal capabilities.

In addition, Schaefer (1987) indicates that the following elements of organization are helpful in clarifying roles, tasks, and the chain of command: (1) *Time* - relative to deadlines, duration of effort, and consumption of resources; (2) *Processes and procedures* - relative to how work is done and how tasks are executed per established arrangements; (3) *Money* - its allocation, transfer, and expenditure; (4) *Product quantity* - how many interim or final products are delivered, and where (i.e., to whom) they are delivered; (5) *Product quality* - the capability of the personnel and other developed resources to function as the program requires; and (6) *Information flow* - with respect to the quantity, quality, and accuracy of information delivery, and in regard to whether the intended targets of the information receive it, and receive it in a form that is decipherable and usable.

Depending on the size of the project to be evaluated, the establishment of an advisory committee may be useful. If it is your own project that is to be evaluated, the establishment of such a committee can be most insightful from the onset. If you have the responsibility for the evaluation of another agency's project, check into whether an advisory committee is in place. If one does not exist, recommend that such a group be formed. Advisory committees, if comprised of key project stakeholders (people who will benefit or be adversely affected by evaluation), decision makers, and consultants can help to ensure that the evaluation proceeds in the "sunshine." That is, the committee can be kept abreast of the process to see that evaluation operates without covert practices, hidden agenda, unethical political maneuvers, or any of the other types of counterproductive activities to which we alluded in Chapter 3.

The Contract/Professional Agreement

The contract to conduct an evaluation of a program is a document that puts definition and dimension to the evaluation to be undertaken. This professional agreement to provide (or receive) evaluation services should be entered into only with the utmost of care and consideration of the parties involved. Although a "handshake" may be the symbol of contractual agreement for a host of informal events that occur in life, it does not work well for formal matters such as work agreements between or among agencies. A contract to conduct an evaluation should be written to protect both the evaluator and the agency. Most governmental agencies and many other organizations will have standard documents that are employed for a variety of contractual arrangements. These standard contracts can, however, be modified through the preparation of an addendum that delineates the specific needs of the parties involved in a given evaluation project.

Stufflebeam (1978) spells out 16 contractual/legal guidelines for executing a program evaluation agreement that contracting parties may wish to consider. These elements are reiterated by French and Kaufman (1981). We will present them here as well, along with our interpretation of the meaning and importance of each one.

Commitment - This element guarantees that the evaluation data are to be used "honorably." In Chapter 3 we alluded to the fact that evaluation results sometimes do not get used, or if they do, they are employed sometimes in an unscrupulous fashion. Prior to beginning the execution of a contract, the evaluator may wish to know how (or "if") results will be used.

Products - Although the meaning of this part of a contract may seem obvious, it is not. The specific products and services that are to be provided by the evaluator to the agency (or program) should be delineated clearly. The lack of care in writing these specifications can result in demands placed on the evaluator for numerous interim reports, follow-up data (after conclusion of the evaluation), additional documentation to support expenditures, and other materials. While receiving requests from agencies for these products and services is not unusual, any specifications or limitations should be spelled out clearly in advance.

Schedule - A schedule should be agreed upon that is realistic, and includes time frames for conducting all foreseen evaluation activities, preparing all interim and final report documents, submitting all bills and expenses, and being reimbursed for services performed.

Finances - There should be agreement concerning a realistic budget. Financial constraints, more often than not, dictate the scope of the evaluation. This point needs to be addressed up front. A "Cadillac" evaluation cannot be carried out on a "Chevrolet" budget. On the other hand, program managers often can detect (and will resent) when the evaluator is trying to "pad" the budget. Personal integrity and common sense need to prevail in budgetary matters. Both parties must be realistic about the scope of the evaluation. The evaluator will want to make sure the budget has flexibility. That is, in the event that personnel services are overbudgeted, and travel, equipment, rented office space, or other matters are underbudgeted, the evaluator wants to be able to shift money around to cover expenses without having to renegotiate the contract. However tempting the opportunity and the money may be, if you do not believe you can deliver the products and services under the constraints of the budget allowed, *do not* enter into the agreement.

Facilities - Contracting parties should agree on office space and equipment that are needed to conduct the study. To understand the pragmatic wisdom of this contractual point, consider the following simple illustration of conflict that occurred in the experience of the present authors:

> A member of a university faculty agreed to oversee a four-community needs assessment concerning public knowledge of epidemiologic factors associated with childhood drownings. A telephone survey was to be conducted. A contract was made between the university and a regional branch of the state health department. Neither party specified from where the telephone calls would be made, out of which office the data collectors would work, or whose telephones would be used to make toll (i.e., long distance) calls. The university faculty member "assumed" that the health department would provide space for the data collectors he hired. Furthermore, he "assumed" that telephones would be available, and that calls could be made from the offices of the health department. The health department made no such assumptions. No budget or specifications concerning space, office furniture, telephones, and telephone service had been made.

Personnel - Parties need to agree about who will perform which evaluation functions. Will *all* evaluative functions be in the hands of the evaluator under contract, will there be multiple evaluation teams, or will some evaluation tasks remain with agency staff?

Protocol - There should be agreement *and* understanding concerning which communication channels are to be used, and which policies and rules are to be observed in carrying out the evaluation.

Security - There may need to be procedures for protecting the data from unauthorized access and use. Security measures help to ensure the integrity of the data, as well as to prevent release of information prematurely to (or by) inappropriate sources.

Informed consent - There should be an agreed upon sequence of steps through which informed consent of individuals providing personal information to the evaluation team will be obtained. The meaning and importance of informed consent are discussed in greater detail in Chapter 3.

Arrangements - Contracting parties should reach agreement about any special conditions or operating procedures for data collection which will be necessary to fulfill the assumptions of the evaluation's sampling and treatment assumptions. Moreover, if the conditions cannot be made available, an alternate arrangement should be specified, or perhaps, a condition for terminating the contract. To illustrate the potential need for this type of a contractual clause, consider the following event brought to the attention of the authors:

A member of a university faculty agreed to be the state health department's chief evaluator of an experimental cocaine addiction intervention program for pregnant women. The program was to be carried out at each of three sites in different parts of the state. The primary objective of the evaluation project was to assess the efficacy of the new treatment procedure using experimental or quasi-experimental procedures (see Chapter 10). The evaluation design required the ability of the three sites, working with the evaluation team, to assign clients randomly to the treatments (conventional treatment versus the new experimental procedure). Early into the intervention, one site decided unilaterally to abandon the new procedure. Not long after, a second site concluded that the randomization procedure was too cumbersome, and questioned the ethics of refusing the offer of the new treatment to some clients just because they were "less random" than other clients. Only one site remained. Ultimately, this site recruited too few clients to its programs to permit the evaluator to have sufficient statistical power to draw defensible conclusions about the efficacy of the intervention. Contingency plans had not been made to address complications in the original design. Nevertheless, the state health department expected an evaluation of the scope that was proposed originally. Both parties were dissatisfied with the turn of events, and the relationship was understandably stressed.

Editing - To avoid subsequent arguments, the parties should reach a decision in advance concerning which group (i.e., agency staff or evaluation staff) will have ultimate editorial authority over the final report. This issue relates directly to some of the issues presented in Chapter 3. It arises whenever the stakeholders in the program under study seek a strongly positive evaluation, but feel that the report places the program or its management in a bad light. Conversely, stakeholders seeking a "hatchet evaluation" (see Chapter 3) may be disappointed by a report that shows good program productivity. The evaluator feels compromised (or should) if there is interference with the data or their interpretation. Conflicts may be resolved if the evaluator is willing to re-examine certain aspects of the data, if requested to do so. Parties are protected if the protocol for such requests is established in the initial contractual agreement, and final editorial authority is specified.

Release of reports - It is vital that there is agreement concerning who may release data, in whole or in part, the format for the release of data, the timing of the release of data, and the parties to whom distribution of any and all reports will be made. As with the issue of security, delineation of this point will designate appropriate responsibility and authority for access to data and related communications.

Value conflicts - Contracting parties should develop a clear understanding concerning how conflicts over the criteria for specifying conclusions and recommendations are to be resolved. As cited above, when, where, and to whom data should be made available may create a difference of opinion between an evaluator and an agency. Conclusions stemming from basic data may incite similar disagreement. Conclusions and subsequent recommendations are no more than interpretations of raw data. But whose interpretation will be used, the evaluator's or the agency's? The issue is settled readily if the agency or institution for whom the evaluation is being performed has final editorial control of the document. While that solution may seem arbitrary, authoritarian, undemocratic, and appear lacking in objectivity, it *does* address the matter. We do not necessarily advocate this position, however direct it may be. We desire simply to point out here that conflicts of this nature do occur, and to offer the recommendation that the issue get addressed early in the process.

Renegotiation - Minor changes in the scope or budget of an evaluation project are to be expected, and have been alluded to above. Moreover, the occasion can arise when significant modification of an evaluation project is necessary. In either case, it is best to have developed and outlined procedures for renegotiating the terms of the formal agreement so that neither party can act in a unilateral or arbitrary fashion.

Spin-off - It may be possible to reach agreement about how the need to conduct an evaluation can be used as an opportunity to "do research" on evaluation, to enhance the audience's ability to develop its own evaluation capabilities, and to increase the audience's appreciation for, or connoisseurship of evaluations. If the chief evaluator is a member of a university faculty, he or she may have students able to receive a rich learning experience from the evaluation. Perhaps a permanent relationship between the university and the agency can be developed whereby students act as interns who perform ongoing evaluations. The idea proposed here is that the opportunity to be involved in a formal evaluation project can lead to much more than just a simple mercenary exchange of money for services, and some agencies are willing to write this element into a contract.

Termination - The time and work dimensions of the evaluator's responsibility to an agency and vice versa should be established in a written agreement, so that both parties know when the contract period is over, and when responsibility for work can be terminated. Moreover, it is important to establish the circumstances under which either party may initiate termination of the contract for reasons other than expiration of the negotiated time period. It is a fact of life that some agreements (like some marriages) were never meant to be, or become unworkable in practice. Circumstances do change, and sometimes these changes require more than a simple renegotiation of terms.

Other Contractual Considerations

Many other factors can affect exchanges that occur between an evaluator and an agency. There is no limit to what can be negotiated between parties or written into formal working agreements. However, two other pertinent issues deserve special consideration here: (1) ownership of data; and (2) terms of publication for the scholarly record.

As was pointed out in Chapter 3, even though an agency program manager may view *all* data generated by the evaluation as belonging to that agency, evaluators do feel a professional responsibility (and sometimes a need) to share findings with other consumers of the evaluation literature. The extent to which evaluators will have access and rights to the data should be established in the terms of the contract. Negative findings about a program's performance may produce a reluctance on the part of the agency to allow itself to be scrutinized before a professional audience. Fortunately, agencies do not necessarily make deliberate efforts to conceal unflattering data about their operation. Program managers and other agency personnel may, in fact, have a profound interest in seeing data published and sharing in the publication experience. Therefore, guidelines for the preparation of manuscripts that use the evaluation data should be formalized. An example of such a simple, but formal agreement outlining some criteria is shown in Figure 4.1.

Members of the HIV/AIDS Prevention Program evaluation team and the Molly County Public Health Department (MCPHD) agree that persons submitting publications and/or abstracts for presentation at professional meetings adhere to the following guidelines:

- A study protocol will be submitted to the MCPHD HIV/AIDS Prevention Program Advisory Committee for approval at least 30 days prior to manuscript submission.
- Authors will reference all relevant previous publications and reports from the MCPHD HIV/AIDS Prevention Program.
- Authors will take necessary steps to ensure the confidentiality of subjects.
- Authors will provide a final copy of the manuscript to the MCPHD HIV/AIDS Prevention Program Advisory Committee for its approval prior to publication.
- All agency persons involved directly in the MCPHD HIV/AIDS Prevention Program will be co-authors of any papers stemming from the evaluation data. Order of authorship will be determined by the principal author's assessment of the amount of effort contributed by each co-author to the publication.
- Any royalties realized from the publication or presentation of data will be revealed to the MCPHD HIV/AIDS Prevention Program Advisory Committee, which will have the authority to decide how the royalties may be assigned.
- Authors will ensure that the contents of publications or presentations are accurate.

Members of the Evaluation Team   **Chairperson MCPHD HIV/AIDS Prevention Program Advisory Committee**

_____

_____   _____

_____   _____

_____   Date

_____

Figure 4.1 Sample Publication Policy

Budget Preparation

When an individual or a group sits down to draft a reply to a **request for proposal** or **RFP**, or prepares an evaluation plan for an agency with whom a working agreement is anticipated, it is customary it seems, to save the budget preparation aspect of the proposal until last. The development of a budget and its justification, are tasks however, that should parallel other proposal writing efforts in magnitude of importance.

Budgets for evaluation of health education programs vary in their amount of detail. While occasionally a funding agency will specify maximum expenditures by budget category, most of the time it is up to the investigator to establish these estimates. Most universities have offices of research and development that specialize in the generation and review of budgets for all sponsored research projects and evaluation contracts. Thus, university personnel have professionals to whom they can turn for assistance. However, there are some fundamentals of budget preparation identified below that should be known by everyone.

A budget for a given project can be divided into two mutually exclusive categories: **direct costs** and **indirect costs**. Direct costs include all personnel and non-personnel expenses related to the project undertaken. Examples of personnel items include *salary and wages*, *employee benefits*, and *consultants*. Examples of some non-personnel costs are *commodities* (e.g., office supplies, equipment, postage), *contractual services* (e.g., advertising for new personnel, rent, computer time, telephone, express mail, FAX services, photocopying, printing and reproduction), and *travel* (e.g., airfares, mileage reimbursement, lodging, meals). Depending on whether equipment and services are purchased or leased (often a function of institutional policy), some items may fall into categories other than as shown above.

Indirect costs (sometimes called **overhead costs**) are charged for services that the contracting institution provides that are not directly related to, but nevertheless, are required for the project to be carried out. These items include such things as environmental management (heating, air conditioning, water, and other utilities), protection and security, custodial services, and equipment maintenance. Indirect costs usually are calculated as a percentage of total direct costs, or occasionally, as a percentage of just salaries and wages (Fink & Kosecoff, 1978). The percentage that is charged can vary widely, and typically is negotiated with the funding agency. The indirect costs ordinarily billed by some universities can be 50 percent or more of the figure for direct costs. Some institutions have percentages that are higher or lower than this number. Funding agencies may have maximum allowable limits for accepting charges for indirect costs as low as zero percent.

The relationship between direct and indirect costs is an important one for a person new to research and evaluation to understand. If an agency awards a $100,000 contract to a university faculty member whose institution has an indirect cost rate of 47 percent, only $53,000 of the $100,000 would go for the delivery of goods and services directly related to the contract. The remaining $47,000 would be "absorbed" by the university for expenses related to administering the grant or contract, and the generation of other services that may or may not be related to the specific project for which the contract was awarded. The institutional *indirect rate* is an important matter to the chief investigator at institution $\dot{A}$. If investigator A's proposal is being considered by agency against that of investigator B's whose institutional indirect rate is only investigator A may be in trouble. If the two proposals are similarly persuasive, knows that for an award of $100,000, proposal B can deliver a $73,000 product, proposal A can deliver only a $53,000 product. Sometimes an institution suc university has to be flexible in its charges for indirect costs to stay competitive in procurement of grants and contracts.

Thus far we have identified some budget categories and listed examples of the items that might be found in these categories. In the text below we will review each one of these elements more closely. It may be helpful to examine the sample budget shown in Figure 4.2 as you read along.

In the general category of direct costs, and under the description of personnel, *salaries and wages* of all full-time and part-time personnel working on the evaluation should be listed in proportion to the amount of time that each individual will devote to the project. The following information can be provided for each position: position title, hourly, daily, monthly, or annual salary, percent of time commitment to the project, length of time to be employed, and the total dollar expense.

Employee benefits also are listed as personnel costs. Ordinarily, benefits are computed as a percentage of salaries and wages, and include monies established by the employer for social security, pensions health care, and other factors.

Finally, under the heading of personnel are *consultants*. Not all projects will have or need consultants, but it often is wise to budget for them. These persons serve as reviewers, advisory committee members, content specialists, or experts in instrument design, data collection, and data analysis. Per diem expenses (food, lodging, ground transportation, and incidental costs) along with travel expenses need to be estimated.

Direct costs also include non-personnel expenditures. *Space* includes the rental cost of facility use on a per square foot basis, along with maintenance and utilities. *Office supplies* literally include all consumable items (paper of all sorts, paper clips, pencils, computer floppy disks, optical scan sheets, printer or typewriter ribbons, etc.). *Equipment* includes all devices that are purchased or rented during the life of the contract. It may include personal computers and printers, photocopiers, FAX machines, telephones, typewriters, and other hardware. *Telephone* expenses include installations costs, monthly local service charges, and charges for long distance calls, and FAX exchanges. *Postage* expenses are all of those costs incurred doing business by mail. *Printing and reproduction* includes all costs accruing from having survey instruments duplicated and collated, having reports reproduced and bound, and other related services. *Travel* expenses are those incurred by any personnel, including air travel, ground mileage, per diem allowances, and so on.

Most funding agencies will ask the person or institution applying for an evaluation contract to provide a **budget justification**. These statements are not always lengthy, but they generally do go beyond a simple remark concerning what a particular piece of equipment will be used for, or what the destination of a given trip is. For example, perhaps you wish to buy a brand new state-of-the-art personal computer for an office using the contract budget. While that may not be an extraordinary request, the persons from the agency reviewing your budget proposal know that most universities and

Direct Costs

I.   *Personnel*

        A.   *Salaries and wages*

1.	Dr. John Michaels, Principal Evaluator (1 year @ $70,000/year @ .40 effort)	$ 28,000
2.	Dr. Jane Richter, Co-evaluator (1 year @ $48,000/year @ .20 effort)	$ 9,600
3.	John Brennan, Data specialist (.50 year @ $30,000/year @ .50 effort)	$ 7,500
4.	Amanda Colin-Austin, Data collector (1 year @ $14,000/year @ .50 effort)	$ 7,000
5.	Rosemary McGill-Edgewood, Secretary (1 year @ $18,000/year @ .20 effort)	$ 3,600
		$ 55,700

        B.   *Employee benefits*

1.	25% of salaries and wages ($55,700)	$ 13,925

        C.   *Consultants*

1.	Elizabeth Grausnick, Curriculum (2 days @ $300/day)	$ 600
2.	Julie Brylawski, Process (4 days @ $150/day)	$ 600
3.	Gail Samuel, Advisory Committee (8 days @ $100/day)	$ 800
4.	Suzanna Henry (8 days @ $100/day)	$ 800
		$ 2,800

Figure 4.2 Sample Budget of A University-based Program Evaluation Project

II.   *Non-personnel*

A.   *Space*

1. Office rent, 120 sq. ft.
(12 months @ $6.00/sq. ft./month $ 8,640

2. Office rent, 120 sq. ft.
(12 months @ $6.00/sq. ft./month $ 8,640

_____

$ 17,280

B.   *Office supplies*

1.   Paper, ribbons, diskettes and
other consumables
(12 months @ $80/month $ 960

C.   *Equipment*

1.   1 IBM-compatible personal computer
with minimum 80 MB hard drive,
with compatible laser printer,
and color monitor $ 2,500
2.   1 computer table
(36" H x 24" W x 56" L) $ 200
3.   4 telephones
(Standard push-button @ $35/each) $ 140
4.   Statistical software
(Brand X Multi-Base with Manual) $ 1,050
5.   Integrated software for
word processing, spreadsheet,
and data base (2 @ $495/each) $ 990

_____

$ 4,880

Figure 4.2 continued

D.   *Telecommunications*

    1.   4 telephone lines installed
           and local service for 1 year $ 800
    2.   4 telephone lines long
           distance service for 1 year $ 2,000
    3.   FAX expenses
           (12 months @ $15/month) $ 180
                                            _____
                                   $ 2,980

E.   *Postage*

    1.   Postage for regular mail service $ 2,200
    2.   Postage for overnight mail
           and other special delivery $ 300
                                              _____
                                   $ 2,500

F.   *Printing and Reproduction*

    1.   Printing of questionnaires,
           interview schedules, reports, etc. $ 5,400
    2.   Other duplication/photocopying
           (80,000 copies @ $0.075/copy) $ 6,000
                                              _____
                                 $ 11,400

G.   *Travel*

    1.   8 trips for principal evaluator
           to agency site, including airfare,
           ground transportation, lodging,
           meals, etc. @ $400/trip $ 3,200
    2.   4 trips for co-evaluator
           to agency site (same expenses) $ 1,600

Figure 4.2 continued

3.	Consultant travel (Grausnick)		
	(2 trips @ $150/trip)		$ 300
4.	Other consultation travel		
	(2 trips @ $150/trip)		$ 300
5.	Other travel for data collection		
	(8 trips @ 90 miles/trip @ $0.25/mile)		$ 180
6.	National and state conference travel		
	(4 @ $800/trip)		$ 3,200

$ 8,780

Subtotal (Direct Costs): *$121,205*

Indirect Costs

48% of direct costs ($121,205)

Subtotal (Indirect Costs): *$ 58,178*

Total Budget Requested $179,383

Figure 4.2 continued

other institutions already have offices with personal computers. Consequently, they may want to know: (1) Is there something special about the proposed evaluation task that requires the requested state-of-the-art personal computer as opposed to last year's model? (2) Is the existing hardware that the institution owns tied up 24 hours a day, thus making the purchase request a necessity? (3) Since the project is of limited duration, could the requested device be leased for a lower price than the one at which it could purchased? These are the kinds of questions to which you may have to address yourself.

It is worthwhile to know that there are at least two ways in which an agency can reimburse an evaluator or the evaluator's institution for services rendered. One mechanism is referred to as a **cost-reimbursement contract**, while the other is called a **fixed price**

contract. There are variations in exact terminology used from one setting to another, but the concepts are the same.

In a cost-reimbursement contract, the evaluator (or his/her firm) may be paid a fee, but is reimbursed primarily just for the actual expenses incurred. In a contract between two state agencies (e.g., state health department and a state university), it is possible that only the actual capital expenses will be reimbursed. In other words, if the actual cost of a completed evaluation was $64,957.34, the institution would get reimbursed that amount, and *only* that amount upon submission of all justifiable bills and expenses.

In a fixed price contract, the evaluator (or his/her institution) agrees to deliver a product or service for an agreed upon price. If the example above had been a fixed price contract of $75,000.00, there would have been a net profit of $10,042.66. Generally speaking, the fixed price method works in the favor of the evaluator unless projected cost estimates are less than actual costs.

Logistics of Data Collection

Evaluation research may employ any of a variety of strategies for data collection. According to Shortell and Richardson (1978):

> The most 'appropriate' method(s) for a given case will depend on the nature of the program being evaluated (objectives, specification of program components, and so on), the variables to be measured, the evaluation design being employed, and the cost and time involved (p.84).

In general terms, data sources can be divided into two main categories: *precollected* and *original* (Shortell & Richardson, 1978). Precollected data are those that come from archival records, administrative audits, anecdotal and other unobtrusive information that serves as social indicators of the baseline condition. Among the most common of the original data gathering techniques are the paper-and-pencil survey or questionnaire, the interview schedule (telephone or face-to-face), direct observations, and physical measures. How does one prepare himself or herself for all of the circumstances, situations, and conditions, that may come into play and threaten the data gathering processes? It is perhaps not at all reassuring to know that you *cannot* plan for *every* contingency. However, there are ways of protecting yourself from disappointment and unnecessary failure and frustration.

One of the best, but frequently underutilized devices for examining logistical issues associated with data collection is performing a pilot study (see Chapter 8). Pilot studies are tremendous tools for testing a procedure, examining an instrument for its shortcomings, or otherwise working out the details of the eventual, larger-scale study. Borg and Gall (1989) identify several clear benefits to be derived from performing pilot studies:

- You can do some preliminary testing of hypotheses that subsequently, can be modified or eliminated. Possibly, new hypotheses that were previously unconsidered will be generated.

- Pilot studies often provide you with ideas and approaches not considered or forseen prior to undertaking the data collection effort.
- You can examine your plan of statistical analysis, or modify data collection procedures to facilitate easier analysis.
- You may decrease the number of errors in data collection as a result of getting acquainted with the factors that can threaten adequate subject recruitment, interviewing, survey administration, or record review.
- You can save yourself time and expense by finding out that what was proposed on paper is impractical to carry out in the time frame or with the financial, personnel, and other resources available.
- You can obtain critical feedback from subjects, data gatherers in the field, observers, and other key people that allows you to make large procedural adjustments or fine tuning adjustments in the way that data are collected.
- Alternative measures can be considered prior to the start of the main study.

Consider some of the logistical issues in carrying out a "simple" survey. Basic to this matter is whether you are going to conduct a paper-and-pencil survey, interview people face-to-face, interview people over the telephone, or collect data via the Internet. How are you going to select a representative sample of people to participate in a study? Do you have the time to gather information from individual interviews or will you have to administer any surveys to groups? Will a previously used instrument be used to collect data, or will one have to be generated specific to the purpose of this investigation? Does the instrument you want to use require purchase or written permission to borrow? How long will the permission process take? Does the time frame for the study allow for instrument development, and pretesting for such things as reliability, validity, readability, and practicality? If human subjects are involved in the evaluation study, how long will the process of going through the institutional review board (IRB) process take? If agencies, schools, or other institutions are to be involved, how will their participation and approval be sought?

The pros and cons of various strategies for conducting your "simple" survey need to be weighed. Mailed surveys are relatively inexpensive to do, can address a wide-range of topics, and reach a broad audience. Moreover, they can be self-administered, done with a large degree of respondent anonymity, and can be completed at the convenience of the respondent. However, these benefits may be offset by the fact that a low response rate may occur, especially if a self-addressed, postage-paid envelope is not enclosed, the appearance of the survey instrument is not "professional-looking," and the number of open-ended responses questions is excessive. Another drawback of mailed surveys is that potential respondents may not understand all of the items asked. Furthermore, the investigator has no assurance that the respondent is actually the person to whom the survey was sent. How long should the investigator wait for responses before proceeding with data analysis? Should reminder postcards (which increase the overall cost of the study) be sent out? Reminders may increase response rate, but will they increase it to the point of (1) justifying the added expense, and (2) justifying the delay in processing data? The investigator must weigh this matter carefully.

Face-to-face interviews are much more personalized than mailed surveys, and permit more in-depth probing for responses. They have greater flexibility than mailed surveys since two-way communication can occur at all times. Such data collection procedures are highly expensive in time and personnel. How many 45-minute interviews can a person comfortably and competently perform in one day? Might the intimacy of a face-to-face interview intimidate the respondent, or could the interviewer's sex, age, race, or mode of dress influence the validity of the respondent's answers to questions? If multiple interviewers are used, they must be trained to do interviews, a tedious process often underestimated by novice investigators. Does one have the time, expertise, and financial resources to accomplish the necessary skills for interviewer training?

The telephone interview for data collection can be an acceptable compromise. Such interviews are less costly than face-to-face interviews, and can be conducted day or night. (This point is important, since there are some areas of a city that one might not want to venture into at night to collect data.) Telephone numbers can be generated randomly, and these numbers can be called an unlimited number of times. Respondents may be more candid in answering questions over the phone than face-to-face. However, not all people have telephones, and some people have unlisted or unavailable telephone numbers (a logistical problem reduced in magnitude by using random digit dialing). Since a growing number of people are screening their calls by means of answering machines, it may be impossible to reach some of the people with whom you wish to speak. Telephone interviewers can be intimidating to residents who fear that the call may be a ruse for a sales pitch or burglary intent. Moreover, there is a practical limit to the amount of time that people will allow themselves to be interviewed on the phone. Consequently, the amount of data that can be collected has time driven boundaries.

We cannot begin to cover all of the issues that will occur in the data collection associated with evaluation research. Each study has its unique features. Careful planning, carrying out of pilot studies, and developing timelines will reduce the potential for facing studies riddled with errors and impediments. In the next section of Chapter 4, we address some project planning tools.

Planning Aides

By now you no doubt have formed the impression that conducting evaluation studies from start to finish can be arduous and laborious tasks. Fortunately, the evaluator has at his or her disposal some planning aides that assist the defining of tasks, the laying out of plans over the life of a project, and the monitoring of progress so that midcourse corrections can be made, if needed. Careful planning and scheduling are beneficial to a project in at least four ways, according to Schaefer (1987):

- They help us to know when each of many actions must be made to happen if our project is to be implemented on time.
- They help us budget funds because they tell us when the resource development activities themselves will have to be paid for, as well as

when cost-consuming resources (staff, rented space) will start requiring payments.

■ They enable us to identify possible savings in time and resources.

■ They give us an approximation of how much management time - even, perhaps, what type of management structure - will be necessary to keep activities on schedule.

A planning and evaluation method sometimes used is the **GOAMs** approach (Office of Substance Abuse Prevention, 1991). GOAMs is an acronym that stands for *g*oals, *o*bjectives, *a*ctivities, and *m*ilestones. It represents a procedure for logically arranging tasks for the planning, implementation, and evaluation of a given intervention. *Goals* are the ends or ultimate outcomes toward which the intervention is directed (e.g., reduce the incidence of HIV/AIDS in adults aged 18-44 years). *Objectives* are statements of specific and measurable outcomes (e.g., among college students, increase the level of use of condoms during first intercourse with a partner to 90% by the year 2005). Each objective should contribute logically to the stated goal. It should specify a single result, but *not* the activities required to attain the objective. *Activities* are the specific tasks that constitute the work of the intervention being planned and developed. They constitute the major work elements required to accomplish the program objectives, and ultimately, the program goals. Activities are of two kinds: *program activities* (e.g., develop the HIV/AIDS program content for persons with a high rate of STD clinic recidivism) and *evaluation activities* (select or develop a pretest/posttest inventory of knowledge concerning HIV/AIDS). *Milestones* are the actual dates by which the listed activities are to be completed. In the process of monitoring progress, target dates and actual dates of completion should be included.

Another method of planning uses the program (or performance) evaluation review technique or **PERT**. According to Rakich, Longest and Darr (1985):

PERT involves identifying the sequence of work activities and three estimates of completion times for each: optimistic, pessimistic, and a probablistic expected time. By diagramming (sequencing) activities on a time axis, it is possible to ascertain the three different time requirements for the work project. This [practice] improves scheduling and allocating resources and control of project completion (p.326).

If PERT seems a bit too involved, a **key activity chart** may be easier to understand. This planning strategy simply identifies the tasks to be performed, the sequence for the activities, and the time period during which the tasks will be done. A sample key activity chart is shown in Figure 4.3. The key activity chart shown here is a simple one just to illustrate the structure of such a planning tool. For instance, on whom is the instrument testing going to be performed? How will these subjects be recruited? At what stage will permission to use human subjects be obtained, and how long will the approval process take? Who will have responsibility for carrying out each of the tasks identified in the key activity chart?

Activities	Dates	Time Allocation
Develop appropriate measures and plan for data gathering	07/01-08/01	30 days
Recruit staff members, conduct interviews, hire, and train	07/15-10/01	75 days
Review literature for existing instrumentation, develop instruments, and conduct field testing	08/01-12/01	120 days
Collect data, perform follow-up activities on subjects, develop codebook	12/01-01/15	45 days
Prepare statistical programs, code data, enter all raw data, conduct analyses	01/01-03/01	60 days
Prepare initial draft of report; share report with advisory committee; conduct internal review of report	03/01-04/15	45 days
Prepare and distribute final report	04/15-06/01	45 days

Figure 4.3 Sample Key Activity Chart

A matter with which many novice evaluators are unfamiliar, and many experienced evaluators forget, is that there almost always is a lag time between the awarding of a contract, and when money actually begins to exchange hands. A contract awarded May 15th to begin July 1st may not have operating funds in the hands of the evaluator by the start-up date. Thus, a 12-month project may need to be planned for over an 11-month time period, or the evaluator may need to be prepared to perform as many low-cost tasks as possible during the early stages of the evaluation. The key activity chart can (and probably should) be meticulously detailed to consider this contingency.

Another illustrative planning tool is the **Gantt chart**, named after the industrial engineer who developed it for use in business. It consists of a matrix of events and time periods that denote the start and end of key project activities (see Figure 4.4).

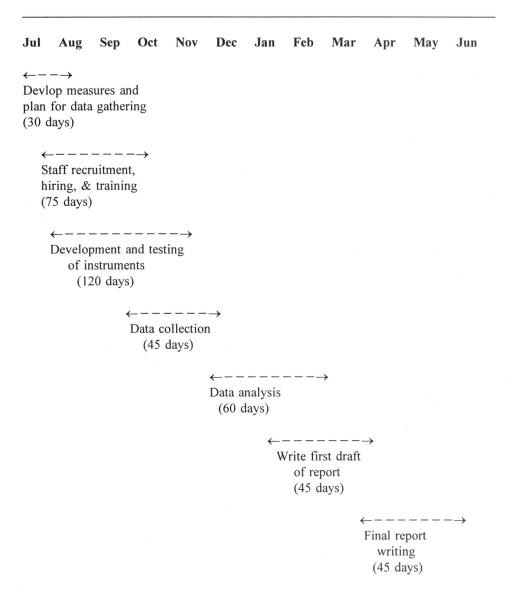

Jul Aug Sep Oct Nov Dec Jan Feb Mar Apr May Jun

←– –→
Devlop measures and
plan for data gathering
(30 days)

←– – – – – – –→
Staff recruitment,
hiring, & training
(75 days)

←– – – – – – – – –→
Development and testing
of instruments
(120 days)

←– – – – – –→
Data collection
(45 days)

←– – – – – – – –→
Data analysis
(60 days)

←– – – – – – –→
Write first draft
of report
(45 days)

←– – – – – – –→
Final report
writing
(45 days)

Figure 4.4 One-Year Program Evaluation Planning Schedule Using A Gantt Chart

The last planning aide that we will consider is the **critical path method** or CPM. CPM lays out all tasks to be performed in a linear fashion, with a careful estimate of the time required for each task to be completed. As you perhaps noticed in Figure 4.3 and Figure 4.4, some activities are overlapping. That is, they are being carried out in a concurrent fashion. CPM seeks the shortest time between project start-up and completion.

Thus, in estimating the time to finish the entire project, CPM would follow the linear path through the activity (among ones occurring in a simultaneous or overlapping fashion) which requires the greatest amount of time to complete before the next sequential activity can be initiated.

Use of Computers in Evaluation

The growth and refinement of computer terchnology over the past two decades has allowed evaluators to make great strides in conceiving, planning, and carrying out evaluation of health education, health promotion, and health services programs. These advances have occurred both in the area of computer hardware and computer software. As Gold (1991) points out:

In 1977, Apple™ and Radio Shack™ computer companies made consumer-oriented microcomputers a reality. However, it was not until the development of Visicalc™ in 1979 by two graduate students at MIT that people bought computers to run an existing piece of software. The microcomputer marketplace changed dramatically again in late 1980 when IBM™ introduced its first personal computer (p.20).

Technological advances of the 1990s allowed smaller, but nevertheless, more powerful and relatively inexpensive personal computers to be available for a variety of uses pertinent to conducting program evaluations. Hardware advances include the development of mass data storage devices, better and more varied input devices, graphical interfaces, voice recognition/output, local and global communications, and laptop computer capability (Gold, 1991).

An outcome of the improvements in computer hardware has been the development and implementation of applications software for administrative and other managerial tasks. Numerous software programs, ranging in both sophistication and cost, are available for activities such as routine record keeping, budgeting, making cost projections and conducting other accounting procedures, taking inventory of supplies. facilitating electronic exchanges of mail, performing word processing, preparing reports, creating graphics displays, managing data bases, carrying out statistical analyses, acquiring data (e.g., random selection and dialing of telephone numbers for surveys), carrying out library data base searches for books, journal articles, reports, government documents, and other literature, and additional activities.

Twenty-five years ago the state-of-the-art in computer technology required that data be keypunched on IBM cards, and read by large mainframe computer systems. The process was slow, cumbersome, and full of potential for making errors. At the dawn of the 21st century, the process is still not error-free, but the potential for error has been reduced. Moreover, the speed with which data can be entered and analyzed has been accelerated. Data can be transferred from paper-and-pencil response instruments onto optical scan sheets and read by scanners using appropriate software. Alternatively, responses can be "bubbled" as they are being gathered by data collectors on optical scan forms, such as during interviews. Respondents to a written survey can be provided with directions for completing a scan form, and thus, save the investigators additional time by filling in the circles or bubbles themselves. Furthermore, a data collector seated at a work station containing a microcomputer and monitor can be gathering interview data over the telephone, and recording the responses simultaneously. Speed and convenience with respect to all of these features will expand dramatically in the next few years.

A critical element of data collection and computer-aided analysis is the preparation of the **codebook** (Bloom, 1986). The codebook contains the procedural key through which raw data become translated for various forms of analysis (such as frequency counts, descriptive statistics, crosstabulations, and other statistical procedures).

Setting up a codebook is not complicated, but requires some forethought about the data to be entered for analysis. How one creates a codebook can be facilitated by considering the questionnaire about breast health shown in Figure 4.5. For each item to be used in the codebook, the coder will need to specify the variable number, the column(s) of the number string in which the variable appears, how many columns a particular variable includes, whether the variable is a numeric variable (identified by the presence of a numeral) or an alpha variable (identified by the presence of a letter), and the code (alpha or numeric) that represents the actual response. For this particular example, all codes are numeric. Codebook formats vary according to the specific statistical analysis software used.

Question 1 on the survey seeks to find out whether or not the respondent had a mammogram performed following a community breast health promotion project. The options are simple in this case. Either she had a mammogram (YES) or else she did not have one (NO). These two responses can be coded "1=YES" and "2=NO" respectively. For Question 1, the bubble labeled "1" would be filled in on an optical scan form if the woman responded affirmatively, and "2" would be completed if she responded negatively. If data were being entered via a microcomputer with a numeric keypad and stored on a floppy disk, the operator would simply enter a "1" or a "2" depending on the response.

Questions 2 through 30 address beliefs, attitudes, and feelings that women have about breast health and breast cancer early detection. Rather than having dichotomous variables as we had in Question 1, these items require one to answer on a five-point, Likert-type scale, ranging from "Strongly Agree" to "Strongly Disagree." Nevertheless, our strategy for coding responses is much like that used in Question 1. This time, our respective codes for each statement will be as follows: 1=Strongly Agree (SA), 2=Agree (A), 3=Neither Agree nor Disagree (N), 4=Disagree (D), and 5=Strongly Disagree (SD). Consequently, if a woman responds "Neither Agree nor Disagree" to Question 7 (Breast cancer would ruin my life) a "3" would be entered to represent that code.

Questions 31-34 are all one-column categorical variables that can be easily coded as shown in the completed codebook shown in Figure 4.6. Question 35 (Age) is a two-column variable (since a respondent's age requires two digits) and is coded in terms of the woman's actual response (e.g., "39"). For some studies in gerontology, it is conceivable that the age variable would have to be in a three-column field to account for centenarians. Furthermore, a study that included persons of all ages might yield coded responses such as 008, 063, and 101. Question 36 (Respondent code) forces us to use a three-column field since there were 556 individual respondents to the survey, each with a unique respondent code ranging from 001 to 556. Note that while variable #8 begins in column 8 and variable #35 begins in column 35, variable #36 begins in column 37. Why? If there were a variable #37, in which column would it begin?

1. Did you have a mammogram (breast x-ray) performed as a result of the Community Breast Screening Project?

   Please circle:　　　**YES　　NO**

For each item 2 through 30, please indicate your level of agreement with the statement shown. **SA**=strongly agree, **A**=agree, **N**=neither agree nor disagree, **D**=disagree, and **SD**=strongly disagree.

2. Early detection of breast cancer increases my chances of having it cured._____
3. Getting a mammogram is a frightening experience._____
4. I believe it is possible to detect breast cancer at an early stage._____
5. The cost of a mammogram is too high for me._____
6. I believe that having a mammogram would give me peace of mind._____
7. Getting breast cancer would ruin my life._____
8. I would not be so anxious about breast cancer if I had a mammogram._____
9. I believe that I will get breast cancer in my lifetime._____
10. I believe that my breast could be saved if cancer is found early._____
11. My doctor has never recommended a mammogram for me._____
12. If left untreated, breast cancer will lead to death._____
13. I personally have known a woman who had breast cancer._____
14. Getting a mammogram is embarrassing for me._____
15. I believe that breast cancer is a serious disease._____
16. As I get older, my chances of getting breast cancer increase._____
17. My family and friends would approve of my getting a mammogram performed._____
18. I do not have time to get a mammogram._____
19. I believe I will get breast cancer in the next five years._____
20. I believe that if my mother or sister had breast cancer, I am more likely to get it._____
21. Getting transportation to a mammography center would be hard for me._____
22. I could get a mammogram performed close to my home._____
23. I believe that having a mammogram is painful._____
24. I am afraid of the radiation from a mammogram._____
25. Losing my breast would change how I feel about myself._____
26. I believe a mammogram is unsafe._____
27. Making an appointment to get a mammogram is difficult._____
28. Losing my breast would change how my husband, boyfriend, or others feel about me._____
29. I worry about getting breast cancer._____
30. Practicing breast self-examination (BSE) is an important activity for me to detect breast changes._____

31. Ethnic background: __Black __White __Hispanic __Other
32. Current marital status: __Married __Divorced __Widowed __Single __Other
33. Annual household income: __<$15,000 __$15,000-$20,000 __$20,000-$30,000 __$30,000-$50,000 __>$50,000
34. Highest educational attainment: __Less than high school __high school graduate __some college __college graduate
35. Age_____
36. Respondent code_____

Figure 4.5 Community Breast Screening Project Survey

1. Did you have a mammogram (breast x-ray) performed as a result of the Community Breast Screening Project?
   Start column=1   No. of columns=1   Type=numeric
   1=yes 2=no

2. Early detection of breast cancer increases my chances of having it cured.
   Start column=2   No. of columns=1   Type=numeric
   1=SA 2=A 3=N 4=D 5=SD

3. Getting a mammogram is a frightening experience.
   Start column=3   No. of columns=1   Type=numeric
   1=SA 2=A 3=N 4=D 5=SD

4. I believe it is possible to detect breast cancer at an early stage.
   Start column=4   No. of columns=1   Type=numeric
   1=SA 2=A 3=N 4=D 5=SD

5. The cost of a mammogram is too high for me.
   Start column=5   No. of columns=1   Type=numeric
   1=SA 2=A 3=N 4=D 5=SD

6. I believe that having a mammogram would give me peace of mind.
   Start column=6   No. of columns=1   Type=numeric
   1=SA 2=A 3=N 4=D 5=SD

7. Getting breast cancer would ruin my life.
   Start column=7   No. of columns=1   Type=numeric
   1=SA 2=A 3=N 4=D 5=SD

8. I would not be so anxious about breast cancer if I had a mammogram.
   Start column=8   No. of columns=1   Type=numeric
   1=SA 2=A 3=N 4=D 5=SD

9. I believe that I will get breast cancer in my lifetime.
   Start column=9   No. of columns=1   Type=numeric
   1=SA 2=A 3=N 4=D 5=SD

10. I believe that my breast could be saved if cancer is found early.
    Start column=10 No. of columns=1   Type=numeric
    1=SA 2=A 3=N 4=D 5=SD

11. My doctor has never recommended a mammogram for me.
    Start column=11 No. of columns=1   Type=numeric
    1=SA 2=A 3=N 4=D 5=SD

12. If left untreated, breast cancer will lead to death.
    Start column=12 No. of columns=1   Type=numeric
    1=SA 2=A 3=N 4=D 5=SD

13. I personally have known a woman who had breast cancer.
    Start column=13 No. of columns=1   Type=numeric
    1=SA 2=A 3=N 4=D 5=SD

14. Getting a mammogram is embarrassing for me.
    Start column=14 No. of columns=1   Type=numeric
    1=SA 2=A 3=N 4=D 5=SD

15. I believe that breast cancer is a serious disease.
    Start column=15 No. of columns=1   Type=numeric
    1=SA 2=A 3=N 4=D 5=SD

16. As I get older, my chances of getting breast cancer increase.
    Start column=16 No. of columns=1   Type=numeric
    1=SA 2=A 3=N 4=D 5=SD

Figure 4.6 Codebook for Community Breast Screening Project Survey

17. My family and friends would approve of my getting a mammogram performed.
    Start column=17 No. of columns=1 Type=numeric
    1=SA 2=A 3=N 4=D 5=SD

18. I do not have time to get a mammogram.
    Start column=18 No. of columns=1 Type=numeric
    1=SA 2=A 3=N 4=D 5=SD

19. I believe I will get breast cancer in the next five years.
    Start column=19 No. of columns=1 Type=numeric
    1=SA 2=A 3=N 4=D 5=SD

20. I believe that if my mother or sister had breast cancer, I am more likely to get it.
    Start column=20 No. of columns=1 Type=numeric
    1=SA 2=A 3=N 4=D 5=SD

21. Getting transportation to a mammography center would be hard for me.
    Start column=21 No. of columns=1 Type=numeric
    1=SA 2=A 3=N 4=D 5=SD

22. I could get a mammogram performed close to my home.
    Start column=22 No. of columns=1 Type=numeric
    1=SA 2=A 3=N 4=D 5=SD

23. I believe that having a mammogram is painful.
    Start column=23 No. of columns=1 Type=numeric
    1=SA 2=A 3=N 4=D 5=SD

24. I am afraid of the radiation from a mammogram.
    Start column=24 No. of columns=1 Type=numeric
    1=SA 2=A 3=N 4=D 5=SD

25. Losing my breast would change how I feel about myself.
    Start column=25 No. of columns=1 Type=numeric
    1=SA 2=A 3=N 4=D 5=SD

26. I believe a mammogram is unsafe.
    Start column=26 No. of columns=1 Type=numeric
    1=SA 2=A 3=N 4=D 5=SD

27. Making an appointment to get a mammogram is difficult.
    Start column=27 No. of columns=1 Type=numeric
    1=SA 2=A 3=N 4=D 5=SD

28. Losing my breast would change how my husband, boyfriend, or others feel about me.
    Start column=28 No. of columns=1 Type=numeric
    1=SA 2=A 3=N 4=D 5=SD

29. I worry about getting breast cancer.
    Start column=29 No. of columns=1 Type=numeric
    1=SA 2=A 3=N 4=D 5=SD

30. Practicing breast self-examination (BSE) is an important activity for me to detect breast changes.
    Start column=30 No. of columns=1 Type=numeric
    1=SA 2=A 3=N 4=D 5=SD

31. Ethnic background:
    Start column=31 No. of columns=1 Type=numeric
    1=Black 2=White 3=Hispanic 4=Other

32. Current marital status:
    Start column=32 No. of columns=1 Type=numeric
    1=Married 2=Divorced 3=Widowed 4=Single 5=Other

33. Annual household income:
    Start column=33 No. of columns=1 Type=numeric
    1=<$15K 2=$15K-$20K 3=$20K-$30K 4=$30K-$50K 5=>$50K

Figure 4.6 Continued

34.   Highest educational attainment:
        Start column=34 No. of columns=1 Type=numeric
        1=Less than high school 2=high school graduate
        3=some college 4=college graduate
35.   Age:
        Start column=35 No. of columns=2 Type=numeric
36.   Respondent code:
        Start column=37 No. of columns=3 Type=numeric

Figure 4.6 Continued

        Invariably, respondents fail to tell you everything that you want to know. That is, subjects skip some items either purposely (because the item is "too personal") or inadvertently (because the item is confusing or the layout of the questionnaire is poor). How does one code missing data? The answer to this question depends on the particular statistical program being used. In some instances the absence of a numeral tells the statistical program to interpret this field as missing. In other instances, the number "9" is used as a conventional code for missing data for a one-column variable, "99" for a two-column variable, and so on. But what if "9" is a legitimate code for a response to an item? Written documentation accompanying the statistical software package or a user familiar with the software is likely to provide you with the best guidance in this instance. (Many high quality statistical software programs exist for use in the social and behavioral sciences. They range in sophistication and complexity, and we advise readers to consult with software users and other experts before selecting a particular statistical package.)

        Examine the strings of numbers on page 82 that represent three of the individual respondent records (respondents 9, 10, and 11) for the Community Breast Screening Project Survey prepared by a data entry person. The computer program would "read" these strings, record the entry according to the instructions it is given by the codebook that was prepared, and yield whatever output analyses are requested. See if you can use the codebook to interpret these records the way that a computer would. For example, can you provide the entire demographic profile for respondent #9 (i.e., code 009)? Does respondent #10 feel that untreated breast cancer will lead to death? Did respondent #11 get a mammogram? What is the annual household income for respondent #11? How does each woman feel about the embarrassment associated with getting a mammogram?

        Let us see how well you did. Respondent #9 is a white, married woman, with an annual household income between $30,000 and $50,000. Moreover, she is a 43-year-old college graduate. To see if respondent #10 views the prognosis for untreated breast cancer as a death sentence, we need to consult the codebook. Upon seeing that this item is a one-column numeric variable beginning in column #12, we count 12 places into the string, and note that this woman "strongly agrees" with the statement. Respondent #11 we find out did not get a mammogram, and it appears that she did not answer the question related to annual household income (since we note no entry). Judging from their responses, all three women seem to find mammograms to be embarrassing, with respondent #10 expressing a little less embarrassment than the other two women.

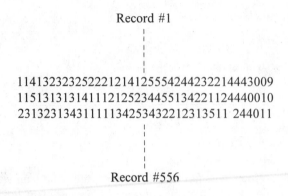

Figure 4.7 Variable String Associated with Breast Cancer Survey

In conclusion, microcomputers are now able to perform sophisticated tasks that 15 or 20 years ago would have been unthinkable by even the most optimistic of investigators. These devices can employ relatively inexpensive software to assist study design, data collection, data storage, data analysis, and report generation.

Summary

Management of tasks is one of the keys to successful evaluation, for it is integral to producing the type of data that is useful to program stakeholders. A meticulously negotiated contract enhances understanding and cooperation between an agency and an evaluation team. Several points can be identified for contracting parties to consider. Careful recruitment, orientation, and training of project staff will enhance understanding of, and commitment to, the evaluative tasks to be performed. Attention to a plan of scheduled activities will minimize resource waste, and provide a mechanism for continuous monitoring and feedback about program progress and program deficiencies. Aides to planning such as the program evaluation review technique, key activity charts, Gantt charts, and the critical path method can assist evaluators in scheduling tasks and monitoring their completion. Budgets must be designed with realistic assessment of the tasks to be performed and the timeline for carrying them out. Specific data collection strategies will depend on the nature of the project and the type of decisions to be made. Computer technology can be of enormous assistance in conducting virtually all phases of an evaluation project from task planning and data collection, to data analysis and report preparation.

Case Study

Taylor, S.M., Ross, N.A., Cummings, K.M., Glasgow, R.E., Goldsmith, C.H., Zanna, M.P., & Corle, D.K. (1998). Community intervention trial for smoking cessation (COMMIT): Changes in community attitudes toward cigarette smoking. *Health Education Research*, *13*(1), 109-122.

In this study, one community within each of eleven matched pairs was randomly assigned to receive a four-year, community-based smoking cessation intervention. The number of surveys conducted was in the tens of thousands. Consider some of the logistics of how this very ambitious study must have been carried out. How were communities contacted? Which individual or key informant within a community would have been the best contact person? Over what length of time might the investigators have decided on the specific communities to include in this study? How were the intervention strategies determined? How was scheduling established? How was the method for survey dissemination, collection, and analysis determined? How do you suppose the investigators determined the time frame for the study? In addition to logistical issues associated with this project, how do you imagine the intended outcomes were predicted? On what basis prior to the intervention might the investigators have concluded the extent to which change in attitude or behavior would occur? Pretend that you were replicating this study in your community. "Walk through" this project under these limited conditions. Try to anticipate the logistical problems *you* might encounter. Develop a key activity or Gantt chart to help you think through your plans.

Student Questions/Activities

1. The Dean of your college wishes to have the health education program evaluated, and have a completed report on her desk in 180 days. She is particularly interested in an evaluation that includes, but is not necessarily limited to, the following information: a) the recruitment and retention of minority students; b) student satisfaction with teaching; c) student academic performance; d) the quality of field experience settings in which students are placed; and e) the scope, quality, and quantity of successfully placed program graduates. The Dean has allocated a maximum of $4,000.00 for the project. Develop a plan for this evaluation that includes the selection of the measures or indicators that will provide the Dean with the feedback she desires. Determine your sources of data and methods of data collection. Are there any points of contract negotiation that may be of relevance to you here? If so, which one(s)? Explain. Suggest the composition of a project advisory committee. Prepare a budget that illustrates the breakdown of the funds the Dean has made available. Finally, using any of the planning charts and techniques discussed in Chapter 4, plan the 180-day project in which you identify the relevant key events and persons responsible for carrying out the necessary tasks and producing the desired end-products.

2.   The State Department of Education, in conjunction with the State Department of Health, has made $100,000.00 available to study the status of health services delivery in the public schools of your state, and your university has been awarded the contract. It is August 1, and these agencies wish to have your final report by next February 1 (just six months away) so that it can be reviewed, and relevant facts can be disseminated to legislators who will be making funding decisions about school health services during the months of April through June. The two cooperating agencies wish to, have data concerning the number of students who are "dropouts" due to health reasons, the number of health screenings (all commonly implemented ones K-12) whose follow-up diagnostic status is known and unknown, the number of physically challenged, and other special needs pupils by grade level, and the range of services they receive, the incidence of absenteeism among the state's public school students, and the number of schools with existing health rooms/nurses' stations, and the outfitting of these facilities. The "political" motive behind this information is to provide legislators with data that will support approval of funds to hire more school nurses. Agency personnel have informed you that the hiring of more school nurses is the conclusion you are to reach. Discuss the probable content of your contract negotiations with these people from the two agencies. Prepare a budget for this project, bearing in mind that your institution has an indirect cost rate of 30% to which it holds steadfastly. Justify your budgetary expenditures. Describe how you would expect to collect data for this project. Identify any staff people that you would expect to employ. List the kinds of people whom you believe would comprise an effective advisory committee. Construct a Gantt chart and a narrative to accompany it that give the details of the project tasks and the personnel who will complete them.

3.   Perform the same task as described in #2 above, except make the project one of 12-month duration. What factors change? Explain.

Recommended Readings

Chambers, L.C., Hoey, J., & Underwood, J. (1998). Integration of service, education, and research in local official public health agencies. *American Journal of Public Health*, *88*(7), 1102-1103.

This brief article iterates some of the logistical challenges when academic public health and public health practitioners form linkages, but also identifies the value that can emerge from such collaboration.

Joint Commission on Accreditation of Healthcare Organizations. (1994). *Forms, Charts, & Other Tools for Performance Improvement*. Oakbrook Terrace, IL: Author.

This handy book of approximately 156 pages is filled with forms and charts that can be used as prototypes for groups and organizations that have simple and complex tasks to perform on a schedule. It is valuable for project logistical planning.

Breckon, D.J. (1997). *Managing Health Promotion Programs*. Gaithersburg, MD: Aspen.

This book addresses many of the tasks in program planning and management with emphasis on logistical concerns. Administrative styles, organizational charts, job descriptions, recruiting and hiring, budgeting, fiscal control, and other issues are presented.

References

Bloom, M. (1986). *The Experience of Research*. New York: MacMillan Publishing Company.

Borg, W.R., & Gall, M.D. (1989). *Educational Research*, 5th edition. New York: Longman.

Fink, A., & Kosecoff, J. (1978). *An Evaluation Primer*. Beverly Hills, CA: Sage Publications.

French, J.F., & Kaufman, N.J. (1983). *Handbook for Prevention Evaluation*. Rockville, MD: (United States Department of Health and Human Services) Public Health Service, (ADM) 83-1145.

Gold, R.S. (1991). *Microcomputer Applications in Health Education*. Dubuque, IA: William C. Brown Publishers.

Office of Substance Abuse Prevention. (1991). *First Pregnant and Postpartum Women and Infants Evaluation Skills Building Workshop*, Washington, D.C.: U.S. Department of Health and Human Services.

Rakich, J.S., Longest, B.B., Jr., & Darr, K. (1985). *Managing Health Services Organizations*, 2nd edition. Philadelphia: W.B. Saunders Company.

Schaefer, M. (1987). *Implementing Changes in Service Programs*. Newbury Park, CA: Sage Publications.

Shortell, S.M., & Richardson, W.C. (1978). *Health Program Evaluation*. St. Louis: C.V. Mosby Company.

Stufflebeam, D.L. (1978). Meta evaluation: An overview. *Evaluation and the Health Professions*, *1*(1), 17-43.

Chapter
5

Introduction to Measurement

Chapter Objectives

After completing this chapter, you should be able to:

1. Identify the major types of instruments used in health education.
2. Describe the four levels of measurement.
3. Describe at least three controversial issues in educational testing.
4. Provide a rationale for multiple measures.
5. Describe how theories, models, frameworks, and curriculum materials can be used as a basis for the development of instrument items.
6. Identify the 13-step process for health education instrument development.

Key Terms

achievement tests
attitudinal inventories
behavioral inventories
biomedical instruments
criterion-referenced tests
health-risk appraisals
high-stakes tests

instrument specifications
interval levels of measurement
nominal levels of measurement
norm-referenced tests
ordinal levels of measurement
ratio scales
triangulation of evidence

Introduction

The selection or development of a data collection instrument is one of the most important elements of the evaluation design. If an instrument is not relevant or appropriate for the target population, one cannot have any confidence in the results of the evaluation. The selection or development of data collection instruments also can be a controversial process. Program administrators may be reluctant for a variety of reasons to have their programs evaluated. Shouting matches can and do break out in meetings over deciding whether it is appropriate to measure behavior and knowledge versus attitudes and skills, when evaluating a health education program. For this reason, evaluators must be both diplomatic and technically careful as they select and develop their instruments.

Health educators involved in evaluations have a wide variety of instruments available for their use. Instruments that measure knowledge, attitudes, behaviors, and biomedical functions are commonly used in health education evaluations. For example, a patient educator evaluating the effectiveness of a hypertension education program might use any combination of the following measures:

- A knowledge test focusing on patient knowledge of the causes and methods of controlling hypertension.
- An attitudinal test measuring the degree to which participants feel they can control their hypertension.
- A behavioral inventory examining patient eating, exercise, and medication patterns.
- A blood pressure cuff, laboratory tests, and scale for weighing the patients.
- An audit of the costs of implementing the program.

It is desirable to evaluate a program using multiple measures. Usually no one test, survey, observational procedure, focus group, or physical examination can be used to evaluate the success of a program adequately.

Contemporary Problems in Measurement

Measurement is a way of life for us. Indeed, one might argue that Americans are obsessed with the notion of measurement. Our children are constantly being tested in our schools (some may argue *over*-tested). When we "work-out," the machines we use for exercise provide us with a number of different measurements, including calories burned, watts generated, speed and distance traveled, and time exercised. The whole notion of total quality improvement is based on comparing a particular organization's performance to accepted standards.

In the field of health education, we also measure things. For example, an evaluator might determine the effectiveness of a program by measuring gains in knowledge and in positive health behaviors as a result of completing a health education course. Measurement instruments are the tools that evaluators use to assess the quality of programs.

Measurement has been defined in similar ways by different researchers. Guilford (1954) indicates that measurement is the description of data in terms of numbers. Nunnally (1978) defines measurement as a system of rules for assigning numbers to objects. Green and Lewis (1986) describe measurement as the process of assigning numbers to objects, events, or people. We propose that measurement is the set of rules used to assign numbers to different objects, events, issues, or people. Through measurement, we can estimate the progress made by our health education programs.

Testing and measurement is not without controversy. For example, our reliance on standardized tests for college admissions is a source of continuous debate. *The Chronicle of Higher Education*, along with many other publications, frequently feature stories about testing. In an article entitled "Moves Against Affirmative Action Fuel Opposition to Standardized Admissions Tests," Mealer (1997) refers to several developments regarding the use of standardized tests:

- A University of California Committee studying Hispanic students recommended to the Board of Regents to stop using the SAT test in the admission procedures.
- Texas lawmakers passed a law that requires public universities to admit all students who graduate in the top 10% of their class, regardless of test scores.
- The president of the American Bar Association has asked law schools in Texas and California to place less emphasis on the Law School Admissions Test.

The national testing movement is another interesting element in our educational process today. One element of this movement is the argument proposed by some educators and politicians that all high school seniors should pass a basic competency test to graduate, under the assumption that there are core skills which all high school graduates should master. Others argue that curriculum diversity or curriculum relevance is desirable. That is, what might be appropriate to teach in a rural farming community might not be appropriate in the inner city. For these reasons, a national test would not be fair. This movement in testing is also felt in the elementary schools. Many students, as young as second graders, are tested using computerized protocols on a weekly basis, concerning basic skills such as reading ability. Parents receive weekly computer-generated reports on their youngster's most recent performance on a test, providing information on reading level, number of items answered correctly on the weekly test, and number of points earned toward a total "reading goal."

Some researchers argue that national testing programs have an impact on the curriculum taught in schools. In other words, teachers may have a tendency to "teach to the test" (Nickerson, 1989). A further problem related to the testing movement is that administrators and school board members will use the test results to compare different schools, school systems, and state systems of education with each other, based on test scores. This approach is problematic for a number of reasons, including the skills and abilities of the students who are in the particular schools, the socio-economic status of the students, as well as the support provided for students from state and local tax funds. In Illinois for example, actual per student funding varies dramatically by school district (from about $3,000 per student per year to about $12,000 per student per year in 1997). The resources provided to each student, therefore, vary substantially by school district. This discrepancy, of course, can affect performance on tests. Yet, one frequently reads in the local papers how different schools "stack up" against each other. The practice of using test scores in this way has been criticized. Clearly, measurement is a controversial and politically explosive issue in the United States, due to the social, legal, and political consequences of decisions based on testing (Linn, 1989; Popham, 1987).

One of the most difficult issues facing those charged with health education program evaluation is the decision concerning "what" to measure. Is it appropriate to measure behavior, skills, attitudes, and knowledge in the evaluation of a program? When should the measurements take place, especially if the program is a multi-year, multiple component program? When and how should the process evaluation take place? Who should have final authority in the design of the data collection instruments? These issues are at the very heart of the evaluation process, and are in general, philosophical in nature. For example, if one believes that in the end, a health education program proves itself by the degree to which youngsters change behavior, then, behavior ought to be measured. On the other hand, if one's philosophy is that health education ought to provide people with decision-making tools and awareness and knowledge of health problems, then the evaluation ought to focus on skills and knowledge.

Several of the problems mentioned above (e.g., SAT exams, law school admission tests) are all related to the unique problems of developing **high stakes tests**. A high stakes test is a test that may have a major impact on the lives of those individuals taking the test as well as an impact on the people who have been charged with teaching or training the test-takers. Examples of high stakes tests include high school graduation tests, examinations that college graduates must pass to teach in a school system (Popham, 1987), medical boards, or an examination to become a certified health education specialist (CHES). High stakes tests must be designed and implemented carefully. They must be fair to those taking the test, as well as fair to those using the test to make decisions.

Levels of Measurement

From the discussion above, one can see that how to assess objects, events, issues, or people is perhaps one of the most controversial aspects of measurement. How should a test that measures the competencies of a health educator be designed? What areas should be covered? What test items should be used? Should there be a practical component requiring individuals to demonstrate their skills? What should the passing score for the test be? Should people be allowed to retake the test if they fail?

A fundamental question concerning measurement is how something is to be measured. Consider a survey item measuring the age of program participants. Figure 5.1 illustrates several methods that might be used by an evaluator to determine age of participants. Each item is a legitimate method of measuring age. A program focusing on human development might use an item that classifies people according to the first method. A pollster may wish to classify people by age groups, while an evaluator working on a research project might want to use actual age for his or her study.

When health educators develop data collection instruments, they must consider the different levels of measurement that can be used when developing items. An understanding of different levels of measurement is important because different statistics are used with different levels of measurement. There are four levels of measurement: nominal, ordinal, interval, and ratio.

Method 1

Which of the following best represents the age of the patient?
a.   infant
b.   child
c.   adolescent
d.   young adult
e.   middle aged
f.   elderly

Method 2

Which age group best represents the age in years of the patient?
a.   0-3
b.   4-11
c.   12-18
d.   19-30
e.   31-60
f.   61+

Method 3

What is the age of the patient in years? _____

Figure 5.1 Sample Items that Measure Age

Nominal levels of measurement categorize individuals, objects, issues, or events into different groups. Commonly used nominal variables found in health education questionnaires are sex and place of residence (north, south, east, or west). These variables in themselves classify an individual with regard to a particular characteristic. However, they do not usually tell us who has more or less of one characteristic than another.

Ordinal levels of measurement rank-order individuals, objects, issues, or events. For example, using an ordinal scale, one may rank all the people in the class from the heaviest to the lightest. From this ranking we would be able to tell who was the heaviest, second heaviest, and third heaviest. However, we would not know how much heavier the person ranked number one would be than the person ranked number two. One commonly used ordinal measure in health education research is the Likert scale, which asks people to identify their attitudes concerning an object, event, issue, or person. An example of a Likert scale item would be:

Smoking cigarettes is dangerous to one's health.

1. Strongly agree
2. Agree
3. Neither agree nor disagree
4. Disagree
5. Strongly disagree

A person who answers "2" more strongly agrees with the idea that smoking is dangerous to one's health than does a person who answers "4," who actually disagrees with the statement.

Interval levels of measurement have the characteristic of rank that appear in ordinal scales, but they also measure the distance between different points on the scale. A commonly used instrument in the health sciences that employs interval scales of measurement is a thermometer with the Celsius or Fahrenheit scale. The difference between 100 degrees and 80 degrees Celsius is 20 degrees, which is the same difference between 50 degrees and 30 degrees. The difference of 20 degrees Celsius is the same amount of difference in both examples, from the chemical and physical perspective concerning how temperature is measured. The differences would not be the same if we, for example, only ranked a large class of students by weight. Even though the difference between the one hundredth person and the eightieth person is 20 rank points, we would not expect that same difference in pounds be present between the fiftieth person and the thirtieth person. One problem with interval scales is that an absolute 0 value is not present. For example, 0 degrees Celsius does not mean there is no temperature present, it is just a point on the scale.

Ratio scales are the most sophisticated levels of measurement. They are characterized by an ability to rank individuals, objects, issues, or events. There is also a known distance between the different rankings, and the 0 value has an absolute meaning. Ratio scales occur frequently in biomedical measurement. Examples of ratio scales include age, height in inches, weight in pounds, or blood pressure. In each of these cases, it is possible to have a 0 value that has meaning.

From a measurement perspective, it is desirable to use the highest level of measurement possible with a given variable. For example, on a questionnaire measuring age, it would be more desirable to obtain the actual age of the respondent in years, rather than obtain age through an ordinal item (e.g., 0-10, 11-20, 21-30 years, and so on). If necessary, one can convert a higher level of measurement to a lower level of measurement. In the age example presented in Figure 5.1, one could take the actual age of the subjects in years (ratio data) and then categorize them according to their ranks (i.e., 0-10, 11-20, 21-30 years). However, one cannot take a lower level of measurement, and convert it to a higher level. Therefore, it is always best to use the highest form of measurement possible for each variable. Of course, certain variables such as sex are categorical in nature; therefore, one would never be able to employ that variable as anything but a categorical measure. (It is statistically possible to manipulate a categorical variable so that it is treated in a ratio manner, through dichotomous scoring, but those procedures are beyond the scope of this discussion.)

Models, Frameworks, Curriculum Materials, and Instrument Development

Program evaluations should always be based on a guiding framework. The framework could be a curriculum outline of goals and objectives for a particular grade level or course, or the framework could be a theoretical model that purports to predict health behaviors. When developing an instrument for evaluation purposes, it is best to design the instrument based on the theory, paradigm, or framework that was used to develop the program. For example, let us say a patient education program was based on the Health Belief Model, a theoretical model designed to describe an individual's perceived benefits and costs and other thought processes, related to engaging in a health behavior (e.g., Rosenstock, 1974). The instrument, therefore, should be comprised of items that reflect important components of the Health Belief Model.

Suppose you have been asked to develop an instrument that examines the effectiveness of a school health education curriculum. Suppose too that one of the data collection techniques you were going to use was to be a survey comprised of knowledge, attitude, and behavior items. The first thing you would do would be to identify the objectives of the curriculum. You would then design a set of items that would match those objectives. You might also want to ensure that some of the items are related to the health objectives for the nation identified in *Healthy People 2000*, the document that guided America's health planning in the 1990s. Figure 5.2 shows how you could identify items related to behaviors identified in *Healthy People 2000* (or possibly, to a specific curriculum). These items were developed in regard to a test that was designed for kindergarten students. Each test item is linked to either a *Healthy People 2000* objective or a specific lesson objective. In addition to being a useful instrument development tool, it is helpful to those asked to evaluate the quality of the test in terms of content validity (see Chapter 7). The example shown is limited to health behaviors. One could, however, develop an instrument that was linked to specific knowledge objectives or attitudinal objectives, or all three domains (knowledge, attitudes, *and* behaviors). The example shown in Figure 5.2, though developed for young children, could be modified for adolescents, young adults, middle-aged adults, or older adults. How might age influence the content of the knowledge, attitudinal, or behavioral items?

Behavioral Questions

1.   Do you eat fruit every day?
     HP 2000 Objective 2.6
2.   Do you eat vegetables every day?
     HP 2000 Objective 2.6
3.   Have you ever tried smoking a cigarette?
     HP 2000 Objectives 3.5 and 4.5
4.   Have you ever tried chewing tobacco or snuff?
     HP 2000 Objectives 3.9 and 4.5
5.   Have you ever tried drinking a can, a glass or a bottle of beer, wine, or liquor?
     HP 2000 Objective 4.5
6.   Have you ever been in a fight where someone was punched, hit, kicked, or hurt
     in some way?
     HP 2000 Objective 7.9
7.   Have you ever carried, used, or shot a gun?
     HP 2000 Objective 7.10
8.   Do you wear a seat belt when you ride in the car?
     HP 2000 Objective 9.12
9.   Do you wear a helmet when you ride your bike?
     HP 2000 Objective 9.13
10. Do you brush your teeth every day?
     HP 2000 Objective 13.1
11. Do you wash your hands after going to the bathroom?
     HP 2000 Objective 20.8

Figure 5.2 Test Item Development Linked to *Healthy People 2000*

The development of the Youth Risk Behavior Surveillance System questionnaire provides an example of an instrument that was developed using a number of different criteria. Kolbe, Kann, and Collins (1993), in their description of the YRBSS, indicate that the overall design of the instrument was based on the leading causes of morbidity and mortality among youth and young adults. The data suggested that the following six areas ought to be the focus of the instrument:

- Unintentional and intentional injury
- Tobacco use
- Alcohol and other drug use
- Sexual behaviors
- Dietary behaviors
- Physical inactivity

A team of specialists from a variety of federal agencies were brought together to assist in the development of the survey. For example, questions related to alcohol and other drug use were developed by experts from the National Institute on Drug Abuse. These specialists helped identify health outcomes related to the risk behaviors, relevant *Healthy People 2000* objectives, priority health behaviors, and questions to be used on the survey. The first draft of the questionnaire was reviewed by representatives from state departments of education as well as survey research specialists. The YRBSS was pilot tested (see Chapter 8) in four waves. Pilot test results were valuable, such as improving the wording of the questions as well as the development of response categories. Pilot testing also identified conditions that would best allow students to be honest in their responses (Kolbe, et al., 1993). Further testing has shown the instrument to have an acceptable level of reliability (Brener, Collins, Kann, Warren, & Williams, 1995).

Types of Measurement Instruments
Used in Health Education

Evaluators use many different types of measures when assessing the quality of health education programs. The most frequently used measures fall under the categories of **achievement tests**, **attitudinal inventories**, **behavioral inventories**, **biomedical instruments**, and **health-risk appraisals**. Achievement tests measure the degree to which an individual has mastered a body of knowledge. Achievement tests are probably the most commonly used measures in health education evaluation today. Examples of these tests are the classroom knowledge tests used to measure the degree to which students have mastered the objectives of instruction. There are two basic forms of achievement tests, **criterion-referenced tests** and **norm-referenced tests**.

Criterion-referenced tests have an absolute pass or fail score. The score needed to pass the test is known as the criterion or cut score. If an individual's score meets or exceeds the criterion, he or she passes. If the score falls below the criterion, he or she fails. The Red Cross CPR certification test is an example of a criterion-referenced test. Norm-referenced tests are used when an individual's score is compared to a group score. College entrance examinations, such as the SAT, are examples of norm-referenced tests. Classroom tests, where the instructor compares student scores with the mean or class rank, are other examples of norm-referenced tests.

Attitudinal inventories measure an individual's attitudes, values, beliefs, or opinions about individuals, objects, issues, or events. The items are usually scaled in both a positive and negative direction, so an individual's responses will indicate whether the respondent feels positively or negatively, or agrees or disagrees, about the idea under study. These types of scales are used frequently in health education evaluation studies designed to measure the degree to which attitudes have changed as a result of participation in the program. For example, an evaluator may be interested in determining how a participant's attitudes have changed concerning working with persons with AIDS, after a program has been implemented that was designed to reduce the fears of individuals from contracting HIV/AIDS through everyday interactions.

Behavioral inventories measure behaviors of individuals. There are two basic types of behavioral inventories: those that are based on self-report items, and those that are based on observation. Examples of behavioral inventories include diet and exercise logs, self-report scales for drug and alcohol use, and observation tests for performance of CPR. (The CPR test is also an example of both an achievement test and a behavioral inventory.)

Biomedical instruments measure physiological functions of the body. Commonly used biomedical instruments include measures for weight, height, blood pressure, and cholesterol levels. Those health educators working in patient education settings frequently use these measures when evaluating the impact of their programs.

Health-risk appraisals are based on an individual's responses to questions concerning his or her personal habits, physiologic status, and medical history (Smith, McKinlay, & McKinlay, 1989). Health-risk appraisals measure an individual's health status at a particular point in time, and then provide the individual with personalized risk estimates that can be explained to individuals, and can be used by educators to develop specific programs for the individual (Kirscht, 1989).

In addition to the teaching function, health-risk appraisals are also used to measure the effectiveness of health promotion programs (Smith, et al., 1989). There is considerable debate concerning the use of these instruments. Nevertheless, they continue to be used by health educators and others today (Kirscht, 1989). Debate centers around the notion that the risk produced through the health-risk appraisals is often based on population statistics rather than an individual's personal characteristics. In addition, research on models of prediction is still in its developmental stages, so interpretations from the models must be made cautiously.

Most likely, an evaluator will select several measures to evaluate the effectiveness of a program. As mentioned earlier, an evaluation of a blood pressure education program might use four or five different measures of program effectiveness. This is desirable because if one uses multiple measures, and obtains similar results using the multiple measures, one will have much more confidence in the results of the evaluation. The use of multiple measures to assess program effects is called **triangulation of evidence**.

Steps in the Development of an Instrument

Once an evaluator has identified the objects, events, issues, or people under study, and has identified a framework for the development of the instrument, he or she can proceed to instrument development itself. The following steps in instrument development focus on the development of knowledge, attitude, or behavioral inventories. It is assumed that if biomedical tests are to be used, existing instruments shall be used, as the development of these instruments is beyond the scope of most health education efforts.

The steps in the development of a health education instrument presented here are based on suggestions from several authors, including Sudman and Bradburn (1986), Green and Lewis (1986), Windsor, et al. (1984), Millman and Greene (1989), and Ebel and Frisbie (1986). These steps are outlined in Figure 5.3.

1. Determine the purpose and objectives of the proposed instrument.
2. Develop instrument specifications.
3. Review existing instruments.
4. Develop new instrument items.
5. Develop directions for administration and examples of how to complete items.
6. Establish procedures used for scoring the instrument.
7. Conduct a preliminary review of the instrument with colleagues.
8. Revise instrument based on review.
9. Pilot test the instrument with twenty to fifty subjects.
10. Conduct item analysis, reliability, and validity studies.
11. Provide instrument specifications and pilot study data to a panel of experts for review.
12. Revise the instrument based on comments from the panel of experts.
13. Determine cut score (for criterion-referenced tests or screening tests).

Figure 5.3 Steps in the Development of an Instrument

Determine the purpose and objectives of the proposed instrument. Millman and Greene (1989) state that: "The first and most important step in educational test development is to delineate the purpose of the test or the nature of the inferences intended from test scores" (p.335). This point makes good sense. If an evaluator is to develop a new data collection instrument, he or she had better be certain of the instrument's purpose (which is based on the purpose of the evaluation study). Otherwise, the evaluator risks developing an instrument that is not relevant to the study -- an expensive mistake!

Develop instrument specifications. **Instrument specifications** define how the evaluator will design the instrument. Common elements of instrument specification include: What is the purpose of the instrument? Who is the audience? What content areas are to be sampled? What types of items are to be used? How many items are to be used? Specifications are useful to both those people charged with designing the instrument and the people who must complete the instrument. This point is especially true in the case of standardized achievement tests (e.g., the SAT), where students may receive a booklet describing the test before it is administered (Ebel & Frisbie, 1986).

Figure 5.4 outlines the major areas to be covered when designing instrument specifications, based on the work of Millman and Green (1989) and Ebel and Frisbie (1986). Instrument purpose(s) and theoretical background, framework, and paradigm refers to the issues generated in step one of the instrument development process. Instrument developers as well as those using the instrument need to know the purpose of the instrument as well as the theory or framework upon which the instrument was designed.

Who will take the instrument? A questionnaire that measures drug abuse among high school students must be designed in a different manner than a questionnaire that measures drug abuse among the elderly. Knowing who the "examinees" are is an important aspect of instrument development.

Time to complete the instrument refers to the amount of time planned for an individual to take the instrument. If there is only ten minutes to complete the instrument, it should be short enough to be completed in this time frame. In general, the shorter, to-the-point instrument will obtain better results. People are much more likely to complete a 15-item survey than they are a 150-item survey.

- Instrument purpose(s) and theoretical background, framework, and paradigm
- Examinees
- Time to complete the instrument
- Instrument delivery system
- Administrators of the instrument
- Content areas to be examined
- Types of items to be used
- Number of items to be used for each content area
- Psychometric characteristics
- Scoring procedures
- Format of instrument
- Methods of reproducing instrument
- Cost to take the instrument
- Cost to administer the instrument

Figure 5.4 Instrument Specifications

Today, there are many forms of instrument delivery systems available, such as traditional paper-and-pencil tests, computer-based tests, simulations, and on-site observation. The instrument's objectives, types of learning, attitudes, or behaviors to be assessed, and the resources available for data collection will all influence the type of delivery system selected. For example, when teaching a unit on CPR, it is best to test the students' knowledge and abilities to carry out the CPR procedures using simulation "dummies" rather than having the students "write out" in essay form the step-by-step procedures for CPR. At times, it may be best to use traditional paper-and-pencil testing methods, and at other times it may be appropriate to use new technologies such as computer-based testing (Sarvela & Noonan, 1988).

Administrators of the instrument must be carefully considered when designing the instrument (Millman & Greene, 1989). If the instrument is being administered on a computer, individuals comfortable and familiar with computers must be selected to administer the instrument. Will the instrument be administered in a group or individual setting? What skills are needed to successfully administer the test? Will the test administrators be proctoring the examination or observing student performance (e.g., CPR examinations)? These issues will strongly influence the design of the instrument.

Content areas to be examined refers to the areas to be covered by the instrument. This specification is linked to the first specification dealing with purpose.

The types of items to be used are also a consideration. Will the items be constructed-response items (e.g., essay or "fill-in" items) or will the items be selected-response (e.g., multiple-choice or true-false)? What scales or levels of measurement will be used?

The number of items to be used for each content area is strongly related to the purpose of the instrument. Areas of more importance will usually have more items assigned to them than areas of lesser importance.

Psychometric characteristics relate to the reliability and validity of the instrument. For achievement tests, difficulty of the test is also considered.

Scoring procedures refer to the number of points assigned to correct or incorrect items, or how many points will be assigned to those who disagree or agree with different statements. Also to be considered here is the method of scoring. For example, will classroom teachers score the instrument, or will an optical scanning form be used?

The format of the instrument considers the physical characteristics of the instrument (e.g., size of print), method of subjects answering the items (writing directly on the form or using an optical scan sheet), flow, expected length in pages, and so on.

Methods of reproducing the instrument consider primarily whether the instrument will be typeset and reproduced by a printer, or will the instrument be generated by a word-processor or typewriter and then photocopied? The better the quality of the reproduction, the better the results obtained from the instrument. If the instrument is on a computer disk, how will it be copied, and for what types of computers will it be used?

The cost to take the instrument must be figured in terms of the amount of money persons are willing to pay for the instrument, as well as intangible costs such as time needed to take the instrument, and distance to be traveled to take the instrument.

The cost to administer the instrument refers to the total design, administration, scoring, and reporting of the instrument's results to the individuals as well as schools, colleges and universities, businesses, or the government.

Review existing instruments. Instrument development is an expensive process. When an evaluator begins a new study, he or she ought to review the literature for all existing instruments that are related to the evaluation study. Computer-assisted literature searches are extremely helpful at this stage. Also, companies frequently publish manuals that review instruments in print.

Demographic items are found on most data collection instruments. Because so many instruments have different forms of demographic items, there is no reason for an evaluator to have to develop a new set of demographic items. A better use of time would be for an evaluator to review several existing questionnaires, and select those demographic items of most use for the evaluation study at hand. Only in rare circumstances should an evaluator have to develop new or unusual demographic items.

An added bonus for using existing instruments, or parts of existing instruments, is that comparisons with the present evaluation study and previous studies are possible. For example, national studies by Johnston, et al. (1993) on high school drug use have generated a tremendous amount of national data concerning drug use behaviors among high school students. Clever evaluators of drug education programs will try to incorporate items from national surveys into their own surveys, so that comparisons can be made between local and national samples. The YRBSS, available from the Centers for Disease Control and Prevention, and described earlier in this chapter, is another instrument with national data to which local data can be compared.

If an evaluator selects items (or uses the whole test or instrument) developed and copyrighted by someone else, it is important to write to write the instrument developer for permission. Most instrument developers in academic settings at public universities will allow others to use their instruments free of charge. Of course, the instrument must be cited in the reference section of the evaluation report. Instruments produced by private companies are usually protected with a copyright that requires a fee. This fee may at first appear expensive. The fee may be relatively small, however, when one considers the development time for designing a reliable and valid questionnaire from scratch. Usually, it is more cost-efficient to pay the fee than to develop a whole new instrument.

Develop new instrument items. At this time, the evaluator should begin to write new items. The items should be written based on the instrument specifications. It is generally suggested that in this stage of item development, one should write twice as many items as outlined in the specification for the final draft of the instrument (Torabi, 1989). Therefore, if the specifications call for a 25-item instrument, initially, 50 items should be written. Pilot study and content validity review procedures will enable you to select those items best suited for your study.

While writing new items it is often helpful to look at different instruments, even if they are measuring totally different issues. For example, an evaluator developing an instrument on frequency of soft drink consumption could use an instrument that focused on frequency of caffeine use as a guide for developing the response possibilities, which will save a considerable amount of time during the initial item generation period. It is also important to review the suggestions of researchers concerning the development of good quality items for your particular subject area. For example, in an experimental trial concerning the development of questions for a dental health survey, researchers found that using the simple phrase "fluoride added to the water" produced 60 percent more correct responses than the phrase "public water fluoridation" (Jobe & Mingay, 1989).

Once the different items have been written, they should be assembled. It is generally recommended that similar items be grouped together. Therefore, one should group all multiple-choice items together, all true-false items together, and so on. Items can also be grouped by similar content areas. In addition, any demographic items asked on the instrument should be placed at the end of the form.

Develop directions for administration and examples of how to complete items. Instruments must have standardized administration procedures so that the data collected will be reliable. Evaluators should outline instructions to those completing the instrument, time limits, resources that can be used to complete the instrument (e.g., if it is an achievement test, can it be of the "open-book" variety?), and the appropriate environment for completing the instrument (American Educational Research Association, et al., 1985). Those administering the instrument also need specific instructions. What will they say to subjects? What types of questions will they answer if the subjects are unclear about something? What types of questions (e.g., understanding a term used in a question) will they not answer, because that is the focus of the examination? Instrument administrators need to know what they should and should not say when answering questions concerning their surveys.

Step-by step instructions for the administration of the instrument are always best. This aspect of the instrument design process is often overlooked, since many people assume that "everyone knows how to fill out a questionnaire." That is an erroneous assumption! It is also important to provide examples of how to complete items. Should the respondents circle the response or fill in a special box? Can they provide more than one response per item? All of these issues must be determined and described on the instrument's cover sheet. Finally, the testing and data collection environment must be outlined to ensure that optimum conditions are present when tests, interviews, and surveys are administered.

Establish procedures used for scoring the instrument. Once the evaluator has drafted and assembled the items, he or she must consider the scoring of the instrument. This matter was initially considered in the item specifications. What will be the value accorded to attitudinal or behavioral items? For example, on a CPR performance test, how many points will the student receive for correctly opening the airway? For attitudinal tests, what might be the points assigned to someone who disagrees with a statement, or agrees with a statement? How about no opinion? With regard to knowledge tests, will each item be worth one point? What if students answer incorrectly? Will they receive zero points, or a penalty for guessing? What if they don't answer a question?

Conduct a preliminary review of the instrument with colleagues. At this time, an evaluator's colleagues should conduct an initial review of the instrument (administration procedures, instructions, and examples, and items). They should look for ease of use, understandability, relevance, wording, grammar, spelling, readability, and flow. Colleagues should use the instrument specifications for this review.

Revise instrument based on review. Based on the review conducted in step 7 (Figure 5.3), the evaluator should revise the instrument as necessary.

Pilot test the instrument with twenty to fifty subjects. Instrument developers should identify twenty to fifty pilot subjects, who are like persons in the target population. It is best when the pilot study participants do not take part in the formal study. Often, an evaluator may try to obtain pilot subjects from a different geographic location, school system, or hospital than from where the actual study will be implemented. Subjects should be administered the instrument as if they were participating in the actual study, and, in addition to gathering data based on their completion on the instruments, evaluators may also ask the pilot subjects to provide feedback similar to that provided by colleagues in step 7.

Conduct item analysis, reliability, and validity studies. The next step is to gather evidence of the instrument's reliability and validity (see Chapter 7). In addition, the evaluator should conduct item analysis procedures such as response selection for attitudinal tests, discrimination indices, and difficulty indices for knowledge tests (see Chapter 6). Pilot test data are used for these analyses (see Chapter 8).

Provide instrument specifications and pilot study data to a panel of experts for review. A panel of experts should review the instrument again, along with the psychometric data developed from the pilot study. This panel should include individuals whose expertise lies in the area of the study, measurement specialists, and professionals familiar with the target audience. For example, if you were developing a health test for kindergarten students, you would have subject matter specialists, measurement specialists, early childhood or elementary education specialists, and a reading specialist, serve as part of your panel of experts. No one professional has all the expertise necessary to develop such a test for kindergarten students. However, by pooling the expertise of several specialists, you will receive the feedback you need to develop a high quality instrument.

Revise the instrument based on comments from the panel of experts. If major changes are made as a result of the pilot test and expert panel review, it may be important to re-pilot test the instrument as well as have a second review by the expert panel.

Determine cut score (for criterion-referenced tests or screening tests). After the evaluator establishes instrument reliability and validity, he or she can develop standards or cut-scores (sometimes called passing scores) for criterion-referenced tests or screening tests. It is important to ensure that the cut-score for passing a test was not set capriciously. Traditional methods, such as Angoff's strategy (1971) for developing cut-scores should be used.

Summary

In this chapter, we discussed current measurement problems facing educators today, and then described the four major forms of measurement. Next, the important issue of the use of multiple measures was described, known as triangulation of evidence. The use of frameworks in developing instruments was indicated. The chapter discussion concluded with a thirteen-step model for the development of health education evaluation instruments. Developing data collection instruments involves a series of systematic steps. The completion of these steps will be discussed in more detail in the next two chapters.

Case Study

Weiler, R.W., Sliepcevich, E.M., & Sarvela, P.D. (1993). Development of the adolescent health concerns inventory. *Health Education Quarterly, 20*(4), 569-583.

Weiler and colleagues describe the procedures used to develop an instrument focusing on the health concerns of adolescents, teachers' beliefs about adolescent health concerns, and parents' beliefs about adolescent health concerns. Results indicated that the instrument subscales had respective Cronbach alphas of .76 to .92. A panel of experts determined that the instrument was content valid, and, factor analysis was used to examine the instrument's construct validity. What were the strengths of the instrument development process? What were the weaknesses? This instrument was originally developed for use by rural students. Would you modify it in any way before you used it with an urban population?

Student Questions/Activities

1. You have been asked to design a set of data collection instruments to evaluate a comprehensive health education program being run in your local elementary schools. The evaluation will include collecting data from multiple stakeholders (students, teachers, parents, community members) and will involve multiple measures (focus groups, surveys, observations, etc.). You have just completed a first draft of the survey and have asked three people to review the instrument (a public health administrator, a reading specialist, and an elementary education specialist). The public health administrator, who is opposed to the behavior items on the survey, circulates the instrument to other people for review without your knowledge, and then reports to your funding agency (the local hospital system that is funding the health education program as well as the evaluation) that you have developed a poor quality instrument. The public health administrator does not tell the unsolicited reviewers about your other data collection techniques. As an evaluator, how will you handle this situation?

2. What was the most important test you have ever taken, or what was the most important test you have ever administered to a group of people? What made this test so important? Do you think it was a fair test?

3. You have been hired as a consultant to evaluate the quality of a diabetes patient education program. What types of measures will you use to assess the effectiveness of the program? Why did you select these measures?

4. What are the benefits of a national standardized test for graduation from high school? What are the disadvantages of such a test? What areas of health education should be covered in the test? Should people fail to graduate high school if they fail to complete the health education component of the test?

5. Identify a current health education problem (e.g., youth drug use, teenage pregnancy, or hypertension). Select a theory that helps explain this problem, and then develop a preliminary set of items that relate to that theory.

Recommended Readings

Pasick, R.J., Sabogal, F., Bird, J.A., et al. (1996). Problems and progress in the translation of health survey questions: The Pathways Experience. *Health Education Quarterly*, *23*(Supplement), S28-S40.

The authors describe the process and challenges faced when translating a questionnaire written in English into Mandarin, Cantonese, Spanish, and Vietnamese. The authors conclude with a "lessons learned" section on translating materials to different languages.

Kann, L., Warren, C.W., Harris, W.A., et al. (1996). Youth Risk Behavior Surveillance – United States, 1995. *Journal of School Health*, *66*(10), 365-377.

The Youth Risk Behavior Surveillance System (YRBSS) was developed by researchers from the Centers for Disease Control and Prevention to track six categories of health behavior: factors related to unintentional and intentional injuries, tobacco, alcohol, and other drug use, sexual behaviors, unhealthy dietary behaviors, and physical inactivity. This paper presents data gathered from the survey in 1995.

Middlestadt, S.E., Bhattacharya, K., Rosenbaum, J., et al. (1996). The use of theory based semi-structured elicitation questionnaires: Formative research for CDC's Prevention marketing initiative. *Public Health Reports, 111*(Supplement 1), 18-27.

The authors describe an open-ended questionnaire, procedures, and results of a study designed to examine condom use among heterosexually active unmarried adults. Results from this qualitative approach can be used in designing health promotion programs as well as quantitative studies.

References

American Educational Research Association, American Psychological Association, National Council on Measurement in Education. (1985). *Standards for Educational and Psychological Testing.* Washington, DC: American Psychological Association.

Angoff, W. (1971). Scales, norms, and equivalent scores. In R.L. Thorndike (Ed.), *Educational Measurement.* Washington, DC: American Council on Measurement.

Brener, N.D., Collins, J.L., Kann, L., Warren, C.W., & Williams, B.I. (1995). Reliability of the Youth Risk Behavior Survey questionnaire. *American Journal of Epidemiology, 141*(6), 575-580.

Ebel, R.L., & Frisbie, D.A.. (1986). *Essentials of Educational Measurement.* Englewood Cliffs, NJ: Prentice Hall.

Green, L.W., & Lewis, F.M. (1986). *Measurement and Evaluation in Health Education and Health Promotion.* Palo Alto, CA: Mayfield.

Guilford, J.P. (1954). *Psychometric Methods*, (2nd ed.). New York: McGraw-Hill.

Jobe, J.B., & Mingay, D.J. (1989). Cognitive research improves questionnaires. *American Journal of Public Health, 79*(8), 1053-1055.

Johnston, L.D., O'Malley, P.M., & Bachman, J.G.. (1993). *National Survey Results on Drug Use from Monitoring the Future Study, 1975-1992. Volume 1, Secondary Students.* Rockville, MD: National Institute on Drug Abuse.

Kirscht, J.P. (1989). Process and measurement issues in health risk appraisal. *American Journal of Public Health, 79*(12), 1598-1599.

Kolbe, L.J., Kann, L., & Collins, J.L. (1993). Overview of the Youth Risk Behavior Surveillance System. *Public Health Reports, 108*(Supplement 1), 2-10.

Linn, R.L. (1989). Current perspectives and future directions. In R.L. Linn (Ed.). *Educational Measurement*, 3rd edition. New York: Macmillan.

Mealer, B. (1997). Moves against affirmative action fuel opposition to standardized admissions tests. *The Chronicle of Higher Education, XLIV*(8), A40-A41.

Millman, J., & Greene, J. (1989). The specification and development of tests of achievement and ability. In R.L. Linn (Ed.). *Educational Measurement*, 3rd edition. New York: Macmillan.

Nickerson, R.S. (1989). New directions in educational assessment. *Educational Researcher*, *18*(9), 3-7.

Nunnally, J.C. (1978). *Psychometric Theory*, 2nd edition. New York: McGraw-Hill.

Popham, W.J. (1987). Preparing policy makers for standard setting on high-stakes tests. *Educational Evaluation and Policy Analysis*, *9*(1), 77-82.

Rosenstock, l.M. (1974). Historical origins of the health belief model. *Health Education Monographs*, *2*, 328-335.

Sarvela, P.D., & Noonan, J.V. (1988). Testing and computer-based instruction: Psychometric considerations. *Educational Technology*, *28*(5), 17-20.

Smith, K.W., McKinlay, S.M., & McKinlay, J.B.. (1989). The reliability of health risk appraisals: A field trial of four instruments. *American Journal of Public Health*, *79*(12), 1603-1607.

Sudman, S., & Bradburn, N.M.. (1986). *Asking Questions*. San Francisco: Jossey-Bass.

Torabi, M. (1989). A cancer prevention knowledge test. *Eta Sigma Gamman*, *20*(2), 13-16.

Windsor, R.A., Baranowski, T., Clark, N., & Cutter, G. (1984). *Evaluation of Health Promotion and Education Programs*. Palo Alto, CA: Mayfield.

6

Types of Measures

Chapter Objectives

After completing this chapter, you should be able to:

1.   Identify commonly used methods of measuring knowledge.
2.   Identify commonly used methods of measuring attitudes.
3.   Identify commonly used methods of measuring behavior.
4.   Identify commonly used methods of measuring health-related fitness.
5.   Describe methods used to collect data from young children.
6.   Identify commonly used tests and procedures in the health care setting.
7.   Set a cut score for an achievement test.
8.   Develop a data collection instrument for use in a health education evaluation study.

Key Terms

authentic measurement
behavioral anchor
behavior rating scales
Bogardus Social Distance scale
constructed-response items
cumulative scale
cut score/passing score
dichotomous items
equal appearing interval scale
foils/distractors
interview/word-of-mouth procedures

item stem
paired comparison/forced-choice technique
portfolio
premises
projective testing
selected-response items
self-report
semantic differential scale
social desirability response bias
summated rating scale
value scale

Introduction

There are many different ways one can evaluate a program. Typically, health education programs focus on one or more of the following areas: knowledge, attitudes, behaviors, or physiological functioning (e.g., blood pressure change as a result of an education program designed to alter behavior). It is critical to match the methods of measurement to the learning or change that is expected as a result of a program. For example, when measuring achievement (e.g., knowledge of different types of foods appropriate for a person with diabetes to eat) a paper-and-pencil test might be appropriate. However, when measuring another type of knowledge, such as proper preparation of foods a person with diabetes should eat, then a performance test might be a more appropriate form of measurement. In this chapter, we will introduce the various measures commonly used in evaluation of health education and promotion programs.

Measuring Knowledge

Probably the area of instruction evaluated most frequently by health educators is the knowledge (cognitive) domain. In the case of program evaluation, an evaluator might be interested in the level of knowledge gained as a result of participating in a health education program. Changes in knowledge are evaluated most frequently by the use of achievement tests.

We all have taken achievement tests. Multiple-choice tests, essay examinations, and performance tests (e.g., CPR tests, skill tests in a high school physical education class, a road test for a driver's license, and so on) are all types of achievement tests that measure the degree of knowledge and skills we have about a certain topic. Knowledge testing is a common occurrence in society.

Health education specialists measure knowledge levels in several ways. The most frequently used approaches employ selected-response and constructed-response items. **Constructed-response items** require test takers to develop their own answers to questions (e.g., short-answer or essay questions). **Selected-response items** ask test takers to choose from among an array of possible answers to questions (e.g., multiple-choice or true-false items).

Constructed-response items are desirable when the learning objectives require subjects to explain, describe, define, state, or write about subjects. If the objective is to have subjects identify, distinguish, or match, then selected-response items are appropriate (Roid & Haladyna, 1982). Other strategies used to measure knowledge include performance tests (such as a test that demonstrates ability to perform CPR). Performance tests are discussed later in this chapter.

Constructed-Response Items. Roid and Haladyna (1982) describe three major types of constructed-response items: *the completion item*, *the short-answer essay item*, and *the extended-answer essay item*. *Completion items* require the subject to provide a key word or phrase to answer a question or complete a sentence. An example of a completion item is as follows:

According to the National Institute on Drug Abuse survey, the most commonly used illegal drug by American youth is _____.

Test developers use *short-answer essay items* to obtain brief responses to questions or instructions. Developers frequently use these items because they can ask more questions in a testing period than they can when using extended-answer essay items. An example of a *short-answer essay* item is:

Give the definition of a controlled substance as described by the Drug Enforcement Administration.

Ebel and Frisbie (1986) provide eight guidelines for writing completion and short-answer essay items:

- Word the question or incomplete statement carefully enough to require a single, unique answer.
- Think of the intended answer first. Then write a question where that answer is the only appropriate response.
- If the item is an incomplete sentence, word it so the blank comes at the end of the sentence.
- Use a direct question, unless the incomplete sentence permits a more concise or clearly defined correct answer.
- Avoid unintended clues in the correct answer.
- Word the item as concisely as possible without losing specificity of response.
- Arrange space for recording answers on the right margin of the question page.
- Avoid using the conventional wording of an important idea as the basis for a short-answer item.

Test developers frequently use *extended-answer essay items* when subjects must synthesize large bodies of knowledge. These item forms are especially desirable when instructors must test general knowledge rather than specific knowledge. An example of an extended-answer essay item is:

Compare and contrast three methods used for promoting smoking cessation. For each method, provide a description of a study that has demonstrated its efficacy.

Ebel and Frisbie (1986) offer six guidelines for writing essay questions:

- Ask questions or set tasks that require the student to demonstrate a command of essential knowledge.
- Ask questions that are determinate, in the sense that experts could agree that one answer is better than another.

- Define the examinee's task as completely and specifically as possible without interfering with measurement of the achievement intended.
- In general, give preference to more specific questions that can be answered more briefly.
- Avoid giving the examinee a choice among optional questions unless special circumstances make such options necessary.
- Test the question by writing an ideal answer to it.

Selected-Response Items. Selected-response items require the test taker to choose the answer to the question from a set of correct and incorrect answers. In the case of large-scale testing programs, such as the test development work conducted by the Educational Testing Service (the developers of the SAT among others), the selected-response item is most frequently used. There are three commonly used selected-response item types: *multiple-choice, true-false,* and *matching* (Roid & Haladyna, 1982).

Multiple-choice test items are the most highly regarded and widely used form of objective test item (Ebel & Frisbie, 1986). Multiple-choice items can be used to measure knowledge, understanding, judgment, problem solving, methods of appropriate action, and making predictions. In addition, multiple-choice items have lower levels of errors due to guessing than other forms of selected-response items, such as true-false items (Ebel & Frisbie, 1986).

A multiple-choice item is comprised of three parts: (1) the **item stem**, which asks the question or starts the statement, (2) the correct answer, and (3) the incorrect answers, known as **foils** or **distractors** (Roid & Haladyna, 1982). An example of a multiple-choice item is as follows:

The chamber of the heart which pumps blood to the rest of the body is:

a. the right atrium
b. the aorta
c. the left ventricle
d. the right ventricle
e. the left atrium

Procedures used to prepare high quality multiple-choice items as recommended by Ebel (1951), Millman and Greene (1989), Ellis, Fredericks and Wulfeck (1979), and Hopkins and Stanley (1981) are found in Figure 6.1.

True-false items are not used by professional test developers as frequently as multiple-choice items because they have a 50 percent guessing rate. Despite this problem, Ebel and Frisbie (1986) argue that when used correctly, true-false items enable the assessment of knowledge in a simple and direct means. An example of a true-false item is as follows:

Cigarette smoking has been associated with the occurrence of heart disease, respiratory disease, and some cancers.

Roid and Haladyna (1982) state several advantages to using true-false items:

- More questions can be used since less time is required to respond.
- True-false items are easy to write.
- A true-false test can have a high level of reliability.
- True-false items take up less space on paper, saving testing materials.
- True-false items can measure a variety of different forms of knowledge.

In preparing true-false items (Ebel & Frisbie, 1986; Roid & Haladyna, 1982):

- Items should test knowledge of important ideas.
- Items should require understanding as well as memory.
- The correct answer should be defensible.
- The correct answer should be obvious only to the examinees who have mastered the material being tested.
- Item should be expressed simply, concisely, and clearly.
- Shades of meaning should be avoided; items should be clearly correct or incorrect.
- Do not use negatives or double negatives in the answers.
- Do not make sentences unnecessarily long.
- Use only a single idea in the item.

Matching items are special forms of multiple-choice items. Roid and Haladyna (1982) indicate that one of the primary advantages of matching items is that they allow one to cover a broad subject matter area, which enhances the content validity of the test. Test developers design matching items by creating lists of **premises** and responses (Ebel & Frisbie, 1986). An example of a matching item is as follows:

Premises	**Responses**
___1. Constructed-Response Item	a. distractor
___2. Incorrect Answer	b. essay item
___3. Selected-Response Item	c. stem
	d. true-false item
	e. valid item

Guidelines for writing matching items (Ebel & Frisbie, 1986) include:

- Items and answers should measure a homogeneous set of content.
- Lists of premises and their associated responses should be short.
- Response options should be more numerous than premises.
- Clear directions should be provided.
- Responses and/or premises should appear in alphabetical order.
- Numerical responses should be arranged from low to high.
- The premise should be longer than the response.

Test items should:

Test important ideas, rather than trivia.

Contain words with precise meanings, avoid ambiguity and nonfunctional words, and have only one interpretation.

Avoid exact textbook wording for the items.

Avoid negatives or double negatives. If used, negatives should be highlighted and grouped together on the test.

Have stems that contain direct questions, incomplete statements, or problem scenarios.

Be grouped together if special tasks are required, and instructions should be presented one time only.

Be grouped by content area or sequence of instruction.

Contain instructions that specify the type of answer required of the respondent.

Focus on a single idea, concept, or problem.

Be independent of each other (e.g., the answer for question 2 should not depend on the answer for question 1).

Be short and written clearly. Awkward or complex sentences should be avoided.

Have a range of difficulty. Level of difficulty of the items should be adapted to the group being tested or the purpose of the test.

Test higher levels of understanding, not just memorization.

Have a stem that is its longest component.

Item responses should:

Have 4 or 5 response options that do not overlap (and only one correct answer).[*]

Be positioned at the end of the item.

Use plausible distractors based on common errors and misconceptions of learners.

Be appropriate for the item so that they are reasonable answers.

Be presented in a logical sequence (e.g., if an answer is in pounds, present options from lightest to heaviest possible weights).

Not use never/always/all of the above/none of the above/A and B only/ etc.

Be grammatically correct, consistent with the stem (e.g., use a(n) to avoid clues through wording or grammar), and be written clearly and concisely.

Have the correct answer randomly assigned to different positions on the test (e.g., avoid having "b" as the correct answer more often than any of the other responses).

Relate to the general content area tested, thus avoiding "easy" distractors.

Be about equal in length. (Correct answers are no longer than incorrect answers).

[*]   Some measurement specialists believe three response options are appropriate and adequate (e.g., Trevisan, Sax, & Michael, 1994).

Figure 6.1 Writing Multiple-Choice Test Items

Reliability and Validity Procedures for Knowledge Items

The method used most frequently for estimating instrument reliability for knowledge items is the internal consistency reliability coefficient. Usually, a KR-20 or Cronbach alpha method is used. Another procedure used to measure internal-consistency reliability with knowledge tests is the Spearman-Brown reliability coefficient. The KR-20 and Spearman-Brown formulas assume that the items are **dichotomous items**, that is, they are scored in a dichotomous fashion (meaning that an item is given a value of 1 when an individual scores a correct response, or a value of 0 when the individual does not answer the item correctly). Most knowledge tests are scored in this manner. Other methods of reliability may also be appropriate. For example, if a health educator is developing two forms of the same test, parallel forms reliability may be appropriate.

The most frequently used method of gathering evidence concerning validity for knowledge tests is content validity. Often, the item-objective format is used, where the test developer is interested in determining how well the test items match the instructional objectives of the curriculum. Reliability and validity procedures are presented in greater depth in Chapter 7.

Measuring Attitudes

Health educators are often asked to address the degree of change in attitude that has taken place when students have participated in health education curriculum exercises. For example, as a result of taking part in a drug education program, did students have more "positive" attitudes about abstaining from drugs? Or, after taking part in a nutrition education program, did students have more positive outlooks on "healthy" eating behaviors? Because health education programs often purport to develop healthy attitudes, they are frequently examined in health education evaluations.

Although it is not always clear as to exactly what we mean by the term "attitude," we spend a great deal of effort trying to measure one. Evaluators can use many different types of items to measure an individual's attitude toward an object, person, issue, or behavior. The following discussion will focus on the more common methods of measuring attitudes.

Summated Rating Scales. A **summated rating scale** is a set of items approximately equal in attitude value, to which subjects respond in terms of degree of agreement or disagreement (Kerlinger, 1973). These scales also are called agreement scales (Henderson, Morris & Fitz-Gibbon, 1978). The Likert scale, a form of a summated rating scale, is probably one of the most commonly used scales by health educators to measure attitudes. When attempting to rank people with regard to a particular attitude, the Likert scale is highly reliable (Miller, 1977). An example of a Likert scale item used to estimate one's attitude about AIDS among health care workers is shown in the following example borrowed from Sarvela and Moore (1989):

I have no sympathy for homosexuals who get AIDS:

a. Strongly agree
b. Agree
c. Don't know
d. Disagree
e. Strongly disagree

Miller (1977) recommends the following steps in developing Likert scale items:

■ Develop, select, and assemble a large number of items related to the attitude studied that are both favorable and unfavorable.

■ Administer the items to a representative sample of the large population.

■ Score the items so that the most favorable attitudes receive the highest values.

■ Score each person's scale by adding up the items.

■ Use discrimination indices to determine which items differentiate most clearly between those people who have favorable and unfavorable responses towards the attitude.

■ Select at least six items with the best discrimination indices to form the scale. An evaluator must make sure that the items selected meet the instrument's specifications to ensure content validity.

Equal Appearing Interval Scales. An **equal appearing interval scale** consists of a set of items designed to measure an individual's attitude toward the object of study, where each item has a scale value indicating a strength of attitude towards the item. The Thurstone scale is a commonly used equal appearing interval scale. Kerlinger (1973) provides an example of a Thurstone scale examining attitudes towards the church:

I believe the church is the greatest institution in America today. (Scale value: .2)
I believe in religion, but I seldom go to church. (Scale value: 5.4)
I think the church is a hindrance to religion for it still depends on magic, superstition, and myth. (Scale value 9.6)

In this scale, the lower the scale value, which was developed by averaging judgments by more than ten judges, (Miller, 1977), the more positive an individual's attitude is towards the church. These items are developed using the following procedures (Miller, 1977):

■ Several hundred statements thought to be related to the attitude under consideration are gathered.

■ A large number of judges (50 to 300) independently assign the statements into 11 groups ranging from most favorable, neutral, to least favorable.

■ The item's value is the median value among those assigned by the judges.

- Statements that are judged differently by many different judges (a wide spread of scores) are discarded because of ambiguity or irrelevance.
- The scale is developed using items that represent broadly favorable, neutral, and unfavorable attitudes (as achieved through judges' consensus).

Value Scale. A **value scale** is a measure of a person's preference for objects of study, such as people, ideas, institutions, behaviors, and things (Kerlinger, 1973). These scales are used frequently when measuring preferences in polling situations. For example, a political pollster may be interested in determining the political climate regarding policy concerning drivers' licenses and 16-year-olds. As a part of the poll, the question might arise: *Do you feel we should reduce or restrict in some way the driving privileges of 16-year-olds?* Common responses for these forms of items include: "yes" and "no," "good" and "bad," and "agree" or "disagree." These items are developed using procedures similar to those for the development of Likert scales. Procedures for the development of value scales are as follows:

- Develop, select, and assemble a large number of items considered related to the attitude studied that are both favorable and unfavorable.
- Administer the items to a representative sample of the target population.
- Score the items so that the most favorable attitudes receive the highest values.
- Use discrimination indices to determine which items differentiate most clearly between those people who have favorable and unfavorable responses towards the attitude.
- Develop the scale using the items with the best discrimination indices.

An evaluator must make sure that the items selected meet the instrument's specifications to ensure content validity.

Other Attitude Item Types. Other forms of scales described by measurement specialists include cummulative scales, semantic differential scales, paired comparison scales, Bogardus Social Distance scales, projective testing, and interviews. A brief description of each of these item types follows.

A **cumulative scale** is comprised of a set of items that are ordered based on difficulty or value-loading (Rubinson & Neutens, 1987). The set of items is designed to measure knowledge or attitude towards one variable. The Guttman scale is the most commonly used cumulative scale. Guttman scale items are designed by arranging a set of items by their degree of positiveness or favorableness towards the variable under study (Mueller, 1986). An example of a Guttman scale from Mueller (1986) is:

- Abortion should be given on demand.
- Abortion is ok for family planning.
- Abortion is ok in cases of rape.
- Abortion is acceptable if the fetus is malformed.
- Abortion is acceptable when a mother's life is in danger.

You can see that an individual who agrees with the first statement will also probably agree with all other statements, whereas a person who agrees with only the last statement will probably not agree with any of the value statements that precede it.

The **semantic differential scale** can provide some interesting insights in health education research and evaluation. McDermott and Gold (1986-1987) used the semantic differential technique to measure attitudes toward the use of contraceptive devices. In their study, they presented a series of 40 bipolar adjectives concerning 10 contraceptive options to 703 university students, asking them to rate each contraceptive from a scale of one to seven, with the bipolar adjectives representing the extremes of the scales. Some of these bipolar adjective scales are shown in Table 6.1 as they might apply to evaluation of condoms.

The method of **paired comparisons** (also called the **forced-choice technique**) enables a respondent to select the more favorable of two choices. After the respondent answers a series of these forced-choice items, he or she receives a score (usually the median) of his or her favorable responses (Kerlinger, 1973; Miller, 1977). An example of a paired comparison item is provided by Dunkel, cited in Kerlinger's discussion on paired comparisons. In this example, people are asked to select from a series of life goal statements, such as the following example:

- Making a place for myself in the world; getting ahead.
- Living the pleasure of the moment.

After answering a series of such items, the investigator can assess the life goals of the respondent.

The **Bogardus Social Distance scale** is used to examine the degree to which people would be comfortable being close to other groups of people. Measuring prejudice is a commonly used example of this scale. An item with a public health perspective dealing with persons with AIDS (PWAs) might be:

- Are you willing to let PWAs live in your country?
- Are you willing to let PWAs live in your community?
- Are you willing to let PWAs live in your neighborhood?
- Are you willing to let PWAs live next door to you?
- Would you allow your child to marry a PWA?

Although used more frequently for psychological research than evaluation of health education programs, **projective testing** is an available procedure that measures a person's attitudes toward an object, or personality functioning (e.g., ego development). A *projective test* is one where examinees must use their own beliefs and attitudes to respond to questions, because there are no response options available for their answer (Mueller, 1986). Commonly used projective tests are the Thematic Apperception Test (TAT) and the Rorschach inkblot test. Other forms of projective testing include writing stories or painting pictures about how examinees feel about certain things, handwriting, telling stories, word association, and having children play with dolls (Kerlinger, 1973; Mueller, 1986).

Table 6.1 Semantic Differential Scales Used to Assess Attitudes about Condoms

clever	1	2	3	4	5	6	7	stupid
non-messy	1	2	3	4	5	6	7	messy
effective	1	2	3	4	5	6	7	ineffective
permanent	1	2	3	4	5	6	7	temporary
painless	1	2	3	4	5	6	7	painful
reliable	1	2	3	4	5	6	7	unreliable
healthy	1	2	3	4	5	6	7	unhealthy
natural	1	2	3	4	5	6	7	unnatural
easy	1	2	3	4	5	6	7	difficult
stress free	1	2	3	4	5	6	7	stressful
moral	1	2	3	4	5	6	7	immoral
efficient	1	2	3	4	5	6	7	inefficient
unobtrusive	1	2	3	4	5	6	7	obtrusive
safe	1	2	3	4	5	6	7	unsafe
fragrant	1	2	3	4	5	6	7	foul
legal	1	2	3	4	5	6	7	illegal
available	1	2	3	4	5	6	7	unavailable
happy	1	2	3	4	5	6	7	sad
non-abrasive	1	2	3	4	5	6	7	abrasive
sufficient	1	2	3	4	5	6	7	insufficient
exciting	1	2	3	4	5	6	7	boring
discreet	1	2	3	4	5	6	7	obvious
harmless	1	2	3	4	5	6	7	harmful
good	1	2	3	4	5	6	7	bad
flexible	1	2	3	4	5	6	7	inflexible
invisible	1	2	3	4	5	6	7	visible
non-distressful	1	2	3	4	5	6	7	distressful
attractive	1	2	3	4	5	6	7	ugly
light	1	2	3	4	5	6	7	heavy
hot	1	2	3	4	5	6	7	cold

Interviews are face-to-face meetings between evaluators and respondents. They are sometimes called **word-of-mouth procedures**, because evaluators record what the respondents say, rather than have respondents write down or check off responses on a questionnaire (Henderson, Morris & Fitz-Gibbon, 1978).

Windsor, et al. (1984) describe several advantages and disadvantages of face-to-face interviews:

- They are extremely useful when subjects cannot read or write.
- They are appropriate when the questions asked are long and complex.
- They are a good data collection method when the content of the study is not specified or not well defined.
- If respondents must be contacted personally, an interview is appropriate.

A main disadvantage is the bias that can occur with regard to the expectations the subjects feel the interviewer has of them. These problems are referred to as social desirability biases. For example, if an interviewer is asking a respondent about drinking and driving, the person might intentionally under-report the frequency of driving after drinking. Another problem with interviews is the issue of interviewer variation, both between different interviewers, and variation by one interviewer from the time the inteview begins to the time when the interview is completed. The problem here is that at different times, or with different people, the same question might be asked in a different manner. Rating reliability checks can be used to reduce this problem (see Chapter 7).

Babbie (1973) provides several guidelines for developing attitudinal items:

- Develop clear items.
- Avoid double-barreled items -- asking two or more questions in one item. For example, a double-barreled item might be: *Do you agree with the enactment of a ban on cigarette smoking in all eating establishments, as well as the enactment of an increased tax on tobacco products to discourage purchases by youth?* In this example, one could agree with the ban on smoking in restaurants, but disagree with the imposition of a tax increase on tobacco products.
- Ensure that the respondent is able to answer items competently. Can they read, are they able to write, do they understand the question, can they accurately provide a response?
- Consider item relevance.
- Keep items short.
- Avoid the use of negative items.
- Avoid biased items.

Reliability and Validity Procedures for Attitudinal Items

As with knowledge items, the instrument developer will often want to use a measure of internal consistency reliability, to ensure that the items in the scale or subscale are measuring the same construct. Probably one of the most frequently used estimates of internal consistency for attitudinal items is *Cronbach's alpha*. If the evaluation program is to be continued over a long period of time, with repeated measures of the object of evaluation, test-retest reliability strategies would also be appropriate. For interviews and observations, inter-rater and intra-rater reliability approaches should be used. Validity procedures include the use of content validity, either with the item-objective approach or the identification of items by their objective. In more elaborate evaluation studies, where the health education treatment is designed to influence some health construct (e.g., health beliefs concerning safer sex), construct validity procedures may be appropriate as well. Where attitudes are designed to predict future attitudes or behaviors, predictive validity studies are indicated. Reliability and validity procedures are presented in much greater depth in Chapter 7.

Measuring Behavior

For certain forms of instructional objectives an evaluator must measure behavior. For example, in a first-aid class, an instructor must observe students performing mouth-to-mouth resuscitation, CPR, putting on splints, and so on. In these cases, paper-and-pencil forms of testing do not adequately or appropriately measure attainment of instructional objectives. If a health educator is measuring the effects of a drug education program, students might be asked to report their behaviors on a questionnaire, since it would not be practical to observe all students regarding their drug use behaviors. These types of questionnaires are called **self-report** questionnaires. Based on these two examples, one can see that behavior can be measured two ways: through self-report or direct observation (Kerlinger, 1973).

Self-Report. With self-report behavioral measurement instruments, the evaluator asks subjects to provide a description of the behavior of interest. A health educator working in cooperation with a hospital's nutrition clinic might ask patients to record everything they have eaten over a two-week period. In addition, the health educator might ask patients to write down their comments after they have eaten something. Duyff's (1997) *Monthly Nutrition Companion* provides a worksheet for people to write in the following regarding food intake on a daily basis:

- Time food was eaten
- Place food was eaten
- Type of food or beverage
- Amount
- Food Group
- Social Situation
- Hunger Level
- Comments

Each day, the person also has a checklist to indicate whether all of the food groups have been eaten, including vitamins, fluids, and so on. In addition, for each day, one records factors relevant to exercise behavior:

- Time of day
- Type of physical activity
- Intensity
- Time spent

The advantages of keeping diaries are that problems with memory and the time events occurred are reduced, and that diaries generally produce higher frequencies of the issue under study than other forms of gathering data. Diary-keeping is not without its problems, though, including:

- The amount of time needed by subjects to maintain diaries.
- The quality of the data varies significantly among subjects.
- Evaluators may have to remind subjects frequently to complete their diaries.
- Evaluators must frequently contact subjects to review the diaries and make sure that they are being completed correctly.
- Keeping a diary may cause change in a subject due to the pressure of having to report behavior and attitudes, subsequently creating a problem in interpreting the generalizability of a program (see Chapter 10).

When developing self-report behavior instruments, it is important for the evaluator to use behavioral anchors. A **behavioral anchor** is a detailed description of the behavior being rated, which does not allow for a lot of interpretation in the response. An example of an item about alcohol use involving behavioral anchors is:

During the last two weeks, on how many days did you have one or more drinks of beer, wine, or liquor (disregarding wine at a religious service)?

a. I did not drink beer, wine, or liquor
b. one day
c. two days
d. three days
e. four or more days

By using behavioral anchors, one can report the behavior accurately in terms of frequency, quantity, and duration. Without behavioral anchors, the respondent is left to his or her own interpretation of the question. For example, if you asked a person to report in a log how much alcohol he or she drank in the last two weeks, he or she might write: "I drank a moderate amount." What one person considers "a moderate amount" another might consider binge drinking. For these reasons, it is best to specify as much as possible the exact behaviors under study.

Observation. Another method of measuring behavior is observing the behavior directly, referred to as a form of obtrusive measurement by Windsor, et al. (1984). Instead of asking college students to report their drinking behaviors, an evaluator could observe students drinking at their favorite bars or pubs. When developing observer scales, Henderson, et al. (1978) recommend that the evaluator outline the following points:

- The number of observations to take place.
- The amount of time to be spent during the observation period.

- A detailed description of what is to be observed, including deciding to what degree the behavior took place.
- The method of recording the behavior or its quality.

An important note of emphasis is needed regarding the third point above. It is necessary for the evaluator to define exactly what is to be observed, and then conduct the observations based on what was decided upon in evaluating, rather than just going to a site and observing individuals. Another important rule of thumb is that it is usually better to observe an individual frequently, for short periods of time, rather than observe an individual once or twice for a long period of time (Noll, Scannell & Craig, 1989).

Behavior rating scales (performance tests) are used by observers to judge the quality of a performance, and to help ensure that all observers use the same criteria in evaluating the performance (Roid & Haladyna, 1982). According to Kerlinger (1973), five general types of rating scales are:

- *Category rating scales*, which enable the judge to pick a category that best represents the behavior being studied.
- *Check list scales*, which are used when a number of observations must be made on a particular performance (Roid & Haladyna, 1982). For example, one could develop a checklist that measured the steps necessary to successfully perform CPR.
- *Forced-choice scales*, which enable the judge to rate the individual using a set of alternatives. Often, the paired comparison approach is used where a judge selects one of two phrases that describe the individual being rated. For example, one may rate a person using the following two phrases: lazy or ambitious. Using a series of items such as this, one could assess the qualities or behaviors in question.
- *Numerical rating scales*, which enable the judge to rate the behavior being studied with each value on the rating scale having a number attached to it.
- *Graphic rating scales*, which are scale lines or bars that have descriptions on the bars.

When using observations in an evaluation study, observers must be trained so there is adequate inter-rater and intra-rater reliability present (see Chapter 7). Otherwise, the reliability of the data collected, and also the validity, would be suspect. Performance tests are usually assessed in terms of their content validity, though, criterion-related validity is sometimes recommended. Another issue is the problem of **social desirability response bias**, and its effects on people's behavior. If subjects know they are being observed, or are completing a self-report survey on an important health behavior, they may behave or report that they behave in a socially desirable manner. That is, if a man being treated for hypertension is being surveyed on his compliance to his doctor's prescribed medications, exercise, and diet, he might answer in socially desirable terms. One way of checking for this phenomenon would be to query his wife or a different "significant other" as well. This person might report his behaviors more accurately, and possibly, be more objective about his actual compliance to the doctor's orders. Of course, when surveying people concerning behaviors that can be assessed physiologically (e.g., substance use), both a survey and lab results could be compared.

Health-Related Physical Fitness Tests

Health promotion and wellness programs emphasize the importance of physical fitness for its positive impact on an individual's total health. Given that emphasis, it is important to understand some of the basic measures of physical fitness. Hastad and Lacy (1994) define health-related fitness as "those aspects of physiological function that offer protection from diseases resulting from a sedentary lifestyle" (p.120). They describe different ways to measure it, including: cardiorespiratory fitness, muscular strength, flexibility, body composition, and laboratory-based testing. Figure 6.2 outlines these types of tests.

Cardiorespiratory Fitness – refers to the ability to exercise for extended periods of time without fatigue. Poor cardiorespiratory fitness is a risk factor for heart disease. It can be measured through laboratory tests such as tests that measure maximal oxygen uptake as well as field tests, such as the 1 or 1.5 mile run, or the step test.

Muscular Strength – refers to the ability of muscles to exert force. Common measurements of muscular strength include sit-ups, pull-ups, and the dynamometer, which measures static strength. In addition, strength can be tested using arm curls, "lat pull downs," bench pressing, and other strength tests and exercises.

Flexibility – refers to range of motion available at a joint or group of joints. People who are highly flexible are generally healthier than those who are not flexible. The sit-and-reach test, the Kraus-Weber Floor Touch, as well as trunk extension, are all methods of measuring flexibility.

Body Composition – usually refers to the percentage of body fat of a person. The most common method of measuring body composition is the skinfold test, which can be applied to the abdomen, calf, chest, scapula, thigh, and triceps. Underwater weighing, discussed below, is extremely accurate.

Laboratory–Based Testing – is the best way to measure health-related fitness. Common lab procedures include underwater weighing of people to determine body composition and measurement of maximal gas uptake. In addition, various blood tests (e.g., cholesterol) and blood pressure, are commonly used when collecting fitness data.

Figure 6.2 Measuring Health-Related Physical Fitness

Adapted from: Hastad, D.N., & Lacy, A.C. (1994). *Measurement and Evaluation in Physical Education and Exercise Science*, 2nd edition. Scottsdale, AZ: Gorsuch Scarisbrick.

A Note on Collecting Data from Young Children

Collecting data from preschool or early elementary students requires special considerations. This point is especially true for health educators, because little health education work has been done with this age group. We strongly recommend that evaluators charged with evaluating health education programs for these populations work carefully with early childhood specialists when developing the assessment measures. Bredekamp and Copple (1997), in their text *Developmentally Appropriate Practice in Early Childhood Programs*, indicate that "assessment of individual children's development and learning is essential for planning and implementing appropriate curriculua" (p.21). They further note that assessing young children is "difficult because their development and learning is rapid, uneven, episodic, and embedded within specific cultural and linguistic contexts" (p.21). Their recommendations are summarized in Figure 6.3. Leavitt and

---

Young children should be assessed in an ongoing, strategic, and purposeful manner. The data should be used to meet the needs of the child, the family, and to evaluate the effects of the curriculum.

Assessment plans ought to reflect progress towards learning and development goals, and the assessment program should be linked to the curriculum planning process.

Assessment of young children should rely on observations of child development, descriptive data, collections of representative work by children, and demonstrations of authentic, not contrived activities. Input from families is important.

Assessments should be used for a specific purpose, with emphasis on the reliability and validity of the assessment procedure.

Decisions that impact on children should never be made on the basis of one assessment.

Developmental assessments and observations should be used to identify special needs children.

Assessment should recognize individual variation, including issues such as the child's use of language, stage of language acquisition, and whether English is used at home.

Assessment should measure not only individual skills but what youngsters can also do with the assistance of others.

Figure 6.3 Guidelines for Assessing Young Children

Adapted from: Bredekamp, S., & Copple, C. (Eds.) (1997). *Developmentally Appropriate Practice in Early Childhood Programs*. Washington, DC: National Association for the Education of Young Children.

Eheart (1991) indicate that assessment of early childhood programs and the children in those programs requires at least four different types of input, including:

- Information from parents.
- Recorded observations of the child at play and in routines.
- Organizing all information into a comprehensive picture of the child.
- Applying the information to curriculum planning.

Points one and two lend themselves nicely to the notion of triangulation of evidence. By getting information from parents, observing the youngster in play, and doing tasks, one has a good idea of how the youngster behaves. Observations (either spontaneous or planned) allow us to develop a picture of the youngster's daily habits as well as interests. This information can be used to develop targeted health education programs for the youngsters. One method mentioned frequently by early childhood specialists organizes information about youngsters in a comprehensive way, and is referred to as the **portfolio**. Wortham (1995) defines a portfolio as "a collection of a child's work and teacher data from informal and performance assessments to evaluate development and learning" (p.203). Portfolios typically contain observation reports, checklists, work samples, records of directed assignments, interviews, and other achievement data. In addition, early childhood authorities focus on the notion of **authentic measurement**, meaning the use of techniques that allow the child to demonstrate the skill or mastery of the concept being measured. Interviews of students, games, directed assignments, and contracts all can be used in authentic measurement (Worthham, 1995).

Common Medical Tests and Procedures

Health educators working in clinic and hospital settings are often asked to use medical data when working with patients. For example, a health educator working in a weight reduction clinic may need to understand basic measures such as height, weight, blood pressure, and pulse. The top 34 diagnoses and services conducted during a six-month period at a large university health service appear in Table 6.2.

When health educators work in patient education settings, it is important that they familiarize themselves with the most commonly conducted diagnostic procedures and services. Often, they will be asked to discuss the health education and health promotion implications of the tests with the patients. Simple procedures such as the measurement of weight, blood pressure, and pulse must be explained to patients, so they understand the significance of the tests. Often, once patients understand the tests, they can better understand the need for changing their behaviors to improve their health status. For example, by understanding the significance of blood pressure, how it is tested, and the need for periodic testing, hypertensive patients may modify less healthy behaviors (e.g., use of salt) and increase more positive behaviors (e.g., exercise and periodic checkups).

Sometimes, health educators will be asked to discuss other types of examinations such as breast or testicular exams. Both of these examination procedures are good examples of how a "test" can be used both as a screening device and a teaching tool. For example, not only could these exams be discussed, but also a general discussion concerning the warning signs of cancer could be implemented as a part of the health

Table 6.2 Frequent Diagnoses and Services Provided By a University Health Service

Rank	Total	Description
1	5432	Unclassified diagnoses
2	3551	Blood pressure
3	2666	Pelvic exam
4	1627	STD check
5	1553	Pap smear
6	1368	R_x refill
7	1279	Breast exam
8	1150	Oral contraceptive refill
9	1140	Immunization
10	1083	Gynecologic, not contraceptive
11	1076	Allergy injection
12	933	Contraceptive consultation
13	869	Other procedure
14	788	Physical exam/evaluation
15	729	Throat culture
16	602	Vaginitis
17	588	Warts unspecified
18	572	Test results
19	542	Ophthalmology
20	471	R_x injection
21	452	Urinary tract infection
22	448	Dermatitis
23	338	Gastro-intestinal other
24	278	Backache
25	236	Headache
26	216	New oral contraceptive
27	205	Major depression
28	203	Pregnancy diagnosed
29	201	Other mental/psychiatric
30	179	Other drug dependence
31	141	Alcoholism
32	127	Acne
33	121	Abdominal pain
34	108	Skin allergy

education program. Where possible, tests *should* not only measure, but also teach.

Another reason health educators should understand commonly used tests and procedures is that they may serve as part of the measures that will be used to evaluate the effectiveness of their programs. Obviously, different clinics and hospitals will conduct some types of tests more frequently than others. One might guess by the diagnoses and procedures described in Table 6.2 that this particular clinic specializes in the treatment of young adults. Health care providers in a geriatric care setting would conduct a different repertoire of procedures. It is the job of health educators to determine what are the most frequently conducted tests, and then familiarize themselves with them.

Determining and Setting Cut Scores

Once an evaluator has developed an achievement test, if it is a mastery learning test, the evaluator must set a **cut score**. A cut score (sometimes called a **passing score**) is the score an individual needs to pass a test. Passing scores are used in criterion-referenced testing situations, where an individual or group's performance is based on satisfactory attainment of previously defined standards.

There are a series of articles devoted to setting cut scores on tests, and for good reason. The setting of a cut score is important from the evaluator's perspective because it involves making decisions about individuals (e.g., Did the person pass or fail the test? Will they become certified health education specialists or not?), and the cut score is important when evaluators assess the quality of instructional material. Setting inappropriately high cut scores may unfairly penalize individuals and may also involve the inaccurate or unfair appraisal of educational materials (Noonan & Sarvela, 1987). In addition, setting cut scores too low might allow unqualified people to pass a test, or allow poorly developed instructional materials to be used on a large scale.

Livingston and Zieky (1982), in their manual entitled *Passing Scores*, emphasize that it is important to use a systematic and psychometrically sound approach to setting a cut score, because "choosing a passing score on a test often leads to controversy" (p.55). Controversy may develop based on the selection of the cut score method, who the judges were who set the cut score, or other issues. The selection of the cut score method is particularly important because different approaches can yield different cut scores for the same test. Noonan and Sarvela (1987), in their comparison of the ISD standard setting approach and the Angoff procedure, found that the ISD approach consistently produced higher standards than did the Angoff procedure. They concluded that the ISD approach may at times unnecessarily penalize students who actually perform at acceptable levels, and may also lead to the unnecessary rejection of sound instructional materials. These ideas reinforce Schrock and Coscarelli's (1990) statement: "There is no simple, cookbook solution to establishing standards for your test, and there is no formula for determining the cut-off score that eliminates the sticky business of human judgment in standard setting procedures!" (p.117).

There are other social and political questions that may arise as a result of setting a cut score on a "high stakes" test. According to Livingston and Zieky (1982), some of these questions include:

- Should there be exceptions to the agreed upon cut score?
- Should people who fail the test be allowed to take it again?
- Should people who pass the test have to retake it at a later date?
- Should an uncertain category be established?
- Should norm information be used to set the cut score?
- Should standards change over time?
- Should different groups have different cut scores?

For these reasons, if the test the evaluator develops is a high stakes test, the cut score decision must be made carefully. One commonly used procedure in setting cut scores is the Angoff method.

Angoff (1971) developed a method of setting cut scores based on a set of judges who estimate the percent of minimally competent examinees who can answer a set of test items correctly. A group of judges independently estimate the percent of minimally competent examinees who would pass each test item. The values for each item are averaged, and an average for all the items is computed. This final average becomes the minimum score individuals are required to achieve in order to pass the test. A simple example of setting a cut score using three judges on a ten-item quiz is shown in Table 6.3.

Table 6.3 Angoff Procedure for Setting Cut scores

Item	Judge 1	Judge 2	Judge 3	Average*
1	75	80	85	80
2	80	80	75	78
3	95	95	95	95
4	60	65	60	62
5	85	85	85	85
6	95	95	90	93
7	50	40	45	45
8	70	70	70	70
9	85	90	85	87
10	100	100	100	100

Cut Score (Based on average of "average" column) = 79.5

* rounded

Psychometric procedures for setting cut scores are appropriate for knowledge tests, although sometimes the standards for achievement must be made on other forms of procedures, not just knowledge tests. For example, in work that may require the use of epidemiologic screening tests, often, the middle most 95 percent of the scores are considered "normal" scores (Mausner & Kramer, 1985). Scores outside the range would not be considered average. If one is working with a blood pressure education program, a goal might be to use the most common range of blood pressures as the standard. Scores outside that range, especially higher scores, would not have met the standard.

Green and Lewis (1986) suggest other approaches for setting standards. They describe standards as the minimum acceptable levels of performance used to judge the quality of professional practice - standards should be stated in as an explicit manner as possible. They describe four ways to setting program standards:

- Historical comparisons with similar programs of the past.
- Normative comparisons with contemporary activities elsewhere.
- Theoretical comparisons with an ideal.
- Consensus among professionals.

Summary

This chapter examined the broad areas related to the measurement of knowledge, attitudes, and behavior of health related issues. Different item types were examined for each area. Strengths and weaknesses of the items were discussed, along with appropriate methods of measuring reliability and validity for each. In addition, some ideas regarding the collection of data from children were presented. A set of commonly used physiological tests and procedures from a health care setting was discussed as well. Finally, the important issue of setting a passing score on a knowledge test was described.

Case Study

Vartiainen, E., Paavola, M., McAlister, A., Puska, P. (1998). Fifteen-year follow-up of smoking prevention effects in the North Karelia Youth Project. *American Journal of Public Health*, *88*(1), 81-85.

Vartiainen and colleagues discuss the long-term effects of a school- and community-based smoking prevention program implemented in Finland. Two surveys were used in the evaluation: a self-administered questionnaire and a survey administered in a local health center by a trained project nurse. They found that lifetime cigarette smoking was 22% lower in the intervention group when compared to the control group. What were the strengths of the data collection design in this study? What were its weaknesses? What difficulties are present when one tries to measure behavior over a 15-year period? What would you add or change regarding the instruments or data collection procedures?

Student Questions/Activities

1. Pick a health behavior that is important for people of all ages (e.g., eating a nutritionally balanced diet). Develop a set of items to be used to measure that behavior for preschool children, elementary school children, high school students, college students, middle aged people, and the elderly. How do your data collection techniques change by age group? What remains the same?

2. Record your own personal dietary and physical fitness behaviors for one week using the items described by Duyff (1997). After one week, think about the following: What did you like about this technique? What didn't you like? Which target populations could use this technique? For which populations would this technique be a difficult one to use?

3. Select a health topic of interest (e.g., youth drug use). Develop a paper-and-pencil instrument that measures knowledge, attitudes, and behaviors related to your topic.

4. Set a cut score for a classroom test or quiz using Angoff's approach for setting standards with three fellow students as judges. Ask a fellow student or colleague to do the same. Were the cut scores set by you and your fellow student/colleague similar?

Recommended Readings

Bentzen, W.R. (1997). *Seeing Young Children: A Guide to Observing and Recording Behavior*, 3rd edition. Boston: Delmar.

Bentzen's text focuses on the procedures and methods used when observing children from newborns through eight-year-olds. In addition to providing an overview and guidelines for observing children, various methodologic issues are presented, including a discussion on sampling as well as various data collection techniques such as checklists, diaries, frequency counts, and anecdotal records. Guidelines for observing various age groups are also provided.

Johnson, R.A., & Gerstein, D.R. (1998). Initiation of use of alcohol, cigarettes, marijuana, cocaine, and other substances in US birth cohorts since 1919. *American Journal of Public Health*, 88(1), 27-33.

Johnson and Gerstein present data collected from the *National Household Surveys on Drug Abuse,* comparing initiation of drug use among cohorts born from 1919 to 1975. They conclude that cohorts born since World War II have had much higher rates of illicit drug use initiation. Two methodological biases related to instrumentation are discussed: bias due to memory errors and bias due to social acceptability and fear of disclosure.

Ransdell, L.B., & McMillen, B. (1997). Uses and limitations of physical activity questionnaires in health education. *Journal of Health Education, 28*(3), 182-186.

In this paper, Ransdell and McMillen discuss reasons why physical activity questionnaires are used, types of questionnaires and their strengths and weaknesses, considerations in questionnaire selection, and application ideas for health education and promotion professionals. They conclude by saying: "Understanding the 'physical activity side' of the target population is the key to planning appropriate intervention activities" (p.185).

References

Angoff, W. (1971). Scales, norms, and equivalent scores. In R.L. Thorndike (Ed.). *Educational Measurement*, 2nd edition. Washington, DC: American Council on Education

Babbie, E.R. (1973). *Survey Research Methods*. Belmont, CA: Wadsworth Publishing Company.

Bredekamp, S., & Copple, C. (Eds.) (1997). *Developmentally Appropriate Practice in Early Childhood Programs*. Washington, DC: National Association for the Education of Young Children.

Duyff, R.L. (1997). *Monthly Nutrition Companion: 31 Days to a Healthier Lifestyle*. Minneapolis: Chronimed Publishing.

Ebel, R.L. (1951). Writing the test item. In E.F. Linquist (Ed.). *Educational Measurement*. Washington, DC: American Council on Education.

Ebel, R.L., & Frisbie, D.A. (1986). *Essentials of Educational Measurement*, 4th edition. Englewood Cliffs, NJ: Prentice-Hall, Inc.

Ellis, J.A., Fredericks, P.S., & Wulfeck, W.H. (1979). *The Instructional Quality Inventory*. Navy Personnel Research Development Center, NPRDC SR 79 – 24: San Diego.

Green, L.W., & Lewis, F.W. (1986). *Measurement and Evaluation in Health Education and Health Promotion*. Palo Alto: Mayfield.

Hastad, D.N., & Lacy, A.C. (1994). *Measurement and Evaluation in Physical Education and Exercise Science*, 2nd edition. Scottsdale, AZ: Gorsuch Scarisbrick.

Henderson, M.E., Morris, L.L, & Fitz–Gibbon, C.T. (1978). *How to Measure Attitudes*. Beverly Hills: Sage.

Hopkins, K.D., & Stanley, J.C. (1981). *Educational and Psychological Measurement and Evaluation*, 6th edition. Englewood Cliffs, NJ: Prentice-Hall, Inc.

Kerlinger, F.N. (1973). *Foundations of Behavioral Research*, 2nd edition. New York: Holt, Rinehart, and Winston.

Leavitt, R.L., & Eheart, B.K. (1991). Assessment in early childhood programs. *Young Children, 46*(5), 4-9.

Livingston, S.A., & Zieky, M.J. (1982). *Passing Scores*. Princeton, NJ: Educational Testing Service.

Mausner, J.S., & Kramer, S. (1985). *Epidemiology: An Introduction Text*, 2nd edition. Philadelphia: Saunders.

McDermott, R.J., & Gold, R.S. (1986/1987). Racial differences in the perception of contraceptive option attributes. *Health Education, 17*(6), 9–14.

Miller, D.C. (1977). *Handbook of Research Design and Social Measurement*, 3rd edition. New York: Longman.

Millman, J., & Greene, J. (1989). The specification and development of tests of achievement and ability. In R.L. Linn (Ed.) *Educational Measurement*, 3rd edition. New York: Macmillan Publishing Company.

Mueller, D.J. (1986). *Measuring Social Attitudes*. New York: Teachers College Press.

Noll, V.H., Scannell, D.P., & Craig, R.C. (1989). *Introduction to Educational Measurement*, 4th edition. New York: University Press of America.

Noonan, J.V., & Sarvela, P.D. (1987). Passing score procedures in instructional systems development. *Performance and Instruction, 26*(9/10), 16-18.

Roid, G.H., & Haladyna, T.M. (1982). *A Technology for Test-item Writing*. New York: Academic Press.

Rubinson, L., & Nuetens, J.J. (1987). *Research Techniques for the Health Sciences*. New York: Macmillan.

Sarvela, P.D., & Moore, J.R. (1989). Nursing home employee attitudes towards AIDS. *Health Values, 13*(2), 11-16.

Schrock, S.A., & Coscarelli, W.C.C. (1990). *Criterion-Referenced Test Development: Technical and Legal Guidelines for Corporate Training*. Reading, MA: Addison-Wesley.

Trevisan, M.S., Sax, G., & Michael, W.B. (1994). Estimating the optimum number of options per item using an incremental option paradigm. *Educational and Psychological Measurement, 54*(1), 86-91.

Windsor, R.A., Baranowski, T. Clark, N., &. Cutter, G. (1984). *Evaluation of Health Promotion and Education Programs*. Palo Alto: Mayfield.

Wortham, S.C. (1995). *Measurement and Evaluation in Early Childhood Education*, 2nd edition. Englewood Cliffs, NJ: Merrill-Prentice Hall.

Reliability and Validity of Measurement

Chapter Objectives

After completing this chapter, you should be able to:

1. Define reliability.
2. Define validity.
3. Compare and contrast the different forms of reliability.
4. Compare and contrast the different forms of validity.
5. Interpret reliability coefficients.
6. Interpret item analyses.
7. Conduct a content validity study.
8. Describe ways to enhance the reliability and validity of instruments.

Key Terms

bogus-pipeline
common-error analysis
construct validity
content validity
criterion-related validity
difficulty index
discrimination index
face validity
internal consistency reliability
inter-rater reliability
intra-rater reliability

item analysis
parallel forms reliability
rater reliability
reliability
response selection analysis
sensitivity
specificity
standard error of measurement
test-retest reliability/stability reliability
validity

Introduction

Imagine that you have just finished a presentation to a group of parents and teachers on a study you conducted in their school concerning student drug and alcohol use. The principal thanks you for your presentation, and asks if there are any questions. The first question asked by a parent is: "How do we know the students are actually reporting what they are or are not doing?" This question is quickly followed by a comment from an elementary school teacher, who indicates that she has looked at the questionnaire, and isn't sure if the students really understood some of the questions. "This is especially true," adds the teacher, "for the children in third- and fourth-grade." In addition, one parent says: "I would bet if you survey these kids again next week you'll get totally different results!" How would you respond to questions like these?

Each of these questions is related in some way to the **reliability** and **validity** of the data collection instrument and the data collection procedures. School principals, teachers, parents, physicians, and researchers rightly ask: "How reliable or valid are the data and their associated interpretations when using various types of evaluation instruments?" In other words, can the stakeholders "trust" the data that come from these types of instruments? Since much of what we think we know about health behavior, especially health behavior of children and youth, is a result of surveys involving self-report (see Chapter 6), reliability and validity are not trivial concerns if responsive health education and promotion programs are going to be crafted based on these data.

To be able to "trust" the data derived from the instruments, evaluators need to conduct reliability and validity studies. Because of the legitimate concerns raised in our introductory example, establishing an instrument's level of reliability and validity is a major element in the health education research and evaluation process. Yet, despite the importance of reliability and validity, experience consistently demonstrates that health-related evaluation and research neglects to study or report the quality of their data collection instruments. For example, in their study of the extent to which reliability and validity evidence is presented in American Psychological Association journals, Qualls and Moss (1996) found that only 20% of the articles provided information on *both* reliability and validity, and just 49% presented information on at least one or the other. Lamp, Price, and Desmond (1989) studied the frequency of investigator reports of reliability and validity in three health education journals. Their findings suggested that: "A lack of research rigor was noted in the three health education journals when rigor is defined as the presence or absence of reported measures of instrument validity and reliability" (p.107). Even though the Lamp, et al. study was conducted more than a decade ago, there is still ample reason to question the extent to which reliability, validity, and other "checks" of data accuracy are carried out today.

An evaluator must be certain that instruments used in evaluation studies yield reliable and valid results. Otherwise, the evaluator cannot have confidence in the study's findings. If one cannot trust the results, what is the value of undertaking the study in the first place, other perhaps, than for "political" purposes (see Chapter 3). Thus, evaluators should attempt not only to estimate the reliability of their instruments, but also their validity. Once the data collection instruments are found to yield reliable and valid data, the evaluator can be confident that the data collected are accurate reflections of the target population's knowledge, attitudes, and behaviors.

Reliability - What Are We Talking About?

Your friend is a reliable worker. What does "reliable" mean? Common traits of a reliable person are consistency (i.e., a hard worker throughout the day, week, month, or year); dependability (i.e., if she says she will do something, she will get it done as expected); stability (i.e., he will come to work day-after-day, and do the job well each day); and carefulness (there will not be a lot of error in the work that the person does).

These same ideas are used by evaluation and measurement specialists when they discuss the **reliability** of data collection instruments. A reliable instrument is one that is consistent, dependable, and stable (Kerlinger, 1973). To groups such as the American Educational Research Association, the American Psychological Association, and the National Council on Measurement in Education (1985) reliability is the degree to which test scores are free from errors of measurement, or it is the degree to which repeated observations of the same characteristic (e.g., knowledge on a health test) yield the same results (Carmine & Zeller, 1979).

Reliability is an important concept for health education evaluators because an evaluator must be sure that the data collection instruments are relatively free from measurement error. It is important to note that there will always be a certain degree of measurement error present. For example, if a person uses a bathroom scale for weighing purposes, the quality of the measurement may be somewhat inaccurate due to problems with springs in the scales, the way the person stands on the scale, or the amount of clothing the person has on. Anyone who has used a scale at home and then used a scale at a medical facility office knows that there can be a large difference in weight between the two scales. The scale at the medical facility would be considered relatively accurate; probably within a quarter of a pound of the person's true weight. This level of accuracy is appropriate for a general assessment of a person's weight. A quarter pound of variability might be intolerable for other types of studies, however. To a chemist, one-quarter of one pound might be a huge margin of error, so more accurate means of measurement would be needed.

This discussion brings to light the notion that reliability is a relative term. Each measurement problem has its own tolerance for measurement error, and it is the job of the evaluator to find an instrument that fits within that level of tolerance. If you were evaluating the effectiveness of a weight-reduction program, a home bathroom scale might not be a sufficiently accurate measurement device. In this instance, you should probably use the balance-beam scale. However, it would be inappropriate to use a chemist's digitized weight scale that reads to one ten-thousandth of a gram, because that level of precision would be more than what was required.

Fundamental to the idea of reliability then, is the concept of measurement error. Nunnally (1978) argues that an individual's *observed score* (the score the instrument produces) is made up of a *true score* (i.e., how much a person would actually weigh if the person was measured with a perfect scale under perfect conditions), and an *error score* (the amount of error that is present due to the unreliability of the measurement instrument). So, for a person weighing 175 pounds at home on the bathroom scale, but 182 pounds using the doctor's calibrated balance-beam scale, you could say that the home scale has a measurement error of about seven pounds.

Just as there is measurement error when we measure the physical characteristics of an individual (e.g., height, weight, blood pressure), there is also measurement error present when we measure a person's knowledge, attitudes, and behaviors. It is because of this fact that we again state the importance of estimating the reliability of all instruments involved in health education program evaluation.

One statistic that measurement specialists have developed to estimate the degree of error is the **standard error of measurement**. It is defined as a statistic that estimates the standard deviation of the distribution of measurement errors around a person's true score (Nunnally, 1978). As Figure 7.1 shows, if we recorded a person's diastolic blood pressure an infinite number of times, we would develop a distribution of errors around the person's true score (in this case, 65).

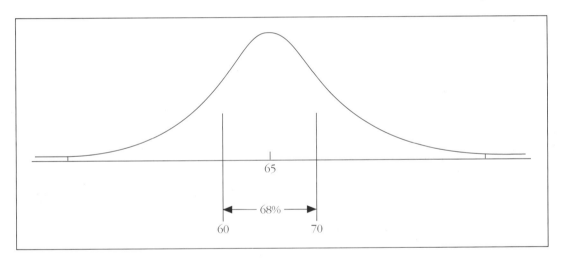

Figure 7.1 The Standard Error of Measurement: Diastolic Blood Pressure of 65 mm Hg with Standard Error of 5 Points

This statistic is used to estimate where a person's true score lies, relative to the observed score. The standard error of measurement is an estimate of the accuracy of the instrument (Ebel & Frisbie, 1986).

We can estimate the reliability of data collection instruments in many ways. The most common procedures are rater reliability, test-retest reliability, parallel forms reliability, and internal consistency reliability.

Reliability and Validity of Measurement   133

Rater Reliability

Rater reliability is associated with the consistent evaluation of an observed event by different individuals (judges), or by the same individual. Most people have seen an athletic event such as figure skating, platform diving, or gymnastics, where a panel of experts judges the quality of an athlete's performance. For example, in international figure skating competition, the skill with which the skater performs a required series of jumps and moves (technical merit), and the ability with which he or she "interprets" the moves, possibly in synchronization with music (artistic quality), is the basis for judging. The performance is evaluated by a panel, with each individual judge awarding a score (from a theoretical minimum of 0.0, to a maximum of 6.0). **Inter-rater reliability** refers to the degree to which two or more raters agree on the characteristics of an observation (Yaremko, Harari, Harrison & Lynn, 1986). For the example above, if a panel of six judges gave a particular figure skater marks on technical merit of 5.9, 5.8, 5.8, 5.9, 5.8, and 5.7, we could say that there was a high degree of inter-rater-reliability. However, if we saw the following pattern of judges' evaluations for artistic quality (5.9, 5.8, 5.2, 5.2, 5.7, 5.8), we might conclude that there was poor inter-rater reliability (and perhaps speculate that a couple of judges might be showing some bias on the basis of the performer's home country). Politics and national loyalties aside, a checklist with agreed upon criteria, along with proper training and experience of judges, helps to ensure that inter-rater reliability for observations is relatively high.

Another form of rater reliability that is important to consider when one individual is conducting a series of ratings over time is **intra-rater reliability**. Intra-rater reliability refers to the degree to which one rater agrees upon the characteristics of an observation repeatedly over time (adapted from Yaremko, et al., 1986). Any teacher who has faced the task of grading a stack of fifty essay exams can relate to this problem. Without proper care and guidelines, it is easy to grade the first person much differently than the fiftieth person, due to rating problems such as fatigue, anger at the students, or perhaps boredom. For these reasons, it is important to have a checklist that outlines how many points each section of the assignment is worth, so that the instructor grades consistently from the first paper to the fiftieth. An example of such a checklist, adapted from Windsor, et al. (1984), and used for an evaluation class project, is found in Figure 7.2.

Rater-reliabilities are most important to estimate when observations are involved in the measurement. Thus, performance tests, such as final examinations for CPR, should be measured for rater-reliability, as should procedures such as observations of individuals in participant-observer studies (see Chapter 11), or essay exams. Inter-rater reliability is established to ensure that multiple observers see and record the same observations, and that once the observations are agreed upon, that the same number of points is awarded for the same behavior by all raters. Rater-reliabilities are most frequently calculated in terms of percent agreement. For example, after conducting a percent agreement check on a CPR test, it might be found that for 90 percent of the items, there was 100 percent agreement among three CPR instructors as to whether the people passed or failed that item (or CPR step). An example of how one can go about estimating inter-rater reliability is found in Figure 7.3.

Student Name: Elizabeth Gwyn   **Identification Number:** 123-456-7890

SECTION	POINTS
ABSTRACT	5
INTRODUCTION	10
Purpose of the Program	
Aims and Objectives	
Description of Participants and Setting	
Program Description	
Nature of the Learning	
Content	
Staffing and Personnel	
REVIEW OF LITERATURE AND EVALUATION QUESTIONS	10
Define the Problem	
Historical Aspects	
Current Research	
Evaluation Questions	
METHOD	20
Sample (e.g., subjects, sampling strategy)	
Instrumentation (e.g., piloting, reliability, validity, readability)	
Research Design (e.g., type, threats to experimental validity)	
Data Collection Procedures (e.g., how data were collected, by whom, etc.)	
Data Analysis Procedures (e.g., statistics used, assumptions, etc.)	
LOGISTICS OF THE EVALUATION	5
Gantt Chart Analysis	
Budget	
Personnel Requirements	
RESULTS	20
Quantitative Findings	
Univariate Analysis	
Bivariate Analysis	
Multivariate Analysis	
Qualitative Findings	
Interviews	
Observations	
DISCUSSION	10
RECOMMENDATIONS	10
REFERENCES	5
APPENDICES	5

Figure 7.2 Checklist for Grading Evaluation Class Project

The basic steps involved in determining rater reliability are as follows:

- Develop or select the instrument to be tested.
- Observe a group of subjects demonstrating the behaviors to be assessed with two or more judges (for inter-rater reliability) or repeatedly by one judge (for intra-rater reliability).
- Score each individual's performance.
- Create a matrix that compares the results of different judges (or different times of judging the same performance by one judge). Attempt to obtain at least 90 percent agreement between the judges on each item.

STUDENTS:

	Klaus Kölsch			Wolf Jever			Paul Bennetov		
	RATER			**RATER**			**RATER**		
	1	2	3	1	2	3	1	2	3
STEP:									
1	P	P	P	P	P	P	P	P	P
2	P	F	P*	P	P	P	F	F	F
3	F	F	F	P	P	P	F	F	F
4	P	P	P	P	P	P	P	P	P
5	P	P	P	P	P	P	F	F	F
6	F	F	F	P	P	P	F	F	F

P=PASS
F=FAIL

The inter-rater reliability for this test, based on these observations would be estimated to be 94 percent, since there was agreement on 17 of the 18 ratings for these three subjects.

* An item with lack of agreement among the judges (raters).

Figure 7.3 Inter-rater Reliability for a New CPR Test

Test-Retest Reliability

Another form of reliability that appears in health education research and evaluation literature is **test-retest reliability**. Test-retest reliability is estimated by correlating the results of a test that has been administered to the same group of people two or more times

(Ferguson, 1981). Alemagno and colleagues (1996) describe the test-retest results of a project that measured substance abuse treatment needs of homeless people. They found that their technique, which utilized cellular telephones to administer a survey, produced high rates of agreement in responses between the first and second time the survey was administered to a group of homeless adults. Rates of agreement for drug use from the first and second testing periods ranged from 83% to 96%.

When an evaluator is involved with a long-term study measuring the subjects several times, it is important to ensure that the measurement instrument is stable over time. Thus, in a weight loss program, if the evaluator weighs a person one day, provided the person has not changed weight, two days later, that person should weigh the same amount as measured two days earlier. In other words, if an individual is measured repeatedly over time, and has not changed in the characteristic being studied, the instrument should produce the same results. Test-retest reliability estimates the stability of the repeated measurements over time. This form of reliability is also called **stability reliability**.

Using test-retest reliability is important when conducting long-term longitudinal studies, because the evaluator must make sure that changes occurring over time are changes that occur in the subject, not in the data collection instrument. For example, test-retest reliability methods might be used in evaluating the effectiveness of a cholesterol-reduction program. It may take a year or more to reduce cholesterol levels and participants may need to follow severe dietary restrictions. As a result, the evaluator might want to measure overall attitudes and well-being at three-month intervals, to detect any reactive anxiety or depression that may have resulted from the dietary restrictions. In this situation, where the instrument might be administered to subjects over a long period of time, the evaluator would want to ensure that the instrument measures the same characteristics consistently over time. Therefore, before the evaluation begins, the evaluator would measure a group of people several times. Provided they have not changed, the data from the administrations should be the same, and test-retest reliability would be established.

The basic steps involved with determining test-retest reliability are as follows:

- Develop or select the instrument to be tested.
- Administer the instrument to a group of subjects twice, at a two-week interval (or longer if appropriate).
- Score each individual's instrument.
- Correlate the results between the two sets of scores. The correlation should be relatively high (.80 or above) in order for the instrument to be considered stable over time.

One problem related to estimating test-retest reliability is that people *really may change* between the first and second administrations of a test. For instance, although age is a "stable" variable, if the test-retest interval is a matter of a few weeks, it is truly possible that some subjects had birthdays. Even more bizarre than that is that for some survey instruments, people might even seem to undergo a "sex change" during the test-retest interval. The probable explanation is that the individual checked the wrong box for "gender" during one of the two times the survey was administered. If such an error is common, it might suggest that more extensive pilot testing of the instrument ought to be done (see Chapter 8) to see if the boxes one is supposed to place a check in need to be delineated more clearly. Sometimes there really will be change in individuals, though. Consequently, if there *is* actual change, the observed test-retest reliability may be low, despite the fact that the test has accurately measured the person. Thus, one must assess the possibility of actual change before bemoaning an unexpectedly low test-retest reliability.

Parallel Forms Reliability

Thousands of people each year take college entrance examinations such as the SAT, ACT, GRE, MAT, or MCAT. These tests are used to make judgments on individuals regarding their suitability or aptitude for entering a particular university or course of study.

Because these tests are so important, measurement specialists develop several forms of the same test. Multiple forms are developed to reduce problems with cheating (the people sitting next to each other rarely have the same form, and if they do, the testing situation is monitored carefully), and to ensure a person does not receive the same test form if he or she opts to retake the test. At any given test site for a large standardized test, proctors may be administering three forms of the same test to the group of people. Approximately one-third will receive form A, one-third form B, and one-third form C.

When developing different forms of the same instrument, one must make sure that the tests are covering the same content areas, and for knowledge tests, make sure the different forms are about the same level of difficulty. Otherwise, if form A is an easier test, those who take form A will get higher grades than those who take form B or form C. **Parallel forms reliability** is defined as the degree to which two or more parallel or equivalent forms of the same test have equal means, standard deviations, and intercorrelations among the items (Ferguson, 1981).

Parallel forms reliability might also be important to establish when an evaluator is using an experimental design to evaluate the quality of a program, where subjects will receive a pretest and a posttest (see Chapter 10). In this situation, one might not want to administer the same form of the test at pretest and posttest time, for fear that the subjects will learn or memorize the answers to the pretest during the course of the experiment. As a consequence of students focusing on the items from the pretest, one could argue that they mastered the specific test items, but not the total domain to be learned. Therefore, parallel forms of a test, if developed, can become a valuable asset for the overall aims of a project.

If the means, standard deviations, and intercorrelations are not exactly the same among different forms of the same test, psychometricians (specially trained educational psychologists) will sometimes *equate* the tests using a series of statistical procedures, to make them statistically equivalent. The demonstration of parallel forms reliability is both difficult and expensive. Nevertheless, it is an important method of estimating reliability in large-scale testing and experimental and quasi-experimental design situations such as are presented in Chapter 10.

The basic steps involved in determining parallel forms reliability are:

- Develop or select two or more forms of the instrument to be tested.
- Administer the instruments to a group of subjects at about the same time (within two or three days).
- Score each individual's instrument.
- Compare the means, standard deviations, and item intercorrelations with each of the test forms.
- If unequal, use an equating procedure to statistically equate the different forms with each other.

Internal Consistency Reliability

Internal consistency reliability examines the average correlation among items in a test. It measures the degree to which the items "hang together," that is, the degree to which items relate to each other (Nunnally, 1978). This form of reliability can be estimated using a number of different procedures, including *Cronbach's alpha* (Cronbach, 1951), the *KR-20* and *KR-21* coefficients (Kuder & Richardson, 1937), and the *Spearman-Brown split-half* reliability procedure (Ebel & Frisbie, 1986).

Each of these procedures measures the degree to which the items are related to each other. There is an inherent notion in testing and measurement that if one is developing an instrument to measure something (e.g., attitudes of health care workers towards working with people with AIDS), the items on the instrument should all be related to each other. Internal consistency reliability measures this relationship, and the coefficient produced using these procedures ranges from a value of 0 (which indicates no reliability) to 1 (which indicates perfect reliability). There are no specific cut-off values for what levels of reliability are acceptable. However, for basic research or evaluation studies, a minimum value of .60 is desirable; for applied studies, a value of .80 or greater is preferred; and, for work that involves clinical decisions (e.g., a test that determines whether a person is mentally competent or not), reliability should exceed .90 (Green & Lewis, 1986; Nunnally, 1978). It should be noted that the value of the coefficient produced is related to the spread of the scores of the group tested. The greater the spread of scores, the higher the value of the internal consistency reliability coefficient.

The Cronbach alpha can be used for many different types of scales (e.g., knowledge tests or Likert scales), whereas the KR-20, the KR-21, and the Spearman-Brown approaches assume that the items on the test are scored dichotomously (each item receives a value of one or zero). Therefore, the KR-20, KR-21, and Spearman-Brown measures are best suited for knowledge tests where each item has only one correct answer.

Another assumption of these statistics is that the items being tested are unidimensional (meaning they cover the same content area). If an evaluator is developing an instrument that covers several different content areas, it will be necessary to estimate the reliability of each content area separately (each individual subscale) rather than the total instrument for the "truest" measure of internal consistency reliability.

A prime example of the use of an internal consistency reliability coefficient is found in a paper by Shannon and associates (1997), who sought to study self-efficacy as a predictor of dietary change among low socio-economic level persons living in the southern United States. They developed a 22-item scale designed to measure the subjects' confidence in making dietary changes. Their instrument had a Cronbach alpha estimate of reliability of .84 for the pre-intervention data, and .83 for the post-intervention data, suggesting good internal consistency reliability.

The basic steps involved in determining internal consistency reliability include:

- Develop or select the instrument to be tested.
- Administer the instrument to a group of at least twenty subjects.
- Score each individual's instrument.
- Use a computer program to assess KR-20 or Cronbach alpha reliability for multiple-choice and true-false tests, or Cronbach's alpha for Likert scales.

One logistical advantage that internal consistency reliability has over other forms of reliability (i.e., test-retest or parallel forms) is that only one administration of one form of the instrument to one group of subjects is needed.

Validity - What Are We Talking About?

Although establishing reliability is an important aspect of the instrument development process, establishing validity is even more important. However, an instrument must first be established as a reliable one before validity studies may be conducted, because an instrument must be reliable for it to provide valid inferences. The opposite is not true however; one can have a reliable instrument, but it may not be a valid measure for a particular study.

Validity refers to the appropriateness, meaningfulness, and usefulness of the specific inferences made from test scores. Validity is the most important consideration in test evaluation. In other words, validity refers to the quality of the data that is derived from the use of the instrument, and the associated "claims" one can make when examining the results based on the findings from the instrument. A "valid" instrument is one that measures what it is supposed to measure. However, an instrument may be a valid means to measure one characteristic for one group of people, but not a valid means of measuring that same characteristic for a different group of people. This phenomenon is what some researchers have described as *situational validity*.

Suppose that we have a valid measure of youth drug abuse (where an instrument might have items concerning alcohol, marijuana, and cocaine use as it relates to peer pressure). Would this same instrument be valid for use with an elderly population? Probably not, because the dynamics surrounding the abuse of drugs by the elderly are different (e.g., mixing prescription drugs with alcohol, abuse of over-the-counter drugs, overuse of alcohol due to depression, and so on). A self-administered instrument might be *valid* for middle school youth, but not primary school pupils and kindergartners, because they cannot read at a level that gives us confidence that questions posed are understood. Validity refers here not only to the items on the instrument, but the administration procedures (e.g., self-administered versus interview).

Validity is a dynamic and evolving concept that changes over time. Using our drug abuse example again, a questionnaire that measured youth drug use in the 1960s might have items concerning drugs such as LSD, mescaline, and PCP. A drug use questionnaire today might include such items as "crack cocaine," a substance that was not used in the 1960s. Instrument validity is dependent on the context and purpose for which the instrument is being used (Smith & Glass, 1987).

Just as there are many types of reliability estimates, there are also many ways of gathering evidence concerning the validity of an instrument and its interpretations. The most frequently used forms of validity in health education evaluation practice are: face validity, content validity, criterion-related validity, and construct validity. In the discussion below, you will read about the meaning and use of each of these basic types of instrument validity.

Face Validity

Face validity is the lowest level of validity that an instrument can possess. An instrument is said to possess face validity *if on the "face" of things, the instrument appears to measure the construct under consideration, and appears to be appropriate for the audience for which it is intended.* An instrument intended to assess dental health knowledge, attitudes, and behaviors among fourth-graders might have the following characteristics:

- It asks about tooth decay.
- It asks about brushing and flossing practices.
- It asks about preventive check-ups.
- It is written with short sentences, large print, and accompanied by sketches and illustrations to assist readers in understanding concepts.

On the surface, an instrument with these characteristics would "appear" to meet the requirements of face validity. Yet, several issues relevant to dental health in children will remain unresolved. Will the instrument convey the relationship between plaque and tooth decay? Will the instrument adequately assess tooth brushing and flossing knowledge and behavior? If a fourth-grader is aware that brushing and flossing should occur after each meal or at least three times per day, does that convey to us any information relevant to the skill and proper technique for performing these tasks? If parents do not partake in, or reinforce preventive check-ups with a dental health professional, is asking about prevention a valid inclusion? The style of presentation (simple words and sentences, "fun" illustrations, and so on) might hold the attention of the "average" fourth-grader, but might not be terribly motivating for peers who are excellent readers or peers with reading and comprehension deficits. The instrument, thus, may work with some members of the audience, but not with group members having other traits and interests.

It should be clear from the example above that possessing face validity may be an important characteristic for an instrument, but certainly not a sufficient one for it to have wide distribution or to have useful interpretation of data made from it. Valid measurement requires other carefully assessed instrument characteristics.

Content Validity

Content validity demonstrates the degree to which the sample of items, tasks, or questions on a test are representative of some defined universe or domain of content (American Educational Research Association, et al., 1985). This method of establishing instrument validity should be used when developing *all* data collection instruments. Often, it is the only form of validity evidence evaluators present. Content validity is especially important with achievement and proficiency testing, and for measures of social behavior (Isaac & Michael, 1985).

Suppose a professor of health education has taught a 16-week course based on a textbook containing 16 chapters. Each week, one chapter was covered in the course. When the professor prepares the final examination, she would need to provide a similar number of items from each chapter (provided each chapter received about the same amount of emphasis in the lectures and discussion). If the professor developed a test where 75 percent of the items were based on four of the chapters, and the other 25 percent of the items were based on the remaining 12 chapters, the test would not be content valid. The items on the test would not be representative of the domain of content covered in the class. From this example, one can see that the most important element related to content validity is *representativeness*. That is, the instrument must examine all the content areas adequately.

Another element related to content validity is the set of *response options* for the items. Although the items may focus on all the domains of concern, the response options afforded those items may be restricted, therefore reducing the content validity of the instrument. Consider the following item designed to measure alcohol use during the previous month:

In the past month, on about how many days did you drink beer, wine, or liquor?

    a. I rarely drink alcohol.
    b. I am a social drinker.
    c. I drank alcohol a couple of times a month.
    d. I drank alcohol a couple of times a week.
    e. I drank more often than this.

The problems with this item should be obvious to you. If a person never drinks, he or she does not have an appropriate answer. Even worse are the problems of defining "social" drinker, and "a couple of times" a month or a week. What one individual may consider "social drinking," another individual may consider heavy alcohol use. A further problem might be that a person who considers himself a social drinker might also respond that he drinks a couple of times a month or a couple of times a week. This item would not be a content valid item for measuring yearly frequency of alcohol use. A better item for asking about this phenomenon would be:

In the past month, on about how many days did you drink beer, wine, or liquor?

a. I drank no beer, wine, or liquor.
b. 1 or 2 days.
c. 3 to 10 days.
d. 11 to 20 days.
e. 21 or more days.

By inspection, one can see that all possible responses to alcohol use are covered in this question, providing a representative and mutually exclusive set of responses regarding alcohol use for all subjects, whether they abstain from alcohol, drink occasionally, or are frequent drinkers. The behavioral anchor (days) is clear, even if the level of consumption during a specific drinking episode is not identified.

Content validity is usually established by a panel of experts. Two approaches are commonly used by measurement specialists: Instructional Quality Inventory (IQI) methods and classification approaches.

The IQI methods have been developed and refined by military testing specialists (Wulfeck, et al., 1978). Using this strategy, experts are asked to assess the degree to which the instrument items match the objectives of the instrument. Experts are given a list of the objectives and the items, and then, using a checklist, are asked to rate the degree to which the items match the objectives. Veneziano and Hooper (1997) describe a typical content validity checklist:

Question as stated:	Appropriate	Inappropriate
Clearly stated:	Yes	No
Response options:	Adequate	Inadequate

Another method is the classification approach for establishing content validity. Using this strategy, a panel of experts is told that the instrument has been designed to cover a certain number of different areas (e.g., drug use, peer pressure to use drugs, self-esteem, and relationships with parents). The panel of judges is then asked to assign the items to each of these four different categories, and on the basis of these assignments, the representativeness and relevance of the items to the instrument's objectives is established (American Educational Research Association, et al., 1985).

Veneziano and Hooper (1997) describe an additional method of establishing content validity, using a more quantitative approach. Their model requires that panel members judge each item on the basis of whether it is "essential," "useful but not essential," or "not necessary." Using this approach, a *Content-Validity Ratio* (CVR) can be developed for the instrument's items, based on the following formula:

$$CVR = (ne - N/2) \div N/2$$

Where: ne = number of panelists indicating "essential"
N = total number of panelists

For example, suppose you have twenty judges rate an instrument. For item one, 15 judges indicate the item is essential. The CVR is calculated as follows:

$$CVR = (15 - 20/2) \div 20/2 = (15 - 10) \div 10 = 5 \div 10 = .50$$

According to the table provided in their paper, with 20 panelists, one would need a CVR of .42 to achieve significance at $p < .05$. In this example, the item would be judged significant. They further propose that all items be analyzed, and that the average CVR of the "retained" items be used to compute the overall content validity of the questionnaire.

Regardless of the approach used, content validity is dependent on the original set of instrument specifications, which outline the objectives of the instrument. If care is taken in the development of the specifications, and if the items match the specifications, evidence of content validity should be present. In addition to the item-objective match, content reviewers should examine the quality of the instrument's directions, cover letter, reading level, and overall print quality (Stacy, 1987).

Criterion-Related Validity

Criterion-related validity demonstrates that test scores are systematically related to one or more outcome criteria (e.g., how well scores on an SAT can predict, and are related to, final college grade point average). The basic question associated with criterion-related validity is: *How accurately can a criterion performance (such as future job success) be predicted from scores on the test?* (American Educational Research Association, et al., 1985). There are two forms of criterion-related validity: *predictive* and *concurrent*.

Predictive validity studies are important to conduct when test designers develop an instrument that makes selection decisions in education and employment. For example, how well do the results on a health risk appraisal predict future health status? Predictive validity studies require measurements to take place at two points in time. Using our health risk appraisal example, a person could be administered a health risk appraisal instrument, and be followed over a course of a ten-year time span. If the original conclusions and predictions derived from the health risk appraisal are true, we would say that the test has a high degree of predictive validity. For instance, if the person has high blood pressure, high blood cholesterol, and is overweight at the time of the health risk appraisal, the results might suggest that if he doesn't change his lifestyle he will have a heart attack within ten years. If over the course of ten years, the person does not change his lifestyle, and does have a heart attack, we would say that the health risk appraisal has good predictive validity. Therefore, predictive validity is established by correlating or comparing the results (or predictions) from the first test, to the results or achievement at a later date (the criterion).

When developing achievement tests, certification tests, and diagnostic clinical tests, criterion-related validity should be based on concurrent validity procedures. Concurrent validity is established when the results of a newly developed instrument (e.g., a drug use questionnaire) are compared to those of an established instrument (e.g., urinalysis test), and found to be similar. In concurrent validity studies, the two instruments are administered at approximately the same time (American Educational Research Association, et al., 1985). In the study described earlier by Alemagno and colleagues (1996), in addition to asking the homeless people about their drug use through a survey, the homeless people also provided a hair sample that was tested for traces of cocaine. Using this strategy, the researchers were able to compare self-reported cocaine use with a biochemical test. The results indicated that there was 78% (95 out of 122 cases) concordance between self-reported use of cocaine and the results of the hair assay, as shown in Table 7.1.

Why would an evaluator be interested in developing a new instrument if there is already an established valid instrument? There are at least three reasons: (1) the new instrument may be less expensive to administer, score, and interpret; (2) the established instrument may be difficult or cumbersome to administer; and (3) the new instrument may be much quicker to administer and interpret.

Table 7.1 Comparison of Self-reported Cocaine Use and Hair Assay Results

		Hair Assay Result		
		Positive	Negative	Total
Self-Report	Negative	23(31%)	44(91%)	67(55%)
	Positive	51(69%)	4 (9%)	55(45%)
Concordance				95/122 (78%)

Adapted from: Alemagno, S.A., Cochran, D., Feucht, T.E., Stephens, R.C., Butts, J.M., & Wolfe, S.A. (1996). Assessing substance abuse treatment needs among the homeless: A telephone-based interactive voice response system. *American Journal of Public Health, 86*(11), 1626-1628.

Concurrent-related validity is established, therefore, when two instruments that measure the same characteristics are administered to the same set of subjects, and the results of the new instrument are compared to the results of the older, more established or valid instrument. If the results of the new instrument are comparable to those of the old instrument, the instrument designers have established concurrent validity, and thus, have increased the versatility of the instrument pool from which future evaluators can select.

Construct Validity

Construct validity focuses on the test score as a measure of the psychological characteristic (i.e., construct) of interest, such as self-esteem (American Educational Research Association, et al., 1985). When assessing construct-related validity, an evaluator attempts to establish evidence that the score derived from the instrument adequately measures the construct under study. Although there are many strategies and methods for assessing construct validity, *convergent* and *discriminant* validity approaches are used frequently (Green & Lewis, 1986).

Convergent validity approaches examine how well constructs relate to each other. For example, results from a newly developed test designed to measure introversion-extroversion would probably be highly correlated to the results of a test dealing with shyness. If one argues that shy people have traits related to introversion, and that indeed turns out to be true, one could suggest that there is evidence of construct validity.

Discriminant validity is supported when items that should *not* be related to each other, are in fact, found to be unrelated. With this form of construct validity, one is attempting to prove that the new construct being tested is distinct and different from previously studied constructs.

One commonly used statistical approach for assessing construct validity is *factor analysis*. Factor analysis is used to measure the intercorrelations of a set of items to each other, and factor scores are developed as a result of these correlational analyses. If items that purport to measure a particular construct are all found to be related to each other, and not at all related to items that had been hypothesized that they would not be related to, evidence for construct validity has been developed. For example, in a study of the construct validity of the dependence syndrome as measured by diagnostic criteria set forth in *DSM-IV*, Feingold and Rounsaville (1995) found that drug dependence items were unidimensional and distinct from variables related to consequences of drug use, such as legal problems. For further information on the use of factor analysis for construct validity studies, including a historical note, consult the article by Thompson and Daniel (1996).

One final note on validity is worth mentioning. When using physiological tests (e.g., blood pressure cuffs, urinalyses, cholesterol screenings), evaluators often speak of the validity of the measures as the sensitivity and specificity of the tests. **Sensitivity** is the ability of a test to correctly identify persons who have the disease or trait under investigation. **Specificity** is defined as the ability of a test to identify correctly those who do not have the disease or characteristic of interest (Lilienfeld & Lilienfeld, 1980).

Methods of Enhancing Reliability and Validity

There are several ways to "build in" reliability and validity when developing measures for evaluation studies. There are also strategies that can be used to improve and enhance the reliability of measures and the validity of the inferences that come forth from the data collected by the instrument. The following areas are covered in this section: methods for improving the reliability of tests, item analysis, bogus pipeline methods, comparisons of results with related governmental data, and social desirability and lie scale techniques.

General Methods for Increasing Reliability

If one conducts a reliability study and finds that the instrument does not meet the standards for reliability, the reliability of the instrument must be improved. Possible solutions to reliability problems are to increase the number of items of the instrument, modify the items that have poor difficulty or discrimination indices, increase agreement among raters on observational criteria, and improve test administration and testing environment conditions.

Regarding rater reliability, Ellis and Wulfeck (1982) describe four errors that can occur when different raters make judgments about the same performance:

- *Error of standards*, which occurs when raters have different standards for what constitutes a "passing" grade.
- *Error of halo*, which occurs when a rater's judgment is biased by his or her general impression of the individual.
- *Logical error*, which occurs when a rater uses a series of rating scales, and gives similar ratings on scales that are not necessarily related.
- *Errors of central tendency*, which occur when raters judge most students to be in the middle of the scale.

For rater reliability, test developers can refine the checklists used for judging pass/fail or other types of scoring. Another important element of rater reliability is to train the raters, so they are in agreement as to what constitutes a pass or fail. Finally, checklists should have behavioral anchors (see Chapter 6) that clearly outline the required behaviors and skills needed to pass the item (Ellis & Wulfeck, 1982).

Item Analysis

Item analysis describes a set of procedures that measurement specialists employ to appraise and improve the quality of their instruments. The most commonly computed analyses are: item difficulty, item discrimination, and response selection.

The **difficulty index** estimates the difficulty of an item on an achievement test (e.g., an item might have a difficulty index of .80, indicating that 80 percent of the subjects answered the item correctly). The difficulty index for a particular item, which is abbreviated as P (proportion correct), is computed according to:

$$P = \text{\# of correct responses} \div \text{total \# of item responses}$$

For example, a middle school health education teacher tested her class of twenty students, and found that for item 1 on the test, 15 students answered it correctly. The difficulty index for that item would be as follows:

$$P = 15 \div 20 = .75$$

Item difficulty indices can range from 0 (everyone got the item wrong) to 1.00 (everyone got the item correct). Difficulty indices help evaluators appraise the degree of difficulty of the test. If the evaluator determines that the test item difficulty indices are low (.30 or less), one could conclude any one of the following:

- There was poor instruction.
- The students are less capable or have not mastered the material.
- The test item was difficult.
- The test item was poorly constructed.

To achieve maximum reliability for a norm-referenced achievement test, the average of the item difficulty indices should be .50 (Guilford, 1954). However, in the typical classroom setting, .50 would be considered a low value of achievement on the item.

The **discrimination index** estimates the power of an item to differentiate those persons who score high on a test from those who score low. For achievement tests, an item discrimination index compares high and low achievers on the test with respect to a particular item in question. For achievement tests, it is desirable to have items that discriminate well between those people who have mastered the material being tested, and those who have *not* mastered the material. This statistic helps determine the discriminating power of each item.

Item discrimination indices range from −1.0 to +1.0. If the value is positive, it suggests that the high achievers had a tendency to pass the item while the low achievers had a tendency to fail the item (in achievement testing, this relationship is desirable). If the value is negative, it means that the high achievers are failing the item, and the low achievers are passing the item (obviously, this situation is not desirable).

Discrimination indices also can be used for attitudinal or behavioral inventories. For example, with a set of items concerning attitudes towards working with a person with AIDS, our evaluator would expect that if a subject was very positive on one item, he or she would probably be positive on the total set of items. When using discrimination indices for attitudinal or behavioral items, an evaluator interprets the values similar to interpreting values for knowledge items. If there is a positive discrimination index between the item and the scale, those who scored high on the item also scored high on the scale as a whole. Those who scored low on the item also scored low on the overall scale.

Response selection analysis examines the response patterns on a wide range of item types, from knowledge items (e.g., multiple-choice or true-false) to attitudinal items (e.g., Likert scales). Response selection analysis examines the percent and/or frequency of responses for each of the possible answers for an item. Response selection analysis can be used to examine responses to many different types of items, not just knowledge items.

Response selection analysis not only has value when creating an instrument for wide dissemination, but also in efforts to improve a test that is administered time after time. When response selection analysis is used for knowledge items, it can: (1) enable investigators to examine the plausibility of the distractors (incorrect responses), and (2) enable investigators to conduct a **common error analysis**, which helps to determine which parts of the curriculum must be revised, or, which parts of the curriculum are confusing or not entirely understood by students. Common error analysis also can be used to develop or select particularly attractive distractors for multiple-choice items.

It is desirable to have items with discrimination indices of .30 or greater. That level of discrimination will also contribute to the reliability of the instrument. When revising preliminary forms of instruments, the instrument developer can select those items with ideal difficulty and discrimination indices, as well as response selection patterns. If an evaluator uses this procedure, it is important to maintain adequate levels of content validity; items should not be selected solely on the basis of item-analytic procedures, as that could possibly create problems related to content validity. The data in Table 7.2 show an example of an item analysis on a preliminary form of a 13-item knowledge test for elementary school aged children.

Table 7.2 Sample Item Analysis from Elementary School Health Quiz (N=160)

Mean = 6.9   Standard Deviation = 2.2   Minimum Score = 2
Maximum Score = 12   Range = 10   Cronbach Alpha = .56

Item Number	Proportion correct	Discrimination Index	Response Selection Analysis (frequency)		
			A	B	C
1	.82	.29	131	25	3
2	.57	.39	40	25	92
3	.84	.20	134	14	11
4	.21	.26	98	33	24
5	.32	.26	52	19	85
6	.22	.21	46	74	35
7	.10	-.05	118	16	23
8	.39	.13	35	62	60
9	.61	.24	98	36	21
10	.97	.14	155	1	3
11	.47	.36	26	53	76
12	.56	.19	21	42	89
13	.80	.19	8	128	23

Bogus-Pipeline

A method that may enhance the results of self-report questionnaires when addressing such areas as illegal drug use is the **bogus-pipeline** approach (Werch, Gorman, Marty, Forbess, & Brown, 1987). With this strategy, individuals are administered a survey, while also asked to provide a physiological specimen (e.g., urine sample, saliva sample). Subjects are advised that survey results will be compared to those of the specimen test (even though they are not, hence the term "bogus-pipeline"). In some settings, this technique may increase the degree to which people will "admit" to illegal behavior. However, the overall utility and ethics of this procedure is debated since its use requires deception (Werch, et al., 1987).

Comparisons with Governmental Data

Another approach for validating survey results is to compare the findings from surveys with relevant commerce data that show actual consumption levels. Hatziandreu, Pierce, Fiore, Grise, Novotny, and Davis (1989) compared self-reported tobacco use with tobacco tax data, and found the comparison to yield similar consumption patterns in the United States. This finding was a positive one for persons who support the efficacy of self-report questionnaires for tobacco use, as the results of self-report surveys are frequently brought under criticism by skeptics.

Social Desirability and Lie Scales

In the study by Shannon, et al. (1997) identified earlier in this chapter, the researchers also included the short form of the Marlow-Crowne Social Desirability Scale. This scale attempts to measure the degree to which respondents provide socially desirable responses to survey instruments. What is a "socially desirable" response? Such responses occur when a person being queried by questionnaire or in an interview is asked about a subject, to which any rational person would successfully guess has a "preferred" answer. Questions such as -- *Do you wash your hands after using the toilet? Do you "buckle up" upon entering a motor vehicle? Do you ever drive a motor vehicle after drinking alcohol?* -- will tempt many people to respond in a socially desirable way, regardless of their actual practice. Gast, Caravella, Sarvela and McDermott (1995) used the Marlow-Crowne scale to help estimate the validity of the Centers for Disease Control and Prevention's (1994) Youth Risk Behavior Surveillance System's (YRBSS) alcohol questions. They found no statistically significant relationship between social desirability scores and self-reports on drinking, providing evidence that YRBSS respondents were accurately reporting frequency and quantity of alcohol use.

Lie scales that estimate the degree of systematic under-reporting or over-reporting of drug use also have been used as a method to enhance the validity of surveys. Sarvela and McClendon (1988) used this approach, adding several "bogus drugs" (drugs that do not exist) to a survey. If persons have a tendency to over-report, they may consistently indicate that they have used a set of bogus drugs (e.g., Sarvorphan, Lowtheral, McClenodines). If a subject positively answers a large number of items related to use of bogus drugs, one can suspect systematic over-reporting, and perhaps, remove the subject from the sample.

Summary

Evaluators must be certain that the instruments they use in their evaluation studies yield reliable and valid results. Otherwise, evaluators and other stakeholders can have no confidence in study findings. Evaluators should attempt to estimate reliability and gather evidence supporting the validity of their instruments for their specific evaluation project. In this chapter, in addition to defining and discussing the importance of reliability and validity, we compared and contrasted the different forms of reliability and validity. The chapter concluded with a discussion concerning various methods that can be to enhance the reliability and validity of results obtained from health education instruments.

Case Study

Snell, W.E., & Johnson, G. (1997). The multidimensional health questionnaire. *American Journal of Health Behavior*, *21*(1), 33-42.

The authors developed a 20-subscale questionnaire to measure psychological constructs related to health, ranging from health anxiety to internal health control. Cronbach alphas for the subscales ranged from .65 to .90. Validity data, based on comparisons of the MHQ and Bausell's measure of health-promoting behaviors, are reported by gender. After reviewing this study, which subscales would you revise? How does content validity affect the decision to remove or modify items from a sub-scale?

Student Questions/Activities

1. Select an instrument you find interesting. Administer the instrument to a group of friends. Two weeks later, administer it to the same group of friends. Were the results the same? To what do you attribute your findings?

2. You have been asked to assess the criterion-related validity of a newly developed instrument that has been designed to predict the future success of recent college graduates in the field of health education. What procedures would you use to assess the criterion-related validity of the test?

3. A newly developed final examination for a general health education course was found to have an internal consistency reliability estimate of .60 using Cronbach's alpha, based on the administration of the instrument to fifty students who recently completed the course. Is this a satisfactory level of reliability? If not,

how would you increase the reliability of the test? What information would you use to decide which items should be kept, modified, or removed?

4.   You have been hired as a consultant to develop a series of tests for elementary school children related to a new school health education curriculum being implemented in the region's schools. Which forms of reliability and validity would you use during the development of the tests? Why would you recommend these different methods?

Recommended Readings

Horowitz, S.M. (1996). Validity of the health risk appraisal for assessing fitness levels. *American Journal of Health Behavior, 20*(3), 98-102.

> Horowitz compares two items measuring physical activity: the CDC Health Risk Appraisal item and an item from the Standard Health Risk Appraisal. Subjects' responses to the questions were compared to subjects' performance on a maximal graded exercise treadmill test using the Balke protocol to estimate maximal oxygen consumption. Results suggested that all three levels of physical activity from the CDC questionnaire had distinctive VO_2max values, whereas levels 1 and 2 in the standard HRA version were not significantly different.

Arday, D.R., Tomar, S.L., Nelson, D.E., Merritt, R.K., Schooley, M.W., & Mowery, P. (1997). State smoking prevalence estimates: A comparison of the Behavioral Risk Factor Surveillance System and Current Population Surveys. *American Journal of Public Health, 87*(10), 1665-1669.

> Arday and colleagues compare results from the BRFSS and the Current Population Survey conducted by the U.S. Bureau of the Census. Results confirmed that BRFSS surveys, conducted by telephone, were similar to the CPS, conducted through household interviews. Although reported BRFSS rates were somewhat lower for men and for African Americans, these differences were not substantial. The authors conclude that the BRFSS provides adequate estimates of smoking rates.

Smith, B.A., Price, J.O., Nicholson, T., & Higgins, C.W. (1998). Health knowledge of predominately Mexican American high school students. *Journal of Health Education, 29*(1), 21-25.

> In this study, Smith, et al. describe the results of a test designed to measure health knowledge among Mexican American youth. In addition to a description of the study design, instrumentation (with a discussion on both test-retest and internal consistency reliability) and analysis procedures, health knowledge is presented, with particular emphasis on test items that high percentages of

students answered correctly, and test items that high percentages of students answered incorrectly.

References

Alemagno, S.A., Cochran, D., Feucht, T.E., Stephens, R.C., Butts, J.M., & Wolfe, S.A. (1996). Assessing substance abuse treatment needs among the homeless: A telephone-based interactive voice response system. *American Journal of Public Health, 86*(11), 1626-1628.

American Educational Research Association, American Psychological Association, & National Council on Measurement in Education. (1985). *Standards for Educational and Psychological Testing.* Washington, DC: American Psychological Association.

Carmine, E.G., & Zeller, R.A. (1979). *Reliability and Validity Assessment.* Beverly Hills: Sage.

Centers for Disease Control and Prevention. (1994). Youth risk behavior surveillance: United States, 1993. *Morbidity and Mortality Weekly Report, 44* (SS-1):1-58.

Cronbach, L.J. (1951). Coefficient alpha and the internal structure of tests. *Psychometrika,* 16, 297-334.

Ebel, R.L., & Frisbie, D.A. (1986). *Essentials of Educational Measurement,* 4th edition. Englewood Cliffs, NJ: Prentice-Hall.

Ellis, J.A., & Wulfeck, W.H. (1982). *Handbook for Testing in Navy Schools.* San Diego: Navy Personnel Research and Development Center.

Feingold, A., & Rounsaville, B. (1995). Construct validity of the dependence syndrome as measured by DSM-IV for different psychoactive substances. *Addiction, 90*(12), 1661-1669.

Ferguson, G.A. (1981). *Statistical Analysis in Psychology and Education,* 5th edition. New York: McGraw-Hill.

Gast, J., Caravella, T., Sarvela, P.D., & McDermott, R.J. (1995). Validation of the CDC's YRBSS Alcohol Questions. *Health Values, 18*(2), 38-43.

Green, L.W., & Lewis, F.M. (1986). *Measurement and Evaluation in Health Education and Health Promotion.* Palo Alto: Mayfield.

Guilford, J.P. (1954). *Psychometric Methods.* New York: McGraw-Hill.

Hatziandreu, E.J., Pierce, J.P. Fiore, M.C., Grise, V., Novotny, T.E., & Davis, R.M. (1989). The reliability of self-reported cigarette consumption in the United States. *American Journal of Public Health, 79*(8), 1020-1023.

Isaac, S., & Michael, W. (1985). *Handbook in Research and Evaluation.* San Diego: EdITS.

Kerlinger, F.N. (1973). *Foundations of Behavioral Research,* 2nd edition. New York: Holt, Rinehart, and Winston.

Kuder, G.F., & Richardson, M.W. (1937). The theory and the estimation of test reliability. *Psychometrika,* 2, 151-160.

Lamp, E., Price, J.H., & Desmond, S.M. (1989). Instrument validity and reliability in three health education journals, 1980-1987. *Journal of School Health, 59*(3), 105-108.

Lilienfeld, A.M., & Lilienfeld, D.E. (1980). *Foundations of Epidemiology*, 2nd edition. New York: Oxford.

Mausner, J.S., & Kramer, S. (1985). *Epidemiology - An Introductory Text,* 2nd edition. Philadelphia: W.B. Saunders.

Nunnally, J.C. (1978). *Psychometric Theory*, 2nd edition. New York: McGraw-Hill.

Qualls, A.L., & Moss, A.D. (1996). The degree of congruence between test standards and test documentation within psychological publications. *Educational and Psychological Measurement, 56*(2), 209-214.

Sarvela, P.D., & McClendon, E.J. (1988). Indicators of rural youth drug use. *Journal of Youth and Adolescence, 17*(4), 337-349.

Shannon, J., Kirkley, B., Ammerman, A., Keyserling, T., Kelsey, K., DeVellis, R., & Simpson, R.J. (1997). Self-efficacy as a predictor of dietary change in a low-socioeconomic-status southern adult population. *Health Education & Behavior, 24*(3), 357-368.

Smith, M., & Glass, G. (1987). *Research and Evaluation in Education and the Social Sciences*. Englewood Cliffs, NJ: Prentice-Hall.

Stacy, R.D. (1987). Instrument evaluation guides for survey research in health education and health promotion. *Health Education, 18(5),* 65-67.

Thompson, B., & Daniel, L.G. (1996). Factor analytic evidence for the construct validity of scores: A historical overview and some guidelines. *Educational and Psychological Measurement, 565*(2), 197-208.

Veneziano, L., & Hooper, J. (1997). A method for quantifying content validity of health-related questionnaires. *American Journal of Health Behavior, 21*(1), 67-70.

Werch, C.E., Gorman, D.R., Marty, P.J., Forbess, J., & Brown, B. (1987). Effects of the bogus-pipeline on enhancing validity of self-reported adolescent drug use measures. *Journal of School Health, 57*(6), 232-236.

Windsor, R.A., Baranowski, T., Clark, N., & Cutter, G. (1984). *Evaluation of Health Promotion and Education Programs*. Palo Alto: Mayfield.

Wulfeck, W.H., Ellis, J.A., Richards, R.E., Wood, N.D., & Merrill, M.D. (1978). The Instructional Quality Inventory. (NPRDC SR 79-3). San Diego: Navy Personnel Research and Development Center.

Yaremko, R.M., Harari, H., Harrison, R.C., & Lynn, E. (1986). *Handbook of Research and Quantitative Methods in Psychology*. Hillsdale, NJ: Lawrence Erlbaum.

Chapter
8

Pilot Testing

Chapter Objectives

After completing this chapter, you should be able to:

1. Identify the purposes of pilot testing.
2. Identify the levels of pilot testing.
3. Describe methods for pilot testing instruments.
4. Describe methods for pilot testing the research design, data collection and analysis procedures.
5. Identify methods used to pilot test curriculum and related educational materials.
6. Identify methods used to pilot test mass media.

Key Terms

alpha test
beta test
cultural sensitivity
cultural tailoring
field test/field study

mini-pilot/prepilot
pilot test/pilot study
preliminary review
readability level

Introduction

The pilot test is the dress rehearsal for the evaluator. Before a new Broadway play is performed for the public, a dress rehearsal takes place. It is at this point when all the musical pieces, dance routines, soliloquies and other aspects of the play are "put together." Often, when one practices for a play, individual scenes are worked on, but the transition from one scene to another, and the total effect of the play, is not experienced until the dress rehearsal. It is the last chance to "fine tune" the play before the public experiences the production. Musical numbers are refined, perhaps changed, shortened, or modified in some other way. Lines are practiced one final time not only to be repeated accurately, but for emotional affect and delivery as well. The dress rehearsal is an essential aspect of the preparation of the play.

As evaluators, our dress rehearsal process is known as the **pilot test** or performing the **pilot study**. When preparing for an evaluation project, developing instruments, determining data collection procedures, and so on, there is much "fine-tuning" to do before we implement the primary study. Pilot tests allow us to make those necessary adjustments. Pilot tests allow us to assess the quality of our instruments, curriculum materials, public service announcements, and other materials and activities before they are reproduced and released on a mass scale.

Pilot testing is important, yet many evaluators, even experienced evaluators, neglect to conduct even simple preliminary reviews of materials. Such neglect is unfortunate because evaluators could correct many mistakes regarding reading levels, multi-cultural sensitivity issues, instructions, data collection procedures, curriculum materials and other things, if they would take the time to conduct a pilot test. As Sudman and Bradburn (1986) suggest regarding instrument development: "If you don't have the resources to pilot test your questionnaire, don't do the study" (p.283). We agree with their statement, and recommend that pilot tests be conducted whenever any evaluation or curriculum development effort takes place.

The Purposes of Pilot Testing

The pilot test (sometimes called the *pilot study*, the *shake-down test*, or the *end-to-end test*) refers to a set of procedures used by evaluators with a small group of subjects to simulate the evaluation study or program that is to be implemented at a later date. A pilot test is conducted to detect any problems with the data collection instruments, data collection procedures, data analysis procedures, curriculum materials and instructional strategies, and mass media. If problems are detected, they can be corrected before the program is implemented on a large scale.

Borg and Gall (1989) identify several reasons for conducting pilot tests:

- Pilot tests allow for an initial testing of hypotheses or ideas, which then enables the evaluator to refine the hypotheses as ideas for the final study.

- Pilot tests produce information evaluators may not have initially considered. This new information may help evaluators expand or reduce the scope of their studies or programs.
- Pilot tests enable evaluators to appraise the data collection and statistical analysis procedures.
- Pilot tests reduce problems with the curriculum because they uncover problems early so there is time to correct them.
- Pilot tests help evaluators decide if it is worthwhile to conduct the present evaluation study; pilot tests may reveal that proposed evaluation designs are not accomplishing the goals of the evaluation projects.
- From pilot test subjects, evaluators can obtain feedback, which will help improve curriculum materials or instruments.
- Evaluators can try out different instruments during pilot tests; evaluators can use the best instruments for the actual study.

To their list we add:

- Pilot tests can help determine the cultural appropriateness of instruments, data collection procedures, curriculum materials, public service announcements, etc.
- Pilot tests help estimate the costs (money, equipment, people, time) of running the actual evaluation study.
- Pilot tests allow for an estimate of the actual costs of running a program over time.
- Pilot tests enable evaluators to assess "political issues" that may be related to implementing the program on a large scale. For example, Thomas, Cahill, and Santilli (1997) describe a pilot test they conducted regarding a computer-based instruction program on sex education. They indicated that "While the field test was successful overall, a number of problems and challenges encountered were relevant to broader dissemination of the intervention. To gain access to local programs, project staff often had to go through gatekeepers at the state or local administrative levels" (p.83).
- Successful pilot testing increases the "marketability" of the health education program, and makes it easier for administrators to allow the program to be implemented at their respective sites (Thomas, et al., 1997).

Pilot testing is sometimes called pretesting. We do not advise using this term for conducting pilot tests, because the term "pretest" has special meaning in experimental and quasi-experimental design (see Chapter 10) as a test or assessment of human subjects prior to their receiving a treatment or intervention.

In the best of circumstances, you should conduct your pilot test in the same manner as the proposed study. Pilot test subjects should be as similar as possible to the subjects who will take part in your actual evaluation project. The evaluator should contact the pilot subjects, administer data collection instruments and treatments, and record and analyze data in as similar a way as possible to the actual study. For example, suppose your task is to evaluate the effects of a cardiovascular disease prevention and health promotion program being implemented through Minnesota's public health departments. You might try to conduct a pilot test in a few counties in Wisconsin, just across the border. For most intents and purposes, the people in Wisconsin will be like those in Minnesota, and thus, would make a good pilot test group for the study. In the pilot test, the people would receive the instruments and treatments in the same way as the Minnesotans will. The study would just be conducted on a smaller scale.

During the pilot test the evaluator will be able observe how well the materials are being used (e.g., whether educational materials are understood and used easily, whether people are able to respond to survey items without needing much clarification about the items) and also gather opinions about the strengths and weaknesses of the instruments, procedures, and curriculum materials through open-ended interviews and other techniques from pilot test subjects.

Levels of Pilot Testing

We categorize pilot tests into four levels. Presented in order of usual occurrence, the levels are:

- *Preliminary review.* Your colleagues help you conduct a **preliminary review**. They will not necessarily represent your target population, yet they will identify major flaws in procedures, instruments, curriculum materials, and so on.
- *Mini-pilot or prepilot.* Once materials and methods have been reviewed by a panel of your colleagues, and you have made the recommended changes, then it is time for a **mini-pilot**, also known as a **prepilot**. Mini-pilots allow the evaluator to test the materials with a small group of subjects. Usually, the evaluator will put together a group of five or six subjects, and have the people work with the materials as they would be used in the actual study. With a mini-pilot, qualitative procedures such as observations, personal interviews, and focus groups with the key stakeholders (e.g., students, teachers, and data collectors) can be used to examine the quality of the materials.
- *Pilot testing.* Once the changes which have been identified through the mini-pilot have been made, then the actual **pilot test** can be conducted. In a pilot test, the evaluator will seek out a sample of subjects which are as similar as possible to the target population, take part in the "dress rehearsal" of the study. Sudman and Bradburn (1986) recommend 20 to 50 subjects for a pilot test. During the pilot test, both qualitative procedures (e.g., observations, interviews, focus groups) as well as quantitative procedures (e.g., utilization of test scores, attrition rates, effect sizes) will be used. Subjects are asked their opinions about the materials, and the performance of the subjects will be monitored.

■   *Field testing.* The **field test** or **field study** is the final pilot test of the materials. Field testing is done in various sites out in the "real world." Up to this point, subjects may be invited to facilities convenient for both the evaluators and the subjects. However, for the final field test, it must be done in the field -- sites like those to be used for the actual study. With a field test, experimental designs or quasi-experimental designs might be used in addition to qualitative procedures. The field test is the "last chance" to catch any problems with the materials being tested. In addition, the field test may be the actual "dress rehearsal." To this point, the pilot testing might have examined bits and pieces of the program, but it may not have put the total program together. This "end-to-end" test is important because it allows people to estimate, not only the complexity, but the time and costs for implementing the program. If we are evaluating a new curriculum, to this point in the pilot testing process, only curriculum developers may have served as instructors. In the field test, the curriculum is implemented by "real live" teachers.

Not all four levels in the pilot testing process will be used for all evaluations. A preliminary review of materials by colleagues is absolutely essential for all evaluation studies, and at a minimum, a mini-pilot or pilot test ought to be conducted. For large scale studies, it would be prudent to utilize all four levels of pilot testing.

A common question is: "Can we use our pilot-test subjects as subjects in our main study?" The quick and simple answer is "no" -- at least not usually. Pilot test subjects should not be used in the main study because these subjects already will have been exposed to the curriculum materials, instruments, and data collection techniques, which may cause a change in the subjects' attitudes, beliefs, behaviors, or knowledge. Their expectations about the project under investigation may be different from those of their peers who have not been exposed previously to the materials and methods. For these reasons, we recommend that pilot subjects be recruited from regions outside the main study area, or at a minimum, not be included in the main study, if the pilot test subjects are from the main study target population region.

Pilot Testing the Research Design

One of the most basic questions to address in a pilot study is whether or not the evaluation design that has been selected for the main study is an appropriate one. For example, suppose an ambitious *Solomon 4-Group Design* (see Chapter 10) was selected to evaluate the effects of a drug education program. How difficult will it be to implement the design? What logistical issues will need to be taken care of so the evaluation will proceed smoothly? Perhaps, after conducting a field test, we find out that using a relatively complex approach such as a *Solomon 4-Group Design* will not work in our study setting. We can then adjust to a simpler design that still employs control and intervention groups.

We might also try out a particular design (e.g., longitudinal design) and determine that we are not getting the number of subjects we need to participate in the pilot test. If we have selected subjects carefully, but still cannot get them to participate, it may suggest that we should take a serious look at selecting another design -perhaps, a case-control design, to address the situation at hand.

Thus, a pilot test will tell us if we have a reasonable chance to implement the type of research design we have selected for the main study. If we cannot implement it successfully in the pilot study, there is little chance that we will be successful in the main study.

Pilot Testing Instruments

Pilot testing instruments is also an important aspect of the instrument design process. When we are pilot testing our instruments, we are trying to determine what is the best method of obtaining information from our subjects? Do they prefer open-ended questions or forced-choice questions? Do they find the instruments easy or difficult to complete? Oganowski, Detert, Bradley, and Schindler (1996) pilot tested a series of instruments to collect data from elementary school children concerning health topics which were covered by teachers. They found that although some items on the questionnaire worked well, four items did not provide verifiable information. In addition, the pilot test indicated that not only did data need to be collected from the youngsters, it also needed to be collected from the teachers, to verify the content areas the youngsters indicated they were exposed to throughout the year. Figure 8.1 outlines issues which must be considered when evaluating data collection instruments.

- cover letters
- directions
- content
- cultural sensitivity
- item appropriateness
- format
- return instructions
- materials needed for instrument completion
- readability
- ease of administration
- reliability and validity

Figure 8.1 Considerations for Pilot Testing Instruments

Cover letter. Cover letters set the tone for the study. They must describe the purpose of the study succinctly, why potential respondents ought to participate, and what benefits the study will yield. In short, a good cover letter arouses interest about the study. In addition, the cover letter should contain a clear statement concerning confidentiality or anonymity of responses (Stacy, 1987). Finally, the cover letter ought to have a human subjects statement in it, indicating that the study has been reviewed and approved by the institutional review board of the sponsoring institution (see Chapter 3).

Directions. Directions must be clear and concise (Stacy, 1987). Subjects must be able to answer each item. That is, they must be in a position to possess the information that is being requested. Moreover, if a subject who is completing a questionnaire has a question, directions must specify to whom the question can be directed. A pilot test will confirm whether the evaluator has addressed the issue of directions adequately.

Content. Content in this case refers primarily to content validity issues (see Chapter 7). Does the questionnaire address the issues of interest in the evaluation adequately? Are items missing or are there items that are redundant or not needed? The overall content of the survey can be refined through pilot test procedures.

Cultural sensitivity. The evaluator must ensure that items are not written in a manner that is offensive to the target audience, and that they are readily understood by the intended audience. In the best scenario, some **cultural tailoring** (Pasick, D'Onofrio & Otero-Sabogal, 1996) is involved whereby members of the intended audience participate in the identification, selection, preparation, and approval of items. The broad issue of **cultural sensitivity** is discussed in greater detail later in this chapter.

Item appropriateness. Items need to be examined carefully during the pilot testing phase. Appropriateness of demographic items, as well as a review of response options to ensure they are mutually exclusive and exhaustive, is critical. In addition, for constructed-response types of items (e.g., fill-in-the blank, essays -- see Chapter 6), adequate space must be provided for responses (Stacy, 1987). Moreover, items should be grouped together by type (e.g., Likert, true-false) as well as by content area. Most importantly, one must be satisfied that the questions and the response options are not too difficult for the intended audience to complete. In preparing items, one must remember that if "you don't ask it now, you can't analyze it later." The converse of this statement is worthy of perhaps even more consideration. That is, if "you aren't going to analyze it, or only think you *might* analyze it, then don't ask it." Information that is valid and reliable, even if limited in scope, is still likely to tell you more than an assortment of items whose value is dubious, and whose inclusion has made the completion process more difficult for potential respondents.

Format. Format refers to the design of the questionnaire. Is it aesthetically pleasing, or is it visually "too busy" with the investigators trying to "cram" too much onto the paper? Have the items and the response options been placed in a way that is "user-friendly?" Is the questionnaire too long given the audience of interest and the method of data collection? How well (i.e., professionally) has the questionnaire been reproduced? With the relative sophistication of today's technology that includes both computer-generated text and graphics, professional looking questionnaires are the norm, and anything of a lesser quality is likely to be regarded as a low priority by potential respondents.

Return instructions. Return instructions are important both for reasons of confidentiality and for ensuring that the evaluator will receive the questionnaires in a timely manner. If you are surveying students in a class, they need to know if they are to return the questionnaire to the instructor, someone other than the instructor, place it in a sealed envelope, or follow some other procedure. If the instrument is to be returned by mail, it should be indicated consistently in several places (e.g., cover letter, directions for completion, at the end of the questionnaire) to where the instrument should be returned. Many a questionnaire has sat uncompleted on a potential respondent's desk because of the lack of clear guidelines as to where and by when the instrument should be returned. Details for handling mailed surveys are covered in Chapter 12.

Materials needed for instrument completion. Essential materials for instrument completion can sometimes be overlooked by even experienced evaluators. If you are using optical scan sheets for instrument completion where respondents "bubble in" their answers, you will need an ample supply of "number 2 pencils." In addition, respondents will need adequate space to complete the forms, adequate lighting to see what they are doing, and adequate privacy to protect confidentiality or anonymity. If people are completing surveys in public places such as shopping malls (or university students standing in a line to pay their fees or complete their course registration process), clipboards may need to be provided to facilitate a successful data collection operation. Once again, pilot testing is the key to uncovering oversights that later on could prove to be confounding embarrassments.

Readability. It is important for the evaluator to know the **readability level** required to complete the instrument under consideration (Stacy, 1987). There are a number of methods used to assess the readability of an instrument, since readability can refer to reading ease, reading interest, or other related constructs. Reading ease is probably the most common element of readability assessed in the pilot testing of instruments. A frequently used procedure for assessing this type of readability is the SMOG index first reported by McLaughlin (1969). The SMOG procedure estimates readability as a "grade level," an important element to know since anything written for general consumption should be no higher than the eighth-grade level, and some written materials being directed at audiences known to be of lower literacy should be a maximum of sixth-grade level. The National Cancer Institute's (1992) use of the SMOG readability analysis is illustrated in Figure 8.2.

Ease of administration. It is essential to assess the ease of administration of the instrument during the pilot test. How easily can the evaluators disseminate the instrument? How easy is it for subjects to complete the instrument? How long does it take on average to complete the instrument? Do subjects have a lot of questions concerning the interpretation of items, or how to complete the items, during the pilot test? The pilot test is the opportunity for the evaluator to ensure that the instrument is as "user-friendly" as possible. Often, if an instrument is difficult to understand, people will not complete it (or they will complete it in a manner that provides erroneous information).

Reliability and Validity. The pilot test provides the evaluator with preliminary data which can be used to assess instrument reliability and validity (see Chapter 7). Data collected from pilot subjects allow for the calculation of reliability coefficients, and reviews by expert panelists permit an assessment of content validity and other relevant instrument characteristics.

The SMOG Readability Formula *

To calculate the SMOG reading grade level, begin with the entire written work that is being assessed, and follow these four steps:

1.   Count off 10 consecutive sentences near the beginning, in the middle, and near the end of the text.
2.   From this sample of 30 sentences, circle [or underscore] all of the words containing three or more syllables (polysyllabic), including repetitions of the same word, and total number of words circled.
3.   Estimate the square root of the total number of polysyllabic words counted. This is done by finding the nearest perfect square, and taking its square root.
4.   Finally, add a constant of three to the square root. This number gives the SMOG grade, or the reading grade level that a person must have reached if he or she is to fully understand the text being assessed.

A few additional guidelines will help to clarify these directions:

- A sentence is defined as a string of words punctuated with a period (.), an exclamation point (!) or a question mark (?).
- Hyphenated words are considered as one word.
- Numbers which are written out should also be considered, and if in numeric form in the text, they should be pronounced to determine if they are polysyllabic.
- Proper nouns, if polysyllabic, should be counted, too.
- Abbreviations should be read as unabbreviated to determine if they are polysyllabic.

Not all pamphlets, fact sheets, or other printed materials contain 30 sentences. To test a text that has fewer than 30 sentences:

- Count all the polysyllabic words in the text.
- Count the number of sentences.
- Find the average number of polysyllabic words per sentence as follows:

Average = Total # of polysyllabic words ÷ Total # of sentences

Figure 8.2 Using the SMOG Readability Method

Adapted from: National Cancer Institute. (1992). *Making Health Communication Programs Work: A Planner's Guide*. Washington, DC: USDHHS, NIH Publication # 92-1493, pp.77-79.

* *This pamphlet is from the American Cancer Society*

- Multiply that average by the number of sentences *short of 30*.
- Add that figure on to the total number of polysyllabic words.
- Find the square root and add the constant of 3.

Perhaps the quickest way to administer the SMOG grading test is by using the SMOG conversion table. Simply count the number of polysyllabic words in your chain of 30 sentences and look up the approximate grade level on the chart. An example of how to use the SMOG Readability Formula and the SMOG Conversion Table is provided.

Example Using the SMOG Readability Formula:
(*Sample only - Information may not be current.*)

(1) In Controlling Cancer — You Make a Difference
(2) The key is action. **(3)** You can help protect yourself against cancer. Act promptly to: **(4)** Prevent some cancers through simple changes in lifestyle. **(5)** Find out about early detection tests in your home. **(6)** Gain peace of mind through regular medical checkups.

Cancers You Should Know About
(7) Lung cancer is the number one cancer among men, both in the number of new cases each year (79,000) and deaths (70,500). **(8)** Rapidly increasing rates are due mainly to cigarette smoking. **(9)** By not smoking, you can largely prevent lung cancer. **(10)** The risk is reduced by smoking less, and by using lower tar and nicotine brands.
But quitting altogether is by far the most effective safeguard. The American Cancer Society offers Quit Smoking Clinics and self-help materials.

Colorectal cancer is second in cancer deaths (25,100) and third in new cases (49,000). When it is found early, chances of cure are good. A regular general physical usually includes a digital examination of the rectum and a guaiac slide test of a stool specimen to check for invisible blood. Now there are also Do-It-Yourself Guaiac Slides for home use. Ask your doctor about them. After you reach the age of 40, your regular check-up may include a "Procto," in which the rectum and part of the colon are inspected through a hollow, lighted tube.

(11) Prostate cancer is second in the number of new cases each year (57,000), and third in deaths (20,600). **(12)** It occurs mainly in men over 60. **(13)** A regular rectal exam of the prostate by your doctor is the best protection.

A Check-Up Pays Off
(14) Be sure to have a regular, general physical including an oral exam. **(15)** It is your best guarantee of good health.

Figure 8.2 Continued

How Cancer Works

(16) If we know something about how cancer works, we can act more <u>effectively</u> to protect ourselves against the disease. Here are the basics:

- **(17)** ■ Cancer spreads; time counts — Cancer is <u>uncontrolled</u> growth of <u>abnormal</u> cells. **(18)** It begins small and if unchecked, spreads. **(19)** If <u>detected</u> in an early, local stage, the chances for cure are best.
- **(20)** ■ Risk <u>increases</u> with age — This is not a reason to worry, but a signal to have more <u>regular</u>, thorough <u>physical</u> check-ups. Your doctor or clinic can advise you on what tests to get and how often they should be performed.
- ■ What you can do — Don't smoke and you will sharply reduce your chances of getting lung cancer. Avoid too much sun, a major cause of skin cancer. Learn cancer's Seven Warning Signals, listed on the back of this leaflet, and see your doctor promptly if they persist. Pain usually is a late symptom of cancer; don't wait for it.

Unproven Remedies

Beware of unproven cancer remedies. They may sound appealing, but they are usually worthless. Relying on them can delay good treatment until it is too late. **(21)** Check with your doctor or the <u>American</u> Cancer <u>Society</u>.

More Information

(22) For more <u>information</u> of any kind about cancer — free of cost, contact your local unit of the <u>American</u> Cancer <u>Society</u>.

Know Cancer's Seven Warning Signals

- **(23)** ■ Change in bowel or bladder habits.
- **(24)** ■ A sore that does not heal.
- **(25)** ■ <u>Unusual</u> bleeding or discharge.
- **(26)** ■ <u>Thickening</u> or lump in breast or elsewhere.
- **(27)** ■ <u>Indigestion</u> or <u>difficulty</u> in <u>swallowing</u>.
- **(28)** ■ <u>Obvious</u> change in wart or mole.
- **(29)** ■ Nagging cough or hoarseness.

(30) If you have a warning signal, see your doctor.

We have calculated the reading level for this example. Compare your results to ours, then check both with the SMOG conversion table.

Figure 8.2 Continued

Readability Test Calculations

Total number of polysyllabic words	=38
Nearest Perfect Square	=36
Square Root	= 6
Constant	= 3
SMOG Reading Grade Level	= 9

SMOG Conversion Table *

Total Polysyllabic Word Counts	Approximate Grade Level ($\pm$ 1.5 Grades)
0-2	4
3-6	5
7-12	6
13-20	7
21-30	8
31-42	9
43-56	10
57-72	11
73-90	12
91-110	13
111-132	14
133-156	15
157-182	16
183-210	17
211-240	18

---

*   Developed by: Harold C. McGraw, Office of Educational Research, Baltimore County Schools, Towson, Maryland.

Figure 8.2 Continued

Pilot Testing Data Collection and Sampling Methods

Another important aspect of the pilot test is the assessment of the appropriateness of the data collection procedures and sampling procedures used in the study. Related to the notion of testing the research design for the main study, a pilot test will be able to help the evaluator estimate how practical the proposed data collection procedures and sampling plan are for the main study. Issues to be considered here include: logistics, procedures for completing forms when personal interviews take place, sampling designs, methods of collecting the data, and response rates.

Logistics

Project logistics refer, in part, to considering the issues related to time, tasks, talents, and equipment needed to implement the study. These issues have been presented in detail in Chapter 4. A few reminders are presented below.

The pilot test will allow the evaluator to determine how long it will take to put the project together. For example, how long will it take to reproduce and collate any questionnaires? If using a mail survey, how long will it take to get the mailing labels together, to send postcards that alert people that a survey will be delivered in a few days, or most importantly, perhaps, how long will it take for a reasonable sample size to be garnered through the mail (or any other method of data collection, for that matter)? Through the pilot test, one is able to determine with reasonable accuracy how much and what kinds of labor are needed to complete the study.

Completing Forms

A basic point of any pilot test is determining how long it will take a subject to complete a questionnaire, and whether any support materials or staff are needed to facilitate the completion of forms. Other considerations may include the content and number of training sessions required for research assistants to complete forms accurately, if they are collecting data from people directly. In addition, the pilot test is the time to ascertain whether people are providing ambiguous information on surveys, or if they are leaving large numbers of items blank (or consistently leaving one item blank), suggesting a need for questionnaire redesign. From the perspective of instrument reliability, pilot tests also allow data collectors to develop consistent approaches for interviewing people, thus increasing the reliability of both data collection procedures and instrumentation.

Sampling Designs

Pilot testing helps to identify the best sampling design for your study (see Chapter 13). If the study depends on data collectors determining who will take part in the study (e.g., if evaluators instruct data collectors to randomly select three city blocks, and then randomly select residents of houses in each block to complete the questionnaire), a pilot test allows evaluators to test the degree to which data collectors are able to implement the sampling design.

Even if the evaluator directly draws the sample of subjects, the pilot test is useful in determining if that sampling procedure is a plausible way of obtaining subjects for the study. For instance, if in using a random sampling design one finds that a particular subgroup is underrepresented in the pilot test (e.g., African American public health workers), then the evaluator may choose to over-sample that group using a weighted stratified random sampling procedure. In doing so, the evaluator might ensure that African American physicians have twice the probability of being selected as non-African American physicians. Performing this step helps to guarantee that an important subgroup's beliefs, attitudes, experiences, and so on are adequately represented in the study.

Data Collection Procedures

A critical decision to be made when planning the evaluation is the determination of the methods to be used to collect data for the study (see Chapter 12). For example, if one is using a questionnaire as an evaluation tool, should the data be collected on site? Should phone interviews be used, or mail surveys? How about e-mail and the Internet? Should we use personal interviews? Each of these methods has its advantages and disadvantages. Personal interviews may allow people to expand on their answers, and clarify any questions the evaluator may have of the subjects. However, personal interviews are costly in terms of time, for both the evaluator and the subject. In addition, people may be reluctant to talk about personal issues (e.g., drinking behavior, sexual behavior) in a personal interview, but in an anonymous paper-and-pencil survey format, feel more comfortable about describing their experiences. Phone surveys might be practical for some groups but not for others. Likewise, using the Internet might a good adaptation for some situations, but certainly not for all situations, topics, and people. Through pilot testing, the evaluator will be able to assess response rates and quality of data, and determine which approach is the best approach for gathering data.

Another issue related to data collection procedures is the time and setting of the study. It is known that many people experience anxiety when visiting their health care provider, and as a result, may find that their blood pressure is higher by a few points than it might be under other circumstances. If one is doing a study with college students, woe to the evaluator who sends out a questionnaire around the time of midterm or final exams. There are simply some times and settings which are better for data collection than other times and settings. A pilot test will help address these issues.

Also related to the topic of data collection is the time it takes to participate in the study. Will it take five or ten minutes to complete the questionnaire, or two hours? This consideration is especially important when gathering data by telephone. Any instrument which takes more than ten minutes to administer over the phone should be revised! Another practical issue related to time is occurs when we are studying youngsters in the school. We must make sure our data collection procedures can be completed in the allotted time frame we have, and, we must make sure that the youngsters have the patience to complete the questionnaire. Whereas a high school senior might be able to spend 30 minutes on an interview or questionnaire, a kindergartner may only be able to focus on the task for five minutes or less!

Pilot tests are useful in helping us estimate response rates for our instruments. If in a pilot test, we find that we only have a 25% response rate, and we need at least 200 subjects to accommodate a particular statistical power, we will either have to survey about 800 subjects to get an acceptable return rate, or, we will have to change our data collection methods.

Pilot Testing Data Analysis Procedures

The pilot test is the ideal opportunity to examine the appropriateness of the proposed data analysis scheme. Using data obtained during the pilot test, evaluators can verify the process used for coding data into the computer, making other coding decisions, and selecting the best data analysis techniques for the study.

Codebooks and data coding. The process for coding data should be pilot tested. How will data be entered into a computer for analysis? Will optical scan sheets be used? What quality control mechanisms will be implemented to ensure data accuracy? Is it better to take the information from the data form directly and enter it into a computer, or is it better to develop an intermediate coding form, and then enter the data into a computer? Some of these decisions are merely a matter of style, but of primary importance is that data are recorded and entered accurately.

Through the pilot test you will find out how long it takes to code a questionnaire or other data form for the computer. Suppose it takes 15 minutes to code one questionnaire, and there are 15,000 questionnaires in all. One needs to be sure that there is enough personnel support to complete the project within the expected time frame. If such a coding procedure is too time-consuming, then it may be wiser to save time by having respondents code their own answers on an optical scan sheet as they complete the survey. This time-saving idea must be weighed against the possibility of adding unnecessary complexity to the respondents' directions, and risking having them perform the coding incorrectly.

An important element of the coding process is the development of the codebook (see Chapter 4). The codebook provides information and descriptions of each variable. The codebook may be thought of as the road map for the data set, and must be useful to persons who were not responsible for the creation of the variables, or for the actual coding.

During the coding process, evaluators must make a series of decisions about the data. For instance, how will "missing data" be coded and treated? How will a response be coded if one gives *two answers* on a survey? What will one code if, on a five-point scale, one marks "3.5" instead of a "3" or a "4" (not an uncommon occurrence)? Will only those persons who have answered every item be included in the analysis, or will all data that *can be used* get considered? What we are talking about here is what are called *decision rules*, which must be thought through prior to the initiation of data entry and analysis. You will want data coders to be making logical and consistent decisions, and the pilot test is a means for anticipating the types of decisions that will need to be made.

For certain kinds of data, special decisions may need to be made. To take a simple example, will some items be combined to form a scale, and thus, yield a scale score rather than just a score for an individual item? What values will be assigned to the item responses? Will all response values be weighed equally? Will some items need to be "reverse coded" to be interpreted? If so, when will that happen — as the data are being entered, or after the data are entered? Figure 8.3 shows how a simple demographic item could be coded two ways, depending on how the data are to be used in the analysis.

Please circle the racial or ethnic group with which you most identify yourself.

> White
> African American
> Hispanic
> Asian
> Native American
> Other

This variable could be coded categorically as one variable:

> 1=White
> 2=African American
> 3=Hispanic
> 4=Asian
> 5=Native American
> 6=Other

Alternatively, this variable could be coded dichotomously as six variables:

1=White 0=non-White	1=Asian 0=non-Asian
1=African American 0=non-African American	1=Native American 0=non-Native American
1=Hispanic 0=non-Hispanic	1=Other 0=non-Other

Figure 8.3 Coding Possibilities for Racial/Ethnic Group Variable

Quality control of the data set. As noted repeatedly, data quality is just about everything to the success of an evaluation. You can use an elaborate sampling design and an elegant data collection instrument, but, if you are not careful in coding data and checking their accuracy, actual results will be compromised. We recommend that a ten percent sample of data be checked for accuracy by comparing what is recorded in the computer data file with the original data forms. If errors are present in the sample, then it is recommended that the entire data set be checked for accuracy before proceeding with analysis and report preparation. The evaluator also can run some preliminary statistical analyses to ensure that all responses have been coded within acceptable bounds of the questions. For example, if item 1 is "gender," and has only two possible coded responses (1=female or 2=male), then there should be a range of only two scores coded into the computer. A "quick and dirty" test of the range of scores allows for inspection of whether the coding is within acceptable ranges. For the "gender" example, any entry except "1" or "2" would suggest an error was made (i.e., a miscode). Similar inspection of each variable will contribute substantially to the quality of the data set.

Data analysis techniques. Once the evaluator develops the codebook, makes coding decisions, codes and checks a sample of data for accuracy, and is satisfied that all things are proceeding smoothly, a trial run of the proposed data analysis can begin. For the evaluator, several questions should come to mind: *Do the data appear to fit the assumptions of the statistical tests which will be run for the main study? Is the proposed statistical software capable of performing the necessary statistical tests, and will your hardware (computer) run the software? Are there alternative analyses possible? Do you have the expertise available to interpret the results of the statistical tests?* The pilot test helps to confirm the best approaches for data analysis given the response patterns of your pilot subjects.

Pilot Testing Curricula

The heart of any health education program is its curriculum materials. All too often, materials are not pilot tested adequately before dissemination to the public. A pilot test of the curriculum materials will help to ensure that they are appropriate for the intended audience in terms of comprehension, clarity, effectiveness, and cultural relevance. The National Cancer Institute (1992) recommends six pilot testing (NCI calls it *pretesting*) methods. The method selected will depend upon context and whether the desired feedback needs to be individual, group, or nonparticipatory. These methods of pilot testing educational materials, including their strengths and limitations, are presented in Figure 8.4.

Another important aspect of pilot testing educational materials is making sure that they are appropriate for various cultural and ethnic groups. Research clearly indicates that however well intentioned we might be, our materials often are inadequate in addressing the needs of, or having the motivational appeal for, selected population subgroups. As Sabogal, et al. (1996) indicate: "Health education materials designed for the general public may be perceived as unattractive, irrelevant, or unclear by members of certain cultural groups" (p.S123). Massett (1996) found in a study of 26 nationally distributed breast cancer education print materials, that "though many of the artifacts displayed elements of cultural competency, all 26 failed to include components essential to reaching and impacting the designated target audience" (p.231). Formative research in the development of materials, as well as in their pilot testing, is ultimately "cost-efficient" (Massett, 1996, p.241). The National Cancer Institute (1992) guidelines for producing materials for ethnic minorities, displayed in Figure 8.5, provide some highlights about preparing materials for special audiences. In presenting them here, we do not intend that these guidelines should be substituted for good formative research, thorough pilot testing, or employing a skilled cultural or medical anthropologist to incorporate the subtle aspects of culture and language that contribute to program success.

I.   Individual

    A.   Self-administered Questionnaires (mailed or personally delivered)

Purpose: to obtain individual reactions to draft materials

Application: print or audiovisual materials

Number of Respondents: enough to see a pattern of response (minimum 20; 100-200 ideal)

Resources Required: list of respondents; draft materials; questionnaire; postage (if mailed); tape recorder or VCR (for audiovisual materials)

Pros: inexpensive; does not require staff time to interact with respondents (if mailed); can be anonymous for respondents; can reach homebound, rural, other difficult to reach groups; easy and usually quick for respondents

Cons: response rate may be low (if mailed); may require follow-up: may take long time to receive sufficient responses; respondents self-select (potential bias); exposure to materials isn't controlled; may not be appropriate for low literacy audiences

    B.   Individual Interviews (phone or in person)

Purpose: probe for individual's responses, beliefs, discuss range of issues

Application: develop hypotheses, messages, potentially motivating strategies; discuss sensitive issues or complex draft materials

Figure 8.4 Summary Pilot Testing Methods for Educational Materials

Adapted from: National Cancer Institute. (1992). *Making Health Communication Programs Work: A Planner's Guide*. Washington, DC: USDHHS, NIH Publication #92-1493, pp. 47-48.

Number of Respondents: Minimum of 10 per type of respondent

Resources Required: list of respondents; discussion guide/questionnaire; trained interviewer; telephone or quiet room; tape recorder

Pros: in-depth responses may differ from first response; can test sensitive or emotional materials; can test more complex/longer materials; can learn more about "hard-to-reach" audiences; can be used with individuals who have limited reading and writing skills

Cons: time consuming to conduct/analyze; expensive, and may yield no firmer conclusion or consensus

C. Central Location Intercept Interviews

Purpose: to obtain more quantitative information about materials/messages

Application: broad range, including concepts, print, audiovisual materials

Number of Respondents: 60-100 per type (enough to establish pattern of response)

Resources Required: structured questionnaire; trained interviewers; access to mall, school, other location; room or other place to interview; tape recorder or VCR (for audiovisual materials)

Pros: can quickly conduct large number of interviews; can provide "reliable" information for decision-making; can test many kinds of materials; quick to analyze closed-ended questions

Cons: short (10 minutes) interviews; incentive/persuasion needed for more time; cannot probe; cannot deal with sensitive issues; sample is restricted to individuals at the location; respondents choose to cooperate and may not be representative

II. Group

A. Focus Group Interviews

Purpose: to obtain in-depth information about beliefs, perceptions, language, interests, concerns

Application: broad; concepts, issues, audiovisual or print materials, logos/other artwork

Number of Respondents: 8-12 per group; minimum of 2 groups per type of respondent

Resources Required: discussion outline; trained moderator; list of respondents; meeting room; tape recorder; VCR (for audiovisual materials)

Figure 8.4 Continued

Pros: group interaction and length of discussion can stimulate more in-depth responses; can discuss concepts prior to materials development; can gather more opinions at once; can complete groups and analyses quickly; can cover multiple topics

Cons: too few respondents for consensus or decision-making; no individual responses (group influence) unless combined with other methods; can be expensive; respondents choose to attend, and may not be typical of the target population

B.   Theater Testing

Purpose: to test audiovisual materials with many respondents at once

Application: present audio or audiovisual materials

Number of Respondents: 60-100 per type (enough to establish pattern of response)

Resources Required: list of respondents; questionnaire; large meeting room; AV equipment

Pros: can test with many respondents at once; large sample may be more productive; can be inexpensive; can analyze quickly

Cons: few open-ended questions possible; can require more elaborate preparation; can be expensive if incentives required

III.   Nonparticipatory

A.   Readability Tests

Purpose: to assess reading comprehension skills required to understand print materials

Application: print materials

Number of Respondents: none

Resources Required: readability formula; 15 minutes

Pros: inexpensive; quick

Cons: "rule of thumb" only/not predictive; does not account for health terminology; no target audience reaction

---

Figure 8.4 Continued

Interaction with the target audience and "intermediaries" familiar with them is especially important when you are targeting ethnic minorities. Remember:

- Use of a language may vary for different cultural groups (e.g., a word may have different meanings to different groups).
- Differences in target groups extend beyond language to include diverse values and customs.
- Different kinds of channels may be credible and most capable of reaching minority audiences.
- Don't assume that "conventional wisdom," published research studies or "common knowledge" will hold true for minority audiences. The degree of assimilation and "mainstreaming" is everchanging, so *current* information will be needed to choose the best channels and message strategies.
- Message appeals should be developed separately for each minority group, since their perceived needs, values, and beliefs may differ from others.
- Print materials should be simply written, reinforced with graphics, and pretested. People perceive graphics and illustrations in different ways, just as their language skills differ.
- Using bilingual materials will assure that intermediaries and family members who are most comfortable with English can help the reader understand the content.
- Print materials should never be simply translated into English; concepts and appeals may differ by culture just as the words do.
- Audiovisual materials or interpersonal communication may be more successful for some messages and audiences.

Figure 8.5 Hints for Producing Materials for Ethnic Minorities

Adapted from: National Cancer Institute. (1992). *Making Health Communication Programs Work: A Planner's Guide*. Washington, DC: USDHHS, p.38.

In addition to the recommendations shown in Figure 8.5, consider the additional suggestions made by Sabogal, et al. (1996) for designing health education materials for special populations:

- Involve the target audience from the beginning of the development of the materials.
- Develop the programs in the native language of the target population.

- Understand and be sensitive to the diversity *within* racial and ethnic groups.
- Decide during the curriculum development process whether the materials should be universal or culture-specific (e.g., should you develop a Hispanic program or specific programs for persons of Mexican descent, Cuban descent, Puerto Rican descent, and so on).
- Deliver messages in innovative ways.
- Use testimonials from people who represent target audiences.
- Use visuals to make important points.
- Work with vendors within the target population.

Pilot Testing Computer-Based Instructional Materials

The usual curriculum quality issues discussed above relate to computer-based instruction as well. For example, materials need to be attractive, factually correct, and designed in a way that is culturally relevant to the target population. Computer-based pilot tests also uncover information not usually expected through other curriculum delivery modalities. Thomas, et al. (1997) found in their field test of a safer sex computer-based curriculum that certain administrators who were approached about the program were wary of computers in general, or thought it inappropriate to make a "game" out of a serious subject like HIV/AIDS. They also found in the field test that several people charged with implementing the program were uncomfortable in troubleshooting problems associated with computer-based instruction.

Hardin and Reis (1997) describe a number of issues that should be considered when developing and evaluating multimedia software. These characteristics are labeled as the four fundamental elements of multimedia development: *audience*, *objectives*, *methods*, and *evaluation*. The careful evaluator will look to see that issues are addressed adequately in the software being evaluated.

Audience. Audience refers to the target group for the computer-based program. Hardin and Reis (1997) suggest that issues such as age, gender, ethnicity, grade level, reading and math skills, motor skills, and learning style preferences ought to be considered during the design process. Particular attention ought to be placed on the cultural sensitivity and relevance of the materials.

Objectives. The goals and objectives of the program should match the instructional needs of the target audience. In addition to ensuring that content is compatible and appropriate for the audience, it is also helpful to know in more detail on what things the program is focusing. For instance, is a hypertension education program focusing on general information about high blood pressure, or is its purpose to change the behavior of a person with hypertension? Both programs focus on the topic of high blood pressure, but each one obviously has unique objectives.

Methods. What instructional methods are employed by the program? Drill and practice exercises might be the protocol when trying to learn the conjugation of verbs in the German language, but more creative, motivating, and exciting instructional techniques might be used to address other educational outcomes. The basic questions of concern are:

What techniques are being used? Are they appropriate for the content being covered? Are they appropriate for the target audience? Will they maintain the interest of the learner? The novelty of computer-based instruction, learning through the World Wide Web, and other technological innovations can only be captured and put to optimal work when the match between method and desired outcome is considered carefully.

Evaluation. The reference here is to the evaluation that took place during materials development. Software developers often use the terms **alpha test** and **beta test**. Alpha testing refers to the initial tests of the program, to make sure it is functioning correctly early in the developmental process. Beta testing refers to testing that occurs much later on, when the program is almost completed and can be reviewed by skilled experts who can fine tune the program. From our perspective, we want to ensure that both formative and summative procedures have been used to evaluate the program and related materials, and that the results of the summative evaluation have been favorable.

Estimating Project Costs

During the pilot test period is also an ideal time to obtain an accurate estimate of the costs for the total project (Aday, 1989). Using pilot test data, evaluators can determine the amount of labor involved in the project, the amount of time that is needed to take the project to completion, and the types and amount of equipment to implement the project.

Thomas, et al. (1997) found that the development of their initial software program (mentioned previously) and two kiosk "delivery systems" cost $58,000. They noted, however, that dissemination costs for the CD-ROM would be $5.00 per disk, and, that utilization of the World Wide Web would reduce costs significantly. Nevertheless, their analysis provides a benchmark for the development costs of their computer-based instruction program. Often, through a pilot test, one finds that the main study is too expensive, and that there will need to be ways to scale down the project. It is better to draw this conclusion during a pilot test than to have to curtail or extinguish a project already in operation.

The Revision Process

Through the pilot test process the evaluator will obtain a wealth of information concerning the curriculum and ancillary educational materials, the data collection instruments, the data collection methods, the overall research or project design, and the computer programs relevant to the project. The evaluator is left with the questions: *When should I make a change in materials or design? On what basis, or according to which criteria, should I make that change?* Generally, one looks at trends in pilot test results to make these decisions. If many people have trouble answering an item on a questionnaire, the item probably needs some fine tuning. If, on the other hand, just one person had trouble with a questionnaire, or with curriculum materials, changes may not be necessary.

With respect to instrument design, Babbie (1973) suggests that question clarity is a major issue to examine when evaluating questionnaire quality. For example, if a large number of people have "filled in" answers *next to* your selected-response items, have ignored items, frequently chosen "other" as their response, or have had to qualify their answers in some way, there is cause for concern, and a need for re-thinking, redesign, and probably, conducting another pilot study. Additionally, if there is little variance in responses to some items, the evaluator may need to change those items in some way to obtain more variation in response patterns.

For curriculum materials, observation in educational settings, as well as interviews with instructors and subjects (students) is likely to produce useful feedback for curriculum improvement. Massive bewilderment of the students accompanied by frustration experienced by teachers as they work through the materials should offer obvious clues concerning areas in need of modification and revision.

According to the National Cancer Institute (1992), pilot testing "cannot absolutely predict or guarantee learning, persuasion, behavior change or other measures of communication effectiveness," and further emphasizes that pilot testing "is not a substitute for experienced judgment. Rather, it can provide additional information from which you can make sound decisions" (p.38). In short, pilot testing provides program developers and evaluators with a wide range of ideas for program improvement, which, when combined with expert judgment, offers the greatest probability of conducting a successful project, and obtaining results that will be utilization-focused, and assist decision makers in making critical program and policy decisions.

Summary

The pilot test is one of the most important elements of the evaluation process. In this chapter, we described the reasons for conducting pilot tests, the different levels of pilot tests, and methods used to pilot test instruments, processes, designs, and analyses. The pilot test is the point where evaluators can detect many of the flaws in data collection instruments and methods, curriculum materials, software programs, or data analysis. It is far less expensive to make changes in plans and materials at this stage than it is after large scale duplication and dissemination have taken place. The chapter concluded with a discussion of methods used to pilot test curriculum materials, including computer-based instructional materials.

Case Study

Oganowski, J.L., Detert, R.A., Bradley, C., & Schindler, J. (1996) The Wisconsin elementary health education pilot project: On-site interviews of student learning and curricular integration. *Journal of Health Education*, *27*(4), 235-241.

Oganowski and colleagues describe a pilot project which examined the impact of health education preparation on experienced elementary school teachers in the delivery of a comprehensive school health elementary education program. Results of the pilot study indicated that those teachers who took part in the program appeared to be implementing a wide range of health education topics in an experiential and integrated manner, and their students were able to recall significantly more health content months later, compared to control group students. What were the strengths of their design? What were the weaknesses? Do you agree with their conclusions?

Student Questions/Activities

1. Select an existing questionnaire available to you on any health issue or problem of interest to you. Pilot test the questionnaire with people who are like those that comprise the target audience. What does the pilot test tell you? What needs to be changed?
2. Using an existing set of curriculum materials, conduct a small pilot test of these materials. What does this pilot test tell you? To what extent do you see a need to add to these materials or make refinements?
3. Conduct a theater test of a health-related video. In terms of the pilot testing process, what were the strengths of performing theater testing? What were the weaknesses?

Recommended Readings

Baldwin, J.A., Rolf, J.E., Johnson, J., Bowers, J., Bennaly, C., & Trotter, R.T. (1996). Developing culturally sensitive HIV/AIDS and substance abuse prevention curricula for Native American youth. *Journal of School Health, 66*(9), 322-327.

> This article describes how researchers and health care professionals worked with several Native American communities to develop an HIV/AIDS and substance abuse prevention partnership. Guidelines which emphasize extensive input from target groups and community members are proposed to assist in the development of materials that are sensitive to the needs and culture of the Native American people.

Turner, A., Singleton, N., Easterbrook, S. (1997). Developing sexual health software incorporating user feedback: A British experience. *Health Education & Behavior, 24*(1), 102-120.

> Turner and colleagues from the Department of Health Policy of the West Sussex Health Authority describe the process used to develop four computer software programs focusing on sexual issues for British youth. The iterative cycle of software development, based on a model of user review, feedback, subsequent program modification, and retesting, was used with approximately 150 youth to develop the programs.

Gilmer, M.J., Speck, B.J., Bradley, C., Harrell, J.S., & Belyea, M. (1996). The Youth Health Survey: Reliability and validity of an instrument for assessing cardiovascular health habits in adolescents. *Journal of School Health, 66,* 106-111.

Gilmer and co-workers describe the development of the Youth Health Survey, including the pilot test results related to reliability and validity of the instrument. They conclude that with minor revisions, the instrument will be appropriate for use in the study of youth risk factors related to cardiovascular disease.

References

Aday, L.A. (1989). *Designing and Conducting Health Surveys.* San Francisco: Jossey-Bass.

Babbie, E.R. (1973). *Survey Research Methods.* Belmont, CA: Wadsworth.

Borg, W.R., & Gall, M.D. (1989). *Educational Research: An Introduction,* 5th edition. White Plains, NY: Longman.

Hardin, P.C., & Reis, J. (1997). Interactive multimedia software design: Concepts, process and evaluation. *Health Education & Behavior, 24*(1), 35-53.

Massett, H.A. (1996). Appropriateness of Hispanic print materials: A content analysis. *Health Education Research: Theory and Practice, 11*(2), 231-242.

McLaughlin, G. (1969). SMOG grading — a new readability formula. *Journal of Reading, 12*(May), 639-646.

National Cancer Institute. (1992). *Making Health Communication Programs Work: A Planner's Guide.* Washington, DC: USDHHS, NIH Publication #92-1493.

Oganowski, J.L., Detert, R.A., Bradley, C., & Schindler, J. (1996). The Wisconsin elementary health education pilot project: On-site interviews of student learning and curricular integration. *Journal of Health Education, 27*(4), 235-241.

Pasick, R.J., D'Onofrio, C.N., & Otero-Sabogal, R. (1996). Similarities and differences across cultures: Questions to inform a third generation of health promotion research. *Health Education Quarterly, 23*(Supplement), S142-S161.

Sabogal, F., Otero-Sabogal, R., Pasick, R.J., Jenkins, C.N.H., & Perez-Stable, E.J. (1996). Printed health education materials for diverse communities: Suggestions learned from the field. *Health Education Quarterly,* 23(supplement), S123-S141.

Stacy, R.D. (1987). Instrument evaluation guides for survey research in health education and health promotion. *Health Education,* 18(5), 65-67.

Sudman, S., & Bradburn, N.M. (1986). *Asking Questions.* San Francisco: Jossey-Bass.

Thomas, R., Cahill, J., & Santilli, L. (1997). Using an interactive computer game to increase skill and self-efficacy regarding safer sex negotiation: Field test results. *Health Education & Behavior, 24*(1), 71-86.

Chapter
9

Needs Assessment and Strategic Planning

Chapter Objectives

After completing this chapter, you should be able to:

1. Define need.
2. Define and provide examples of needs assessments.
3. Define and provide examples of strategic and tactical plans.
4. Describe the reasons why we conduct needs assessments and develop strategic and tactical plans.
5. Identify and describe five types of needs assessment/strategic planning models.
6. Identify five data sets to be used in needs/assessment strategic planning activities.
7. Identify data collection techniques commonly used in strategic planning activities.
8. Design and implement a needs assessment for a local health department and develop a strategic and tactical plan for the program.

Key Terms

APEX-PH model
benchmarks
community analysis
need
needs assessment

PATCH model
PRECEDE-PROCEED model
strategic planning
SWOT analysis
tactical planning

Introduction

Suppose you move to a new town and visit a new primary care provider. It is common on an initial visit with a new provider that she or he will want to give you a "physical." That is, the provider will take a detailed health history, perhaps run some basic tests, and discuss with you your goals regarding the care she or he will provide. Perhaps you have some health related goals you wish to discuss at your initial visit (e.g., lose weight, start an exercise program, etc.). Perhaps, additional goals will come forth as a result of your physical examination (e.g., reduce intake of high fat foods due to a high cholesterol count). In a sense, when you visit your provider, you have some ideas about where you want to go regarding your personal health, and after the examination, the provider will provide you with additional input (e.g., you may think you have a cholesterol problem, but after testing, you may find that your cholesterol level is ok). By pooling your ideas and values with those of your health care provider, along with the results of the tests, you will come up with a treatment plan.

What is described above is analogous to the process of conducting needs assessments and developing strategic and tactical plans for communities. In the **needs assessment** process, we are actually giving a "physical" to the community. We run some basic tests (often in the form of analyses of epidemiologic data), and we solicit opinions from various community stakeholders through a variety of methods (e.g., surveys, focus groups, personal interviews) to identify the basic needs and problems of the community of interest. On the basis of this needs assessment, we develop a strategic plan which describes our goals for the program. From the strategic plan comes forth the tactical plan, which describes how we are going to attain our goals. The strategic and tactical plans are analogous to the treatment plan which you and your health care provider develop.

The determination of need as well as goals, objectives, and strategies to achieve those goals, is a value-laden process. Different people value different things. Therefore, the planning process must be thought of as a technical, as well as a political, process. Because of the political nature of planning, it is essential that program stakeholders be involved in the process from the initial design of the needs assessment to the final crafting of the tactical plan. Without input from stakeholders, the program is doomed to failure.

An Example of a Strategic Plan: *Healthy People 2000*

A strategic plan which received a decade of considerable attention is the *Healthy People 2000: National Health Promotion and Disease Prevention Objectives*, developed by the U.S. Department of Health and Human Services (1990). This planning document set forth the public health agenda for the United States until the year 2000. The plan drove state and local prioritization processes, funding decisions for grant-related efforts, as well as research agendas throughout the 1990's for the entire nation.

Healthy People 2000 was developed using a wide variety of sources, ranging from drug and alcohol surveys to maternal and child health data. To develop the objectives, experts representing almost 300 national organizations (e.g., the American Public Health Association, the American Medical Association), as well as staff from state health departments and the Institute of Medicine of the National Academy of Sciences, held eight regional hearings throughout the United States. Over 700 individuals and organizations attended these hearings. Once developed, over 10,000 people provided comments regarding the preliminary objectives.

Three broad goals came forth from the plan: to increase the span of healthy life for all Americans, to reduce health disparities among Americans, and to achieve access to preventive services for all Americans. From these three goals, a series of 22 priority areas, along with associated objectives, were developed (Figure 9.1).

For example, in the priority area related to tobacco use, one objective was:

Reduce cigarette smoking to a prevalence of no more than 15 percent among people aged 20 and older. (Baseline: 29 percent in 1987, 32 percent for men and 27 percent for women).

The objective is broken down further according to special target populations as shown in Figure 9.2. From this example, one can see that there is a set of objectives for the nation. Then, special sub-objectives for specific populations are identified. These types of objectives can be used to help create **benchmarks**, which can be used to compare future performance of a program in reference to an objective. In a sense, a benchmark is a special type of an objective. Accountants create benchmarks based on previous performance or expected future performance for companies and other organizations (Larson, Spoede & Miller, 1994). We, too, can use benchmarks in the development and evaluation of health education programs, and *Healthy People 2000*, along with other state and regional data, provide many objectives which can be used to craft the benchmarks.

Healthy People 2000 objectives are used by state and local health agencies as the basis for various initiatives. Upon review of relevant epidemiologic data, state public health planners can identify which objectives are being met, and in which regions of the state. Moreover, they can identify which objectives are not being met. For example, a certain region of the state may have a low teen birth rate (relative to *Healthy People 2000* objectives), yet high maternal smoking rates. Obviously, in that situation, resources should focus on the maternal smoking rates, while programs which have successfully maintained a low rate of teen pregnancy should be continued, but perhaps, with less emphasis than ones that address maternal smoking rate. In the end, this practice will be a judgment call, based on values. Having to make such a call underscores the importance of receiving stakeholder input in the planning process. In addition, these objectives can be used, not only to provide the focus for public health education programs, but also for evaluating the effectiveness of the programs, once they have been implemented. Health objectives for the coming decade, the successor to *Healthy People 2000*, are due to be published before the onset of the 21st century. The lessons learned in the previous decade have sparked much interest in the process for determining the health objectives through the year 2010, as well as the strategies for assessing their progress. As public health education professionals, you will, no doubt, play a role in this critical assessment process as you pursue your respective careers.

Health Promotion

1.	Physical Activity and Fitness
2.	Nutrition
3.	Tobacco
4.	Alcohol and Other Drugs
5.	Family Planning
6.	Mental Health and Mental Disorders
7.	Violent and Abusive Behavior
8.	Educational and Community-Based Programs

Health Protection

9.	Unintentional Injuries
10.	Occupational Safety and Health
11.	Environmental Health
12.	Food and Drug Safety
13.	Oral Health

Preventive Services

14.	Maternal and Infant Health
15.	Heart Disease and Stroke
16.	Cancer
17.	Diabetes and Chronic Disabling Conditions
18.	HIV Infection
19.	Sexually Transmitted Diseases
20.	Immunization and Infectious Diseases
21.	Clinical Preventive Services

Surveillance and Data Systems

22.	Surveillance and Data Systems

Age-Related Objectives

Children
Adolescents and Young Adults
Adults
Older Adults

Figure 9.1 *Healthy People 2000* Priority Areas

Source: U.S. Department of Health and Human Services. (1990). *Health People 2000*. Washington DC: Author.

Needs Assessment and Strategic Planning

Target Group	Population Prevalence 1987*	Target Prevalence 2000
People with high school education or less aged 20 and older	34%	20%
Blue collar workers aged 20 or older	36%	20%
Military personnel	42%	20%
Blacks aged 20 and older	34%	18%
Hispanics aged 20 and older	33%	18%
American Indians/Alaska Natives	42%-70%	20%
Southeast Asia men	55%	20%
Women of reproductive age	29%	12%
Pregnant women	25%	10%
Women who use oral contraceptives	36%	10%

Figure 9.2 *Healthy People 2000* Special Target Populations for Cigarette Smoking

* Some baseline prevalence data based on particular age groups, different tribes, or years other than 1987.

Definitions and Purposes of Needs Assessments and Strategic Plans

Needs assessments, as well as their associated strategic plans, are developed to address the notion of need. In that spirit, the fundamentals of assessing needs and developing plans are the same regardless of discipline. Whether one is trying to identify a market need from a business point of view, or a health need from a health educator's perspective, the general task is to identify needs, and then develop plans to address those needs.

What is a **need**? Needs are terms that are used rather loosely in everyday use. From a professional's point of view, we must be precise in differentiating needs from other things, such as wants or desires. *Webster's Third New International Dictionary* (1971) defines need in many ways:

- a necessary duty
- a want of something requisite, desirable, or useful
- a physiological or psychological requirement for the maintenance of homeostasis of an organism
- a condition requiring supply or relief
- want of the means of subsistence

Each of these definitions is in some way related to identifying health needs in populations. However, the fourth definition, focusing on "a condition requiring supply or relief" is probably best suited for our definition of needs assessment. McKillip (1987) argues that a need is "a value judgment that some group has a problem that can be solved" (p.10). He strongly emphasizes the notion that a need is a value judgment. This perspective suggests that what some people believe would be a need, others would not view in that way. Politics will enter into the equation of need, too, because of the differences in values among people. McKillip (1987) also differentiates among needs, wants, and demands. He suggests that a *want* is something for which people are willing to pay, while a *demand* is something for which people are willing to march!

From a public health perspective, needs are usually developed on the basis of normative data, or on projected socially desirable states for the target population being assessed. For example, one common approach to assessing needs by public health planners, is to compare data from the target population (e.g., county rates or special population rates of a disease) to those of neighboring counties, populations, or states. By comparing rates, one can determine if the target county's rates are higher (or lower) than desired rates. If a discrepancy is present, one might say there is a need for a program. For example, in the *Healthier People in Wisconsin* document produced by the Wisconsin Department of Health and Social Services (1990), data suggested that although infant mortality rates were 7.7 per 1,000 births among Whites, infant mortality rates were 17.3 per 1,000 births among Blacks. The Native American infant mortality rate was 20.7 per 1,000 births. These data strongly suggest that additional or revised prenatal care programs are needed for Black and Native American parents in the state of Wisconsin.

These prenatal data could also be used when employing the social definition of need as well. For instance, *Healthy People 2000* calls for a reduction in infant mortality deaths to 7 per 1,000 live births by the year 2000. In Wisconsin, rates among Whites were almost at the desired benchmark, whereas Black and Native American rates were much higher. Using the social definition of need would also suggest that Black and Native American prenatal care programs are in great need.

When conducting an assessment, a problem often arises when the target population is "healthier" than the comparison populations (either neighboring populations or an agreed upon standard). Do findings such as these suggest that the programs should be discontinued? That is a difficult judgment call by planners, because if a program is discontinued, the health of the population may deteriorate. However, if a target population is doing well in one area, and poorly in another, it may suggest that funds need to be reallocated to the problem areas. Again, values will be important in making this judgment.

What are the purposes of needs assessments and strategic plans? Kaufman (1988) suggests that needs assessments serve two functions: (1) they identify gaps between current results and required results; and, (2) they place those needs (gaps in results) in a priority order. **Strategic planning** is conducted to help organizations make decisions and actions that shape and guide what the organization is, what it does, and why it does it (Bryson, 1988). **Tactical planning** helps an organization decide how to implement the strategic plan (Eldert, 1996). A needs assessment should precede a strategic plan, and, both of these steps should occur prior to developing the tactical plan. Developing a strategic plan without first conducting a needs assessment is not a good idea! Developing a strategic plan without tactical considerations also represents poor decision making.

Several educators, public policy specialists, and health specialists have proposed reasons for conducting needs assessments and developing strategic plans (Bryson, 1988; Kaufman, 1988; McKillip, 1987; Stufflebeam, McCormick, Brinkerhoff & Nelson, 1988). A set of 11 reasons for conducting needs assessments and strategic plans, based on a synthesis of these writings, appears in Figure 9.3.

- To provide descriptive information concerning the target population.
- To identify target population needs (as well as "non-needs").
- To establish priorities, goals, and objectives.
- To provide descriptive information concerning other organizations in the target region that can help meet the needs of the population.
- To identify types and amounts of resources to be used to address priority needs (both internal and external to the organization).
- To provide a "blueprint" for the design, development, and implementation of a program.
- To provide benchmarks to be used in the evaluation of a program.
- To provide a systematic basis for which organizational decisions are made.
- To serve as a public relations tool.
- To create an awareness of a health problem.
- To provide defensible programmatic goals for an organization.

Figure 9.3 Reasons for Conducting Needs Assessments and Developing Strategic and Tactical Plans

Needs Assessment and Planning Models

A number of different types of needs assessment and strategic planning models have been proposed which are helpful to planners of health education and health promotion programs. It is our belief that a pragmatic and eclectic approach is ideal. Therefore, we believe that combining the best elements of different models is the preferred strategy when conducting a needs assessment.

According to any of the following models, the geographic region and target population must first be established before one begins to collect data. Sometimes this step is a relatively easy process. For example, if you are working in a county health department, the county will be the geographic region of your study, and the county residents (or some subset of its residents, e.g., pregnant women) will be your target population. However, for some types of projects, geographic or population boundaries are not so distinct. You may be the community health educator for a local hospital. What are the boundaries of your target area? Does the hospital serve all people, or does it have a specialized population for service? At first, these questions appear rudimentary. However, it has been our experience that many hours are spent looking at a map to determine the target areas for the needs assessment before data collection is initiated. These discussions must take place before the project is started.

Once geography and population characteristics are identified, the actual data collection can begin. It is always helpful to use a framework when collecting the data. Hence, the following models are provided to give some idea as to how you can structure your needs assessment, and strategic and tactical planning process.

Dignan and Carr's Model of Community Analysis

Dignan and Carr (1987) present a needs assessment model, which they describe as **community analysis**. This model details the various types of data which should be collected during a comprehensive needs assessment study. It outlines the different types of information, especially quantitative forms of data, which are useful in the needs assessment process. In all, they identify six categories of information are collected in the model:

Boundary information
- physical differences in health-related variables
- social differences in health-related variables

Backdrop information
- geographic characteristics
- business and commerce in the region
- demographic characteristics of the population
- social and political structure

Community health status
- vital statistics
- morbidity data

Community health care system
- manpower
- organization of service delivery

Community social assistance system
- participation in federal programs
- participation in local programs

Community diagnosis
- identify major health issues, their antecedents, methods to address the problems (using information described above)

Dignan and Carr's framework is an excellent way to begin thinking about the types of data which should be collected in a comprehensive needs assessment project. For example, people often fail to think in terms of "backdrop information," such as geography, business, and industry, but these factors contribute greatly to a community's health, both in a positive and a negative manner. It is well known that certain cancers cluster in particular geographic regions. The formation of these clusters is related to many factors, ranging from exposure to sunlight, to the industries and occupations in the region (Braus, 1996). By starting with this list, one can begin to identify the type of information that is needed, along with the sources of the information.

PRECEDE-PROCEED

This classic health education and health promotion needs assessment model was developed by Green, Kreuter, Deeds and Partridge (1980). Known originally as PRECEDE (predisposing, reinforcing, and enabling causes in educational diagnosis and evaluation), the model provided a solid conceptual and methodologic approach for the collection and analysis of needs assessment and program planning information. Since that time, this model has been refined, and published as the PRECEDE-PROCEED model (Green & Kreuter, 1991). In the revised version of the model, PRECEDE refers to *predisposing, reinforcing, and enabling constructs in educational/environmental diagnosis and evaluation.* PROCEED stands for *policy, regulatory, and organizational constructs in educational and environmental development.*

The **PRECEDE-PROCEED model** is comprised of nine components: social diagnosis, epidemiologic diagnosis, behavioral and environmental diagnosis, educational and organizational diagnosis, administrative and policy diagnosis, implementation, process evaluation, impact evaluation, and outcome evaluation. The model is unique in that it details all aspects of program administration, from the initial needs assessment aspects of program development to implementation, and to the final evaluation aspects of a program. This model emphasizes the importance of considering the evaluation activity up-front, during the needs assessment phase of program development.

PRECEDE-PROCEED begins with an assessment of the "quality of life" of the people being studied in the needs assessment. This social diagnosis examines a variety of indicators which can be used as measures of quality of life. These indicators include variables such as absenteeism rates, crime, crowding, illegitimacy, unemployment, and welfare rates. In addition to these variables, more qualitative variables are examined, such as the population's happiness, self-esteem, and hostility. Through an examination of these variables and others, an evaluation of the target population's quality of life can be made.

Next, the epidemiologic diagnosis takes place. The purpose of this phase is to study those health issues which have a major impact on the quality of life of the target population. Data collected in this phase include morbidity, mortality, and fertility variables. Other data which can be collected and analyzed include disability, discomfort, fitness, and risk factor data (e.g., CDC Behavioral Risk Factor Surveillance System data). These indicators are studied in relation to distribution, duration, prevalence, incidence, intensity, longevity, and functional level.

In the behavioral and environmental diagnosis phase of the assessment, behavioral as well as environmental factors related to the health status of the population are examined. This phase includes health behavior issues such as compliance to physician recommendations, consumption patterns, coping issues, prevention activities, self-care, and health care utilization of the population. The physical, economic, services, and social environments are also assessed at this time.

The process moves next to focus on educational and organizational diagnosis. In this phase, predisposing, reinforcing, and enabling factors related to health behavior, as well as the environment, are diagnosed. Predisposing factors include knowledge, attitudes, beliefs, values, and perceptions. Reinforcing factors are attitudes and behaviors of peers, parents, employers, as well as health personnel, while enabling factors relate to the availability and accessibility of resources, referral practices, rules or laws, and skills.

Next, an assessment of administrative and policy issues occurs. In this phase, the components of an effective program are developed and implemented on the basis of the data collected through the first four phases of the assessment. Public policy issues are also examined. Many of the gains made recently in public health have been related to public policy. For example, the reduction in drinking and driving rates, as well as decline in smoking rates are attributable, in part, to aggressive public policy measures implemented at the federal, state, and local levels. Public policy is an area that health educators often ignore, yet, increasingly, will be called upon to help shape.

The next phases, implementation, process evaluation, impact evaluation, and outcome evaluation, all relate to conducting the program, as well as the assessment of the program while the program is running, its immediate impact, and its long term impact. Although these aspects of the model are not directly related to the needs assessment process from a program development perspective, they play an important part in the needs assessment process. When evaluation is considered during the program's planning phase, it helps program developers focus on the goals and objectives of the program. Also, it ensures that the evaluation of the program will be less controversial because performance benchmarks were agreed upon up front, during the planning phase of the project.

PATCH

The **PATCH model** was developed by researchers from the Centers for Disease Control and Prevention. PATCH is an acronym for *planned approach to community health*, which is a process that enables community members to plan, implement, and evaluate programs which are related to significant health problems in their community. With a special emphasis on community development activities, the goal of PATCH is to reduce the prevalence of risk factors for the leading causes of morbidity and mortality in the target community (CDC, 1994).

The five "critical elements" of PATCH include:

- community participation.
- data (which guide program development).
- development of comprehensive health promotion strategies (based on data).
- evaluation.
- capacity building in the community that facilitates implementation of health promotion programs.

Implementation of PATCH requires three main partners: the state health agency, the local community (comprised of a community group and a steering committee, organized by a local coordinator), and staff from the CDC, who provide training for, and technical assistance to, the state and local partners.

PATCH has been implemented successfully in many areas in the country (e.g., Sarasota County, Florida), yet it does not exist uniformly in all states and communities. The strength of the model lies in its reliance on community participation, and the fact that it is data-driven. Emphasized by the model is that data should be used in the identification and prioritization of health problems, and, that data should help guide the development of the health promotion interventions.

APEX-PH

Another CDC-derived model, developed in partnership with the National Association of County Health Officials (NACHO), the American Public Health Association (APHA), and several other organizations, is **APEX-PH**. APEX-PH stands for *Assessment Protocol for Excellence in Public Health*. Similar to the PATCH process, APEX-PH utilizes community groups to prioritize health problems for the local health department. In addition, APEX-PH pays special attention to the organizational capacity of the public health department. Therefore, APEX-PH is designed around two major tasks: (1) assessment of the organizational capacity of the health department, and (2) an assessment of prevailing health problems in the community, and the development of a plan to address them (NACHO, 1991). A major strength of the APEX-PH process is the emphasis, not only on the needs assessment and strategic planning aspects of health promotion programming, but also on the methods used to address the problems. This strategy includes outlining who will carry out which tasks, by when, and, with what desired results. The APEX-PH protocol emphasizes both strategic and tactical planning.

An often overlooked aspect of any strategic planning or needs assessment process is the assessment of the organization's strengths and weaknesses in relation to the mission of that organization. In the organizational capacity assessment, the organization examines its strengths and weaknesses using a specific set of indicators outlined in the APEX-PH manual. These indicators examine areas such as legal authority for the health department to operate, intergovernmental relations, community relations, and public policy development. Departmental staff members engage in a self-study, and rate the department according to a large set of variables based on the indicators (and others) listed above. On the basis of this assessment, strengths and weaknesses are identified, and an action plan is developed to address those issues needing remediation. The goals and objectives for each problem area are outlined, as well as who is to address the goals. The methods to be used to address the goal, and, a projection of when the goal will be reached, are also outlined.

The second component of the APEX-PH process is the development of a community health plan. This plan is developed through a series of steps, including collecting and analyzing health-related data, forming a community group, having the group identify and prioritize health problems, and analyze those health problems in terms of their risk factors, creating an inventory of community health resources, and developing a community health plan. Similar to the PATCH process, community groups review data and prioritize health problems to be addressed by the health department. A detailed analysis of the causes of those health problems takes place which helps in the design of the health promotion interventions. The inventory of community resources, agencies, and programs which potentially can partner with the local health department are also identified in the process. Such identification will minimize unnecessary overlap and duplication of effort. Thus, if a local community group identifies lung cancer as a major health problem in the community, then smoking prevention and cessation programs should be in place. If the American Cancer Society or one of the local hospitals already has a cessation program in place, then, the health department does not need to develop a new one. Instead, the health department staff can concentrate on other activities. Using all of these data points, a community health plan is developed. Like the organizational capacity assessment, this plan will include a detailed set of goals and objectives to be addressed (the strategic plan) as well as the methods which will be used to address the problem (the tactical plan).

A modified version of the APEX-PH model was implemented and completed by all 86 health departments in Illinois in 1994. This project, known as IPLAN (Illinois Project for Local Assessment of Needs) required each of the health departments to undergo an internal organizational capacity assessment, and, to conduct a community assessment and develop a community health plan. Approximately 1200 community leaders and residents took part in the community assessment process, and, statewide, 325 community health priorities were identified. IPLAN was seen by local health departments as a productive set of activities. It provided focus for Illinois communities regarding *Healthy People 2000* objectives, and allowed for community participation in the development and implementation of public health programs (Illinois Department of Public Health, 1994).

Bryson's Strategic Planning Model

Although not a model developed specifically for health education or public health purposes, Bryson's (1988) eight-point model of strategic planning provides an adaptable framework for anyone who is beginning a strategic planning project. The model includes:

- *Initiate and agree on a strategic planning process* - This step refers to having a series of discussions with leaders in an organization regarding the purposes and methods to be used in the strategic planning process.
- *Identify organizational mandates* - Planners must identify the things an organization must do. For example, a health department must collect data on certain reportable diseases, and then forward that information to the state health department. A high school must teach certain subjects to meet the state standards for the youngsters to graduate. On the surface, these mandates may seem obvious. However, through a careful analysis of organizational mandates, one might find out that the organization is not doing what it is mandated to do, and, is doing things it is not supposed or required to do.
- *Clarify organizational missions and values* - Leaders must review the organization's mission statement and determine what social and political needs the organization is supposed to meet. Other issues to consider include a common understanding of the organization's philosophy, what makes the organization unique, and how the organization responds to stakeholders.
- *Assess the external environment* - This phase relates to the process of identifying opportunities for, and threats to, the organization. This analysis includes scanning the political, economic, social, and technological forces and trends in the environment, as well as identifying the interests of program stakeholders.
- *Assess the internal environment* - In addition to an examination of the external environment, organizations must look internally at their strengths and weaknesses. What are the strong points about the organization? What are its weak points?
- *Identify the strategic issues facing the organization* - Based on the information collected in the first five steps of the process, the organization must then develop a succinct list of strategic issue statements, list the factors that make it an issue, and, describe the consequences of failing to address the issue.
- *Formulate strategies to manage the issues* - To address the issues identified in the previous step, policies, programs, and actions should be developed, and appropriate resources should be assigned.
- *Establish an effective organizational vision for the future* - This step is the most important element of Bryson's model. It is a statement describing what the organization should look like in five years, or when it is deemed successful. Much has been written about organizational

vision and vision statements. Bryson considers Martin Luther King's "I have a dream" speech as an outstanding example of a vision of success.

Bryson's model depends heavily on the quality of the analysis which is conducted in steps four and five. These steps constitute what is commonly referred to as a **SWOT analysis,** an assessment of the *strengths* and *weaknesses* within an organization, and the *opportunities* and *threats* with which the organization is confronted. An honest and thorough assessment of these issues allows for the development of a responsive strategic plan. Organizations probably need to perform a SWOT analysis on some recurring basis, both to assess progress, as well as to survey the extent to which circumstances that affect the elements of the SWOT analysis have changed.

A Note on Tactical Planning

Though there has been reference to tactical planning in this chapter, little has been written about it in the field of health education. In some planning textbooks, the tactical plan is called the "work plan." In general, tactical plans focus on how the strategic plan will be implemented. The occasionally heard phrase, "the devil is in the details," was probably thought up by someone who was familiar with the problems of tactical planning.

At the meeting of the National Association of College and University Business Officers, Eldert (1996) suggested that tactical plans:

- identify the people responsible for attaining each program objective.
- describe the methods used to address the objectives, including the mix of staffing, purchased services, supplies, equipment, and other activity-related revenue and allocations.
- identify the expected timing of the activities.
- match expected sources to uses.

In addition, tactical plans that are developed should be in line with the tactical planning policies of the organization, and represent the best approach to achieving the objectives of the strategic plan (Eldert, 1996). The development of the tactical plan must involve those persons responsible for implementing the strategic plan, and must allow for discussion concerning the best methods to address programmatic objectives, and do so in the most cost-effective manner.

Sources of Needs Assessment and Strategic Planning Data

There are two sources of data which can be used when conducting needs assessments and developing strategic and tactical plans: *existing data* and *investigator-collected data*. The advantage of existing data is simple − they already exist, may be easily accessed, and in many cases, are of high quality and allow for analysis of large geographic regions. For example, health statistics collected and compiled by health departments are reported on an annual basis, and provide information for developing the health profiles of the communities. Census data are also widely available, and provide a wealth of statistics. In addition, these data are often available without charge or for a nominal fee.

Sometimes there are problems with existing data. Census data, for instance, are only collected once every ten years, and in some instances, may be too old for useful assessments or predictions. Existing data also may not be related directly to the problem of primary interest. Finally, some existing data may not accurately reflect the population due to methodologic issues associated with the research design and means of data collection (McKenzie & Smeltzer, 1997). Despite these disadvantages, good planners use existing data, and interpret them in light of their limitations.

Investigator-generated data can be advantageous in that they are collected and analyzed specifically for the purpose of the current study. If, for example, one is studying drug and alcohol use in two rural counties, there may not be any data available. The absence of existing data may necessitate first-hand data collection. Second, if data *are* available, they may not be useful for the target population with respect to geography, age, or other important variables of interest. There is no better way to get up-to-date and relevant information for your study than to collect it yourself. The problem is, collecting data for each study is an expensive undertaking. In addition, as with existing data, newly collected data are only as good as the methods used to generate them. Thus, sampling, instrumentation, data collection procedures, and analysis and interpretation must all be done well to have valid and reliable data from which good decisions can be made.

Existing Data

There are many sources of data and a well-versed health educator should know from where these data can be obtained. A case study will illustrate the utility of *existing data*, or, as we referred to them in Chapter 6, *precollected data*. Below, we will describe how existing data were used in the IPLAN project referred to earlier (Illinois Department of Public Health, 1994). The data set that was developed for the health departments was comprised of six data groupings: ·

- Demographic and socioeconomic data
- General health and access to care
- Maternal and child health
- Chronic disease
- Infectious disease
- Environmental, occupational, and injury control

Each of these data groupings contained a number of variables. For the first data group (demographic and socioeconomic data), variables included population size, distribution by age, and proportion of the population that was at or below the poverty level. For the health-related variables (e.g., lung cancer rate) data were available at the county level, at the state level, and at the national level. In addition, data for premature death, sorted by various ethnic groups, were also present. These data were used by health officers to determine how their counties compared to neighboring counties, the state, and the nation, and also to make comparisons to the health objectives for the nation by the year 2000.

Data for the IPLAN data system were taken from 15 sources:

- Illinois Department of Public Health
- Illinois Environmental Protection Agency
- Illinois State Board of Education
- Illinois Department of Public Aid
- Illinois Department of Employment Security
- Illinois Health Care Cost Containment Council
- Illinois Criminal Justice Information Authority
- Illinois Department of Transportation
- Illinois Behavior Risk Factor Surveillance System
- Illinois State Police
- National Center for Health Statistics
- U.S. Bureau of the Census
- U.S. Department of Agriculture
- U.S. Health Care Financing Administration
- U.S. General Accounting Office

Each of these agencies supplied Illinois health departments with information that was used in their community assessment to develop their health priorities. All states have similar agencies charged with collecting health and safety-related data.

IPLAN data were used not only for county assessments, but for statewide assessments as well. For example, Leitner and colleagues (1996) used the IPLAN data set to develop a 31-variable model to determine health needs related to primary care in rural Illinois. By using the array of variables employed in the model, they were able to identify those counties which appeared to have the most need for primary care programs.

The most important existing data for health planners, especially those planning for county or larger populations, are the data from the U.S. Bureau of the Census. Demographic data comprise the foundation of any large-scale strategic plan, because it is important to be able to describe and predict the size and composition of the target population. At a minimum, one needs to know population size, the breakdown of the population by age and sex, and the ethnicity of the population. Ethnicity is of particular importance in areas where people do not speak English as a first language, because health promotion programs need to be delivered in the language of the population.

It is important to note that many of the data sets we have talked about are now available "on-line" through the Internet. Both the U.S. Bureau of the Census and the Centers for Disease Control and Prevention have data sets readily available for planning purposes. These data are convenient, accurate, and available at no cost.

Once program planners have identified the exact geographic location of the target population, and can describe its demographic characteristics, they can move on to the various health-related indices, economic indices, and other variables of interest. With regard to health data, there are at least five "rules of thumb" which must be remembered in the interpretation process:

- Infectious disease data are often "under-reported" (e.g., chicken-pox prevalence data are almost always higher than the stated values, because many people don't bring their children to see the family doctor when the youngsters have chicken pox. Also, though it is a reportable disease, physicians sometimes don't report cases).

- Reporting rates for various infectious diseases vary by local health department. For example, in a university town, there may be a tremendous emphasis placed on reporting sexually transmitted diseases. This careful reporting may make one particular county appear to have higher rates of a disease than another county, because that county may not choose to emphasize such careful surveillance and reporting.

- Different states may report different diseases in different ways. For example, if one is examining lung cancer rates, one must make sure that other cancers of the respiratory system are not included in the number. Consultation with epidemiologists will help ensure that you are comparing "apples to apples" not "apples to oranges."

- Different counties or regions of study vary according to certain demographic characteristics. For instance, a county in Florida with a large retirement population will have higher rates of some chronic diseases than a county with a relatively young population. Generally, it is best to use age-adjusted rates when comparing data from various regions. *Never* compare one type of rate (e.g., age-adjusted rate) with another rate (e.g., crude rate).

- The actual utility of some indices that are available is questioned at times by various authorities. The Kessner Index, which examines various dimensions of prenatal care, is viewed by some authorities (e.g., Mahan, 1996) with some skepticism. These types of debates are important, and should be considered when planners interpret data sets.

Investigator Collected Data

Numerous methods are employed to collect data directly from people, i.e., *investigator collected data*, or as we referred to them in Chapter 6, *original data*. Probably the most popular approaches are focus groups, the nominal group process, and surveys. Discussed in detail in other chapters, these methods are used to gather both qualitative and quantitative information from the target population.

A method used less frequently by health educators is "consensus building." An example of this approach is described by deHaven-Smith and Wodraska (1996), and is based on the American Assembly process developed by Dwight D. Eisenhower while he was President of Columbia University. The strategy brings together 65 to 75 stakeholders to discuss a specific policy issue. A modified, ordered version of the procedure includes:

1. A steering committee is formed to select topics for discussion, assist in the preparation of papers (see #2), as well as to select other assembly participants.
2. Experts write background papers related to the issue.
3. At the assembly, the people are divided into small groups to discuss the issues.
4. A facilitator and recorder are assigned to each small group.
5. The assembly can meet several times over a period of time. In deHaven-Smith's example, participants met over a 15-month period. Longer time periods or shorter time periods may be necessary depending on the specific tasks to be accomplished.
6. Each group addresses the same questions. At the end of the assemblies, the steering committee synthesizes the small groups' work into a final report.
7. Open forums are held throughout the target region to obtain additional stakeholder input on the problem.
8. A final "plenary" session is held with all assembly participants to agree on the final report.

As a result of testing this process, deHaven-Smith and Wodraska (1996) advise:

- Start discussions with very general issues, and then work to specific issues.
- The process is as important as the decisions that come forth from the process.
- The authority of the steering committee must be respected.
- The public forums and the process of seeking council from stakeholders is essential.
- An outside facilitator is important.

Linking the Budget to the Plan

A critical error is to develop a strategic plan without considering the impact of programs on the organization's overall budget. As organizations commonly say: "We cannot be all things to all people." Strategic plans can and should help guide the budgetary process. Programmatic areas which are high priorities for the organization ordinarily receive funding priority.

There are no formulae or equations which can be used when making final budgetary decisions for programs. The process requires good judgment. However, a strategic plan, with lists of priority areas, the tactics which will be used to address the priorities, as well as the resources needed for the priority areas, will provide considerable guidance in the development of a budget.

Summary

In this chapter we described the processes used to conduct needs assessments as well as to develop strategic and tactical plans. We believe that the most successful needs assessments are those which utilize a wide variety of stakeholders in providing input for the program. When using a stakeholder-based approach in concert with solid grounding in health status data, programs can be developed, implemented, and defended. Once a solid needs assessment has been conducted, a strategic plan outlining programmatic goals and objectives can be developed. Finally, the tactical plan, describing how goals and objectives will be met, can be synthesized.

Case Study

Morrison, C. (1996). Using PRECEDE to predict breast self-examination in older, lower-income women. *American Journal of Health Behavior*, *20*(2), 3-14.

In this paper, Morrison describes the use of the elements of the first part of Green and Kreuter's PRECEDE-PROCEED model, to predict breast self-examination among older, lower income women. How would you use these findings to develop an intervention program for this target population? Describe how you would continue her study through the PROCEED aspects of Green and Kreuter's model. Select another health problem (e.g., heart disease, skin cancer), and sketch out the variables of relevance for each phase of the PRECEDE-PROCEED model.

Student Questions/Activities

1. Consider each of the needs assessment/strategic planning models described in this chapter. Select a topic of interest (e.g., youth tobacco use) and develop a needs assessment plan using two of the models. Compare and contrast the plans resulting from the two models.

2. Suppose that you have been asked to work with a community group in an APEX-PH type setting to prioritize community health problems which will be addressed by the local health department. Suppose you work as a health educator at this health department. The group has reviewed the epidemiologic data, and has begun to prioritize the health problems. Although the teen birth rate in your county is low compared to state and national figures, the community group insists that teenage pregnancy is a major problem, and wants to make it a high priority in your community health plan. At the same time, your lung cancer rates are very high, yet the community group does not want to address this problem. What will you do? How would you go about getting the group to change its mind regarding priorities? Would you try? Explain.

3. Suppose that you have been hired recently as a new administrator of a local health department which has recently had a series of employee dismissals, as well

as misunderstandings with other area health care and social service providers. The county board has recently raised some questions as to what the mission of the health department is, and whether the health department's health education and health promotion role duplicates the roles of a rather aggressive community education program sponsored by the local hospital. Describe a SWOT analysis in this environment, and how the SWOT analysis would help you to define (or redefine) your health education department's mission?

Recommended Readings

Green, L.W., & Kreuter, M.W. (1991). *Health Promotion Planning: An Educational and Environmental Approach*, 2nd edition. Mountain View, CA: Mayfield.

This textbook is considered a classic by some authorities as it relates to the planning, implementation, and evaluation of health education and health promotion programs. The text details the different phases of the model, as well as describes the model's application in the development of high quality health education programs.

Lamm, R.D. (1996). The ethics of excess. *Public Health Reports, 111*, 218-223.

In this article, former Colorado governor Richard Lamm describes the "excessive" capacity we have in the United States in terms of excess physicians, excess institutional capacity (too many hospital beds, intensive care beds, etc.), and too much medical technology ("The United States has far more medical technology than it can effectively utilize." p.222). Excessive capacity suggests that resources are being used in certain areas (e.g., hospital beds) when in fact the resources could be used for other things (e.g., prenatal care programs for women).

Thacker, S.B., Stroup, D.F., Parrish, R.G., & Anderson, H.A. (1996). Surveillance in environmental public health: Issues, systems, and sources. *American Journal of Public Health, 86*(5), 633-638.

The environment can have a profound impact on a population's health status. This article describes an environmental public health surveillance system, current and projected environmental health surveillance needs, and a wide array of data sources. These data can be used to develop, as well as to evaluate, health education programs.

References

Braus, P. (1996). Why does cancer cluster? *American Demographics*, March, 36-41.

Bryson, J.M. (1988). *Strategic Planning for Public and Nonprofit Organizations.* San Francisco: Jossey-Bass.

Centers for Disease Control and Prevention. (1994). *Planned Approach to Community Health: A Guide for Local Coordinators.* Atlanta: Division of Chronic Disease Control and Community Intervention, National Center for Chronic Disease Control and Health Promotion.

deHaven-Smith, L., & Wodraska, J.R. (1996). Consensus-building for integrated resources planning. *Public Administration Review, 56*(4), 367-371.

Department of Health and Human Services. (1990). *Healthy People 2000: National Health Promotion and Disease Prevention Objectives.* Washington, DC: Author.

Dignan, M., & Carr, P. (1987). *Program Planning for Health Education and Health Promotion.* Philadelphia: Lea and Febiger.

Eldert, J. deB. (1996). *Long Range Evolution and Linking Strategies to Budgets.* National Association of College and University Business Officers Meeting on Strategic Planning and Budgeting in the Information Age. New Orleans, November 25-26, 1996.

Green, L.W., & Kreuter, M.W. (1991). *Health Promotion Planning: An Educational and Environmental Approach*, 2nd edition. Mountain View, CA: Mayfield.

Green, L.W., Kreuter, M.W., Deeds, S.G., & Partridge, K.B. (1980). *Health Education Planning: a Diagnostic Approach.* Palo Alto: Mayfield.

Illinois Department of Public Health. (1994). *IPLAN User's Guide.* Springfield, IL: Office of Epidemiology and Health Systems Development.

Kaufman, R. (1988). Needs assessment: A menu. *Educational Technology, 28,* 21-23.

Larson, K.D., Spoede, C.W., & Miller, P.B.W. (1994). Fundamentals of Financial and Managerial Accounting. Boston: Irwin.

Leitner, D.W., Gast, J.A., Sarvela, P.D., Ring, M.C., & Newell, L.A. (1996). An epidemiologic approach to assessing primary care needs in rural Illinois. *The Journal of Rural Health, 12*(2), 110-119.

Mahan, C.S. (1996). Prenatal care indices: How useful? *Public Health Reports, 111,* 419.

McKillip, J. (1987). *Need Analysis.* Beverly Hills: Sage.

McKenzie, J.F., & Smeltzer, J.L. (1997). *Planning, Implementing and Evaluating Health Promotion Programs: A Primer,* 2nd edition. Boston: Allyn and Bacon.

National Association of County Health Officials (1991). *Assessment Protocol for Excellence in Public Health.* Washington, DC: Author.

Stufflebeam, D.L., McCormick, C.H., Brinkerhoff, R.O., & Nelson, C.O. (1985). *Conducting Educational Needs Assessments.* Boston: Kluwer-Nijhoff.

Webster's Third New International Dictionary. (1971). Springfield, MA: Merriam Co.

Wisconsin Department of Health and Social Services. (1990). *Healthier People in Wisconsin.* Madison: Division of Health.

10

Quantitative Evaluation: Methods and Designs

Chapter Objectives

After completing this chapter, you should be able to:

1. Define internal and external validity.
2. Identify several threats to internal and external validity.
3. Describe designs that reduce or eliminate some of the threats to internal and external validity.
4. List the properties of quantitative evaluation.
5. Analyze the strengths and weaknesses of several quantitative research and evaluation designs.

Key Terms

dependent variable
external validity
hypothesis
independent variable
internal validity

posttest
pretest
quasi-experimental design
true experimental design

Introduction

Evaluation designs can be divided into two types: *quantitative* and *qualitative*. In this chapter we will look at the nature of quantitative designs, and their utility for the evaluator of health education and promotion programs. As we will demonstrate, the evaluator often wants to answer questions like: How effective is program A as opposed to program B? Was the intervention employed actually responsible for the results that were achieved (or were there other influential factors)? Would the program under consideration that appears to be effective also work in other settings, at other times, and with other people? These questions and related ones are addressed, in part, through rigorous quantitative designs that may be simple in some instances, and quite complex in others. This chapter will introduce you to some of the commonly employed quantitative evaluative procedures, and provide you with some easy-to-follow illustrations of these designs in practice. In the next chapter, we will look at the use of qualitative procedures, a series of contrasting procedures for carrying out evaluation studies.

Theory of Quantitative Evaluation

In simple terms, quantitative studies attempt to "quantify" things for us. Schofield and Anderson (1984) provide a more elaborate definition that may be useful. According to these authors, quantitative inquiry:

focuses on the testing of specific hypotheses that are smaller parts of some larger theoretical perspective. This approach follows the traditional natural science model more closely than qualitative research, emphasizing experimental design and statistical methods of analysis. Quantitative research emphasizes standardization, precision, objectivity, and reliability of measurement as well as replicability and generalizability of findings. Thus, quantitative research is characterized not only by a focus on producing numbers but on generating numbers which are suitable for statistical tests (pp.8-9).

The evolution and popularity of quantitative inquiry in the 1950s and 1960s was a function of the fact that many people who served as program evaluators during this time period were educational and psychological researchers, people who worked in the experimental tradition (Worthen & Sanders, 1987). Subsequent work by Campbell and Stanley (1966) helped to crystalize the experimental and quasi-experimental style of investigation.

Two questions of utmost importance in most program evaluations are: (1) To what extent can the observed outcomes be attributed to the program that was implemented? and (2) To what extent can the results be generalized to other times, to other settings, and to other subjects? Quantitative measures can be employed successfully to help us answer questions such as these. However, before proceeding with learning about experimental and quasi-experimental evaluation techniques, it is important for us to look at two very critical concepts: internal and external validity.

Internal and External Validity

The first of these two questions identified above brings into focus an issue known as **internal validity**, or the extent to which we can presume causality, i.e., that the effects identified were really attributable to the program, and not to extraneous factors or other explanations relevant to the evaluation design. Put another way, how much confidence can we have that the program or intervention actually was responsible for producing the results that were achieved? Initially, this question may seem a bit preposterous. A layperson in fact might be inclined to ask: "Well, what else besides the treatment could have made the difference?" As we will see, numerous alternative explanations (besides the benefit of a planned intervention) cannot be ruled out. The validity of one's conclusion about the causal nature of a particular intervention might indeed be threatened.

Our second question forces us to confront the issue of **external validity**, or the ability of our evaluation design to allow us to generalize the results of a particular intervention to other persons, settings, and times. While both internal and external validity are important concepts, the former is probably of greater concern at the onset. After all, if we are unable to demonstrate with confidence that our program was responsible for producing a given result, there is not much point in asking if the results are generalizable, or if the program can achieve similar outcomes beyond the setting in which it was tested.

Threats to Internal Validity

In their classic work, Campbell and Stanley (1966) identified seven factors that can threaten an evaluation design's internal validity, i.e., an evaluator's ability to show a causal relationship between two phenomena (treatment and effects). That is, certain events can take place that affect the program's outcomes, and become confused with the true influence of the program. The text below describes these confounding influences in general, and more specifically, provides some examples of how they can interfere with evaluation of health program interventions.

Contemporary history. Historical threats are events that occur at the same time as the program and which can inadvertently, become part of the program (Fink & Kosecoff, 1978). Suppose one were interested in evaluating knowledge gains concerning HIV/AIDS arising from the introduction of a new sex education curriculum in an intervention school versus those in a school where no such program was in place. Any true influences of the educational intervention might be obscured if, during program delivery, one of the major television networks broadcasts a highly publicized program on HIV/AIDS, a well known personality is diagnosed as being infected with the AIDS virus, or the Surgeon General of the United States is quoted frequently in the press about risk behaviors associated with contracting HIV. If knowledge of HIV/AIDS in the intervention school increased over that of the comparison school, one could not be certain that the knowledge gains were due to the influence of the formal educational intervention, other concurrent events, or a combination of these factors. If students in both educational settings showed similar knowledge gains, the true impact of the intended intervention (which might be high under ordinary circumstances) would be obscured by the real, but "chance" occurrence of a powerful media event. If evaluators are aware of the competing event, they may be in a position to try to separate out the effects of the intended intervention, or to attempt to repeat the intervention on another occasion, thereby putting themselves in a better position to make an evaluative judgment about the program in question. A more insidious situation occurs, however, if evaluators are unaware of any competing event (a real possibility) and draw conclusions based on what are assumed to be the true effects of the intended intervention alone. Thus, history constitutes a potentially serious threat to internal validity.

Subject maturation. Results achieved from an intervention also can be influenced by changes (physical or psychological) going on with the subjects participating in a given program. Whereas history is a threat occurring from external events, maturation arises from events taking place within the person. Suppose a class of elementary school pupils performs poorly on a general test of health knowledge at the beginning of a school year, but is exposed subsequently to health education. The pupils might perform better at the end of the school year for at least two reasons. (There might in fact be several explanations, but for our purposes here, let us just consider the issue at hand.) In the more desirable case, the health education program might be a good one, and thus, be responsible for the apparent achievement of the class. Alternative (and quite feasible) interpretations can be advanced, however. Perhaps the pupils became better readers during the school year. Now that they can read and understand test items better (a maturation in reading skill), they are in an improved position to select correct responses. Maybe pupils matured with respect to test anxiety -- being less anxious they can respond to test items without interference of their emotions. Any maturational change in skill, wisdom, physical strength, or other abilities can account for gains that might be incorrectly attributed to the intervention.

Pretesting effects. To demonstrate improvement in performance, especially in the cognitive domain, it is a common practice to **pretest** subjects on items of interest. It is possible, however, for a pretest to serve as a kind of intervention in and of itself. A test about factors affecting cholesterol level in the blood given prior to a heart health promotion program can provide a learning cue for subjects. Even a person who did not know the correct answers, and in fact, was oblivious to the whole subject of cholesterol, might begin to "tune in" to information about cholesterol that is encountered in everyday life, and related to concepts presented in the test. Upon repeating the test, the person performs better -- whether or not the formal educational intervention was ever presented. The simple practice of taking a test can prove beneficial as well, since subjects will be more familiar with the test when they are confronted by it the second time (**posttest**). Pretesting does not *always* mean that posttest scores might be better, even in the absence of an intervention. To the contrary, pretesting can create such anxiety in subjects that they do much worse on posttest (Shortell & Richardson, 1978). Unless the evaluation design takes the possible confounding factor of pretesting into consideration, its possible contribution to program results cannot be overlooked.

Instrumentation. According to Fink and Kosecoff (1978), "Instrumentation threats are due to changes in the calibration of an instrument, or changes in the observers, scores, or measuring instrument used from one time to the next" (p.14). If from the time of pretest to time of posttest, questions are altered, interviewers pose questions in a different style (more emphatic or less emphatic), or interviewers (the people themselves) change, the data collection process has been modified. Such modification can affect internal validity. Other examples of instrumentation effects abound. The interpretation of the benefit of a program designed to promote weight loss could be influenced profoundly if a scale's calibration is changed. (Note how your bathroom scale can vary 1-2 pounds or more with repeated weighings occurring just seconds apart. Obviously one would want to use a more accurate scale if interested in true changes in weight over time.) Other common instruments prone to measurement error are some types of skin-fold calipers, blood pressure cuffs (and the people who use them), and people in general. A laboratory technician reading the meniscus of a test tube may change his or her line of sight from one time to the next, or worse, two different technicians may implement conflicting procedures for examining the level of fluid in a test tube. Different readings are recorded despite the fact that the level of fluid has not changed. One has to wonder, too, if a judge viewing such Olympic sporting events as figure skating, gymnastics, or platform diving views the twentieth competitor with the same criteria and accuracy as the first. Does a fatigue factor set in? Does a person become less discriminating or more discriminating? All of these examples illustrate the principle of instrument-related measurement error and its potential impact on internal validity.

Statistical regression toward the mean. It is a statistical fact that when persons are selected to participate in a program on the basis of previous testing (extreme high scores versus extreme low scores), high achievers may perform less well as a group on follow-up testing, while low achievers may be inclined to perform better. The net result is that each group's performance (measured in mean score) begins to edge toward the mean of the overall group of subjects. Why? Measurement error is the most likely interpretation. According to Shortell and Richardson (1978):

The more deviant a set of scores in the sense of being selected for extremely high or low values, the larger the error measurement they will contain. Intuitively, we know the extremely low scorers have had unusually bad luck (large negative errors), while the extremely high scorers have had unusually good luck (large positive error). But because such luck is not likely to hold up over time, we expect on a posttest to find the low scores improving somewhat on the average and the high scores declining somewhat (p.40).

Put simply, people who initially perform at the extreme high end of a range have nowhere to go but down, and vice versa. Attributing changes under these conditions to the influence of a treatment or intervention is almost certain to be incorrect (French & Kaufman, 1981).

Selection bias with respect to subjects. Suppose we evaluated the benefit of an aerobics program on certain cardiovascular and respiratory fitness by offering it to one group of subjects but not to a second group. Our thought would be that having the second group would allow us to make a performance comparison to the program recipients after the aerobics program had been operating for a reasonable length of time. However, if the fitness levels of individuals in each of the two groups were not equivalent at the beginning, how would we know if the program we introduced was responsible for differences we measured later on? In fact, we could never know with certainty. Inherent differences between the groups due to age, gender, previous activity level, and other factors might offer a better explanation for disparate fitness performances. It is crucial to establish group equivalence at the onset to eliminate selection bias as a threat to internal validity. Means for demonstrating group equivalence are discussed later in this chapter.

Subject mortality or differential attrition. Subject mortality (also known as differential attrition) refers to the fact that when two or more groups of subjects of approximately equal numbers are compared, it is possible for any true group differences at posttest to be confounded if group sizes are altered differentially during the course of the study. Fink and Kosecoff (1978) provide the following illustration:

For an evaluation that compared a new asthma treatment with the traditional treatment, the 60 patients who volunteered for each group were asked to visit the clinic at the end of their treatment program for a mini-physical examination. Fifty-seven patients from the traditional group and 43 from the treatment group came for the examination, but the evaluator could not be sure if any changes in health status were the result of the treatment or the result of changes in the groups due to their differing drop-out rates (p.14).

In the example above, suppose the overall health status of the 43 patients in the treatment group appeared to be significantly better than that of their study counterparts. Such a conclusion truly would be erroneous if the drop-outs in the treatment group actually experienced severe symptoms of ill health (unknown to the evaluator), were too weak to come for the physical examination, or dropped out due to having experienced a fatal asthma attack (perhaps from a reaction to the medication), and thus, experienced literal mortality!

Consider another illustration of the problem of subject attrition. Suppose a group of subjects receiving a stress management program was examined with respect to a comparison group receiving no stress management program. What could one conclude if subjects voluntarily dropped out of the intervention group in large numbers? Was the program too stressful? Were the subjects assigned to the intervention different from those assigned to the comparison group in that they were more "stressed," and therefore, prone to dropping out due to not perceiving themselves to have time in their frenzied schedules to attend the program? The real effects of the program could be masked because of the composition of the group.

Interactions of internal validity threats. It is possible for some of the individual threats to internal validity cited above to interact with one another and yield further confounding effects on our ability to draw an accurate conclusion about the value of an intervention. For instance, there can be an interaction between selection and maturation. This phenomenon is possible when groups receiving a treatment are maturing at different rates. When middle class and lower class children are compared at two different times on a test of cardiovascular disease knowledge, children from more affluent families may perform better on posttest. Middle class children may gain at a faster rate, perhaps due to motivational factors, the influence of cultural exposures, being better readers, or other variables. Issues of cardiovascular health may be more relevant to middle class children who perhaps have a greater likelihood of being exposed to a wider variety of foods, including "health" foods, participating in certain competitive sports, aerobic programs, and related activities than lower class children whose interests and opportunities may be considerably different.

Selection and history also can produce an interaction effect. Each group receiving a particular intervention may experience a unique local history that influences its receptivity to an intervention, and as a consequence, its subsequent performance. Suppose two geographically distinct communities are introduced to a high school-based program to promote responsible alcohol use. Imagine the program's receptivity (and potential confounding influence of this receptivity) in a community that recently has had five teenagers killed in a tragic automobile accident linked to a drinking episode, versus another participating community where no such event took place. The program's apparent performance in the more sensitized community could cause evaluators to make an exaggerated judgment or recommendation that was not a true representation of the program's most likely impact if implemented in a less sensitized setting.

As one further illustration of interaction, selection and instrumentation can produce confounding effects together. This phenomenon occurs whenever an instrument cannot record any more true gains in one of the groups (called "ceiling effects"), or when more scores from one group are clustered around the low end of a scale that is unable to record further declines (called "floor effects"). A bathroom scale that tops out at 250 pounds illustrates the principle of a ceiling effect. It would not be possible for a football player on a special diet (not steroids!) to know his true gains from the program once he exceeded the 250-lb. mark.

Fortunately, as we shall see later in this chapter, evaluators can examine programs using designs that measure or control for most of the threats to internal validity that Campbell and Stanley (1966) described. As investigators became more and more familiar with the concept of internal validity, and learned how to protect themselves from drawing erroneous conclusions, new problems arose, however. Other issues that affected internal validity needed to be addressed, especially where experimental designs were concerned in the evaluation process. Cook and Campbell (1979) identified several other factors that can affect the evaluator's ability to prove the existence of a causal relationship between a treatment and observed effects. The unfortunate nature of these factors is that typical experimental and quasi-experimental designs do not permit the evaluator to control for their potential influences easily. These additional issues are discussed below.

Ambiguity about the direction of the causal influence. Which event came first? Did "A" cause "B" to happen, or did "B" lead to "A" taking place? This question is of importance almost any time one is dealing with correlational data, i.e., when the occurrence of one event seems to be associated with the occurrence of another event. The existence of correlation between two events is not proof that "A" causes "B" or vice versa. To illustrate, we know from correlational data that in persons with a particular predisposition, a diet high in sodium can exacerbate existing hypertension. One may be able to argue with equal vigor, though, that people with high blood pressure experience a craving for sodium. Both situations may make one's hypertension worse. Directionality cannot be assumed. Perhaps a more familiar illustration of this principal is helpful. The authors of this textbook are willing to bet that you and most of your fellow students get up in the morning and immediately perform at least one of the following five activities: (a) use the bathroom; (b) take a shower; (c) eat breakfast; (d) engage in toothbrushing; or (e) some other highly specific and predictable activity. Correlational data would suggest a strong association between sunrise and one or more of the events listed above. Could one conclude that the rising of the sun "causes" toothbrushing? No more so than one could conclude satisfactorily that the intention to brush one's teeth "causes" the sun to rise. The direction of the causal influence is ambiguous.

If the relationship between two events is examined using a two-tailed statistical test, and yields a statistic that exceeds the critical value ($p < .05$), one can only conclude that the events are related in some way. If one wishes to test whether the relationship is in a particular direction, the more statistically powerful one-tailed test must be used. If for some reason you have to use a two-tailed test, be alerted to the fact that you may not be able to determine directionality.

Diffusion, imitation of the treatment by the control group, or the school bus effect. When evaluators compare a group that received a particular intervention with a group that did not, they have set up a simple experimental condition. However, if people in the treatment group can speak to, and interact with people to whom they are being compared, there is the chance that one of the things they can talk about is the intervention itself. Information that was intended for the treatment group thus "diffuses" to persons outside of the treatment group. When the two groups are subsequently tested, the performance of the non-treatment group is similar to that of the group receiving the intervention. The treatment, in a sense, has been imitated. In school settings, where one classroom of pupils receives an intervention, and a second class acts as a control group, this phenomenon is routinely referred to as the *school bus effect*. Since these children doubtlessly encounter one another in everyday activities (such as riding the school bus together), opportunities to share information occur. As you may have concluded already, it is a risky idea (in terms of internal validity) to use two groups in close proximity. Thus, evaluators using two neighborhoods that are next to each other, two states that border on one another, or two shifts of workers in the same industrial setting, also may risk a diffusion problem, if one is serving the role of comparison group for the other.

Compensatory rivalry by those receiving a less favorable treatment - the "John Henry" effect. Somewhere in American folklore you will find the story of John Henry, the "steel driving man" who drove railroad spikes in the days of the American frontier. Supposedly, John Henry and his cohorts, about to be put out of business because of the speed of the newly invented steam-driven raildriver, set up a challenge of "man versus machine." As legend has it, John Henry, who was the champion of his trade, raced the machine, working at a speed in excess of his normal capacity. John Henry won the challenge, but collapsed and died -- or so the story goes.

Sometimes in investigative settings, people who are not receiving a particular intervention find out, perhaps causing them to work harder. As a result, they perform at a level beyond their normal capacity, as John Henry did in the story above. They may do as well as, or even outperform the treatment group when both are tested. Possible beneficial effects of the intervention are masked, making the treatment appear less promising than it in fact may be. Such an occurrence is common in worksite settings where persons in different departments or who work on different shifts are assigned to different interventions.

Resentful demoralization by those receiving a less favorable treatment. This threat to internal validity is virtually the opposite of the "John Henry" effect. An intervention may appear to be beneficial, but only because persons in the control group found out, became angry or demoralized, and just plain gave up trying. People who lose heart see their productivity decline, giving the appearance that an opposing treatment is considerably better than it might actually be. The potential for "resentful demoralization" is present in worksite, school, and other settings where evaluations are carried out.

Compensatory equalization of treatments. For logistical, as well as for ethical reasons, comparison groups sometimes are offered an intervention supposedly unrelated to the one the evaluator is examining in the treatment group. Suppose in the town of Lake Mills, the pupils at Sonnemann Middle School are provided with the "Growing Healthy" curriculum, while the pupils at the McCormack Middle School receive the Gustafson Reading Improvement Program. Each school acts as a reciprocal control group for the other. However, as a result of the special reading program, the pupils at McCormack Middle School read a multitude of materials, allowing them to improve their vocabulary, verbal abilities, powers of reasoning, and other skills (possibly including matters related to health knowledge). Moreover, when tested with the pupils from Sonnemann Middle School about health concepts, their enhanced reading skills help them to perform about as well as the pupils who were exposed to "Growing Healthy." Inadvertently, exposure to a reading enhancement program has compensated for any deficit in health-related learning activities.

Threats to External Validity

So far, our discussion has focused on factors that affect the internal validity of the evaluation design. Often the evaluator and program stakeholders are concerned about the relevance of the program's effects beyond the confines of the setting in which the evaluation was conducted. To which other populations of subjects, settings, times, and variables can the findings be generalized? When seeking to maximize external validity of a design, the evaluator examines the threats to representativeness identified below.

Interaction effects of selection biases and treatment. The characteristics of subjects selected to take part in a program determine, in part, how extensively the findings can be generalized. Seventh-grade pupils from Marquette Middle School who are exposed to the intervention may not be typical of 7th-graders everywhere. Freshmen students in Psychology 101 at a large midwestern university may not be representative of university students nationwide, of students at the same institution, or even of all freshmen at that school. Some special trait of the program participants (e.g., very high or very low IQ), or unique feature of the setting where the program is conducted can prevent the evaluator from saying that results elsewhere will be similar. Wright (1979) sees the problem of external validity as largely being one of choosing good samples. Sampling is indeed an important feature of making generalizations, and is discussed in detail in Chapter 13.

Reactive interaction effect of pretesting. Being given a pretest may limit the generalizability of some evaluation findings. Pretesting that occurs in a group selected for treatment prior to the actual presentation of an intervention may cause people to react in a way that affects their response to the intervention. Unless persons outside the original investigative setting are pretested similarly, their response to the intervention may be different. Two examples will illustrate this point.

First, let us suppose that one was asked to evaluate the effect of a new diet and aerobic exercise program on weight loss and body composition. As part of being in the program, all participants are weighed at the beginning of the program and at regular intervals thereafter. It is possible that any subsequent weight loss might be motivated by the combination of being weighed and then participating in the program, rather than by the program alone (Fink & Kosecoff, 1978). Getting weighed may sensitize subjects to the intervention, and make them unrepresentative of the larger population of subjects to whom the evaluator wishes to make inferences. Persons in other settings, and at other times, who are not weighed before program onset, may respond differently.

As a second illustration of this phenomenon, suppose that high school seniors are pretested about their feelings toward persons with a gay or lesbian sexual orientation. As part of an intervention to help students become more accepting of the lifestyle of homosexuals, the students view a socio-drama with a sexual orientation discrimination theme. Students' responses to the posttest may not reflect the effect of the intervention as much as it reflects increased sensitivity to homosexuality that taking the pretest caused. The pretest may have alerted students to moral questions, issues, problems, or other variables that ordinarily would have gone unnoticed. The effect of the intervention may not be representative of its effect for high school seniors who participate without being pretested.

Reactive effects of procedures (situational effects). Workers or students participating in a new or innovative program may be excited about that fact, or simply aware of being evaluated because of the presence of observers, the battery of tests, or other factors. Therefore, they behave in ways that deviate from their normal pattern. If the procedures surrounding the intervention (rather than the intervention itself) alter the participants' behavior, the evaluator cannot conclude that the treatment effect for the participants will be the same for subjects exposed to the treatment in settings that are more "natural" and less investigative in nature.

A famous example of "reactivity" to innovation occurred as part of the Hawthorne studies at the Western Electric Company in Chicago during the 1920s. In this industrial efficiency study, it was demonstrated that the selection of a group of workers for a special project in which their work environment was altered, and during which their work performance was evaluated, caused profound behavioral change. Regardless of how the work environment was modified (made more pleasant or less pleasant) productivity increased, presumably because of the novelty and the awareness of being studied. Since the time of this study, the phenomenon of having subjects act differently as a result of their knowing they are part of an evaluation study has been called the *Hawthorne effect*.

Interaction with history. Sometimes a unique "local history" can influence the perceived effectiveness of a particular intervention. Consider the possible results in two communities that are exposed to a heavy media campaign to promote breast and cervical cancer screening. Suppose community "A" has been exposed in recent years to prostate and colo-rectal cancer screening programs, or a toxic waste site in the community has been linked to a special occurrence of cancer in the population. Also, suppose that community "B" has no previous history of involvement in cancer awareness programs. In which community is the new breast and cervical cancer program more likely to "take hold"? No one can say for sure but there is good reason to suspect that the impact of the very same program in the two settings could be quite different. Which result indicates the true "generalizability" of the program?

Non-experimental Evaluation Designs

A number of investigative "designs" in health education are seriously flawed. Their flaws do not allow us to draw the kinds of conclusions that are necessary to make a decision as to whether a particular intervention produced the observed effect (internal validity), or whether the program can be transported to other places and populations (external validity). Below, we describe some of these "weak" designs that still comprise some research and evaluation studies in health education and health promotion.

The one-shot case study. Imagine that you have just come on board as the health education specialist responsible for prenatal education at a large urban hospital. You learn that an educational intervention designed to improve the knowledge of low literacy, high risk pregnant women was implemented during the previous month. This program consists of four fifty-minute sessions about pregnancy, labor and delivery, breastfeeding, and infant care. According to one of your new colleagues at the hospital, the results are very encouraging. By all appearances, the women are quite knowledgeable in these areas, and the health education staff is ready to implement this intervention on a large-scale basis. You learn that program participants' knowledge of these areas was not tested prior to the initiation of the educational sessions, but was tested upon completion of the last session.

The study design presented above is known as the one-shot case study, and can be represented diagrammatically by

$$X \qquad O$$

where "X" represents the intervention (also called the "program" or the "treatment"), and "O" represents the observation (also called the "measurement" or the "test"). Upon examining the design (and knowing about the threats to internal validity) you begin to become concerned that the value of the program may be far less than what meets the eye. Before reading on, can you spot some of the potential threats to internal validity?

To conclude that the program contributed to the favorable knowledge pattern of the group tested could be erroneous. Since no measurement was made prior to the program, it is possible that the group was well informed before the onset of the program. (While we are told they are a low literacy group, perhaps they have had considerable experience in childbearing or child care.) Even if there was a change that occurred, could we automatically attribute it to the education classes? The apparent change in knowledge among the program participants could be explained by history. Seeing a television program, talking about prenatal events and child care with friends, or even receiving medical attention during the prenatal visits could have contributed to changes in knowledge. Maturation also could have affected participants' knowledge about pregnancy and childbirth, especially if the intervention that took place occurred over several weeks or months. It is conceivable that the women became more motivated or changed psychologically as their pregnancies progressed, thus making them more receptive to the educational program. Can you think of any additional factors that might explain the observations that were made following the program and thus, might threaten internal validity?

The one-group pretest-posttest design. In the example discussed above, suppose the women *had* been tested on their knowledge of program content prior to the program's implementation. A diagram of this design is represented by

$$O_1 \quad X \quad O_2$$

where "O_1" represents the mean pretest score for the group, "X" represents the intervention, and "O_2" is the mean posttest score for the group. This design provides some improvement over the one-shot case study in that this situation allows us to look at the pretest-posttest difference in the group mean. However, sources of error are possible. One has no assurance that "X" is the major factor influencing any O_1-O_2 difference. History and maturation are plausible explanations for a posttest improvement, as they were for the one-shot case study. Testing effects may also explain the improvement at O_2 if the pretest served as an intervention itself for the women. We assume that the pretest and posttest instruments were identical, but if they were not the same, or the circumstances of administering them changed, this alteration of procedure could explain the O_1-O_2 difference. We must assume here that all of the subjects who took the pretest also took the posttest. But what if some of the women dropped out of the program before it concluded? What if the women who dropped out were persons who performed poorly on the pretest, leaving only the better achievers (or the persons already equipped with the most knowledge before the intervention) to take the posttest? Bias due to subject mortality could easily explain posttest improvement.

The static group comparison. Continuing with this same example, suppose we had two groups of women, one of which received the prenatal classes, the other of which did not. We can diagram this scenario as

$$X \quad O$$
$$O$$

where "X" is the prenatal intervention received by one group, and "O" represents an observation (a test of knowledge in this case). Upon completion of testing, the investigator concludes that the mean score of the group of women receiving prenatal education was significantly higher than the mean score of the comparison group. Now does this "proof" signify that the program is truly effective? In fact, it does not demonstrate this relationship since there was no pretest given. How could the investigator possibly know whether or not the intervention group's knowledge of pregnancy and childbirth was higher before the intervention even occurred. The posttest scores that were recorded might reflect nothing more than the differences that existed prior to the intervention. The education program may have contributed little or nothing to the eventual outcome. Despite clear and obvious shortcomings to this type of design, some investigators make use of it in assessing programs, and attribute more value to it than is deserved. Thus, they also risk drawing invalid and erroneous conclusions from studies.

Experimental and Quasi-experimental Methods and Designs

An *experiment* is a study in which the investigator controls or manipulates one or more factors or **independent variables**, and observes the effects of this manipulation on **dependent variables**, those events, outcomes, or phenomena that are under observation, but not manipulation. The investigator advances a **hypothesis** about what is believed to be the probable relationship between the independent and dependent variable. "The dependent variable is so named because its value is hypothesized to depend upon, and vary with, the value of the independent variable" (Ary, Jacobs & Razavieh, 1990, p.299). To illustrate, consider that an evaluator was interested in the effect of different interventions on knowledge of cigarette smoking and tobacco use in general. The investigator might manipulate the intervention by changing the content of the program (i.e., varying the independent variable) to identify the effect upon knowledge about tobacco, the dependent variable. If all groups of subjects receiving the interventions had equivalent levels of knowledge about tobacco initially, the investigator would be in a good position to determine which one of the programs (i.e., which variation of the independent variable) was most successful in bringing about cognitive changes. According to Best and Kahn (1989):

Experimental design is the blueprint of the procedures that enable the researcher to test hypotheses by reaching valid conclusions about relationships between independent and dependent variables. Selection of a particular design is based upon the purposes of the experiment, the type of variables to be manipulated, and the conditions or limiting factors under which it is conducted. The design deals with such practical problems as how subjects are to be assigned to experimental and control groups, the way variables are to be manipulated and controlled, the way extraneous variables are to be controlled, how observations are to be made, and the type of statistical analysis to be employed in interpreting data relationships. The adequacy of experimental designs is judged by the degree to which they eliminate or minimize threats to experimental validity (pp.123-124).

Green and Gordon (1982) write that the "ideal design for the evaluation of anything, including health education, is the true experimental design" (p.5). Moreover, they identify five essential elements of the experimental design: a sample of program recipients that is representative of the target population (see Chapter 13); pretests (measures preceding the educational program or intervention); a control or comparison group that does not receive the intervention under study; random assignment of the study participants to experimental and control groups; and, posttests to measure the effects at the conclusion of the intervention.

True experimental designs employ random assignment of persons to experimental and control (or comparison) groups. Randomization is the means by which assurance is provided that the groups are equivalent prior to implementation of a treatment or intervention. In the real world, it is not always possible to assign people to groups randomly. For example, while investigators may have access to students in a school, they may not have the luxury of selecting individual students for assignment to groups. Intact groups of students (i.e., classrooms) may be all that is at an investigator's disposal. In this situation, investigators are said to be using a **quasi-experimental design**. Let us look at some of the frequently employed experimental approaches.

Randomized control group pretest-posttest design. This design selects subjects and assigns them to experimental or control groups randomly, and pretests each group. One of the groups is exposed to the intervention while the other is not. Posttest measures are taken, and an appropriate statistical procedure is employed (see Chapter 14) to check whether the difference in posttest performance is statistically significant. This design is illustrated below, with "R" indicating that randomization has been employed, and "O" and "X" representing the observational measure and intervention respectively. "E" represents the experimental or intervention group, while "C" is the control group.

		Pretest	Intervention	Posttest
R	E	O_1	X	O_2
R	C	O_1		O_2

In some circumstances, it may be desirable to compare two or more variations ("a" and "b") of the experimental group. This situation might produce the design illustrated shown below.

		Pretest	Intervention	Posttest
R	E1	O_1	X_a	O_2
R	E2	O_1	X_b	O_2
R	C	O_1		O_2

Are these designs powerful ones? The answer is "Yes," and "No," where internal validity is concerned. Extraneous variables that occur between O_1 and O_2 (e.g., history, maturation) are controlled for since all groups should be affected similarly. Likewise, pretesting effects produce no issue since *all* groups are pretested. Differential selection is controlled for by the randomization procedure. Even statistical regression is controlled for according to Isaac and Michael (1971) "...when extreme scorers from the same population are randomly assigned to groups, statistical regression will occur but it will occur equally with all groups" (p.39).

What is *not* controlled for are the variations within the educational sessions themselves (i.e., room conditions, personalities and idiosyncrasies of program facilitators/teachers, use of unidentical language and explanations, etc.). The effects of these kinds of situational variations can be minimized by randomly assigning subjects, times, places, and instructors (if possible).

The randomized control group pretest-posttest design does not control for any of the threats to external validity. Thus, interactions between "X" and pretesting, selection, history, and reactive effects of the experimental procedures could invalidate results, and make generalizations tenuous. Review the threats to external validity discussed earlier if you are unsure about the reasons for lack of generalizability.

The randomized Solomon four-group design. This design is one of the most powerful of the true experimental designs because it allows the investigator not only to control for many confounding influences, but to measure their effects as well. For instance, the effects of history, maturation, and pretesting can be both controlled for, and measured. The Solomon four-group design can be displayed schematically as shown below.

Group		Pretest	Intervention	Posttest
1	R Pretested E	O_1	X	O_2
2	R Pretested C	O_1		O_2
3	R Unpretested E		X	O_2
4	R Unpretested C			O_2

This design overcomes the external validity issue related to pretesting by employing unpretested groups 3 and 4. Moreover, since random assignment is used, it can be assumed that pretest scores for groups 3 and 4 are similar to those of groups 1 and 2. Since pretesting is not done on groups 3 and 4, no interaction between X and O_1 can be reflected in the posttest measure.

One can measure the effect of X all by itself by looking at the difference of the posttest scores of groups 3 and 4 (i.e., Group 3 O_2 - Group 4 O_2). What would one have to do to find the effect of pretesting alone? the effect of the interaction of pretesting and X?

The randomized posttest only control group design. While there is no argument concerning the design validity of the Solomon four-group approach, it is a tedious design to carry out. One must have access to a large group of subjects to construct four groups. Furthermore, it is a labor-intensive design since there is a great deal of program delivery and measurement effort (2 pretests, 2 interventions, 4 posttests), as well as the ethical dilemma of how to handle unexposed control groups (see Chapter 3).

$$R \quad E \quad X \quad O_2$$

$$R \quad C \quad \quad O_2$$

As can be seen in the schematic above, the randomized posttest only control group design reduces one's workload without sacrificing much in the way of validity. It controls for the confounding influences of history, maturation, and pretesting (although it does not allow one to measure these effects directly). Since randomization is employed, pretests are unnecessary as it can be assumed that groups are equivalent at the start of the program. Moreover, there can be no interaction effects between pretesting and treatment, since no pretest is given. When resources do not permit four groups to be used, or when confounding factors need only to be controlled for and not measured, this design is a valuable alternative. It is also a preferred design when one wishes to explore the possible impact of an intervention that is new or innovative, or when circumstances are such that rapid feedback is desired, and more complex designs prove to be expensive or unwieldy.

The nonrandomized pretest-posttest control group design. This approach is quasi-experimental in nature since it does not use a randomizing procedure. In the "real world," evaluators are forced to make these kinds of compromises for administrative or other reasons. Intervention and control groups may be *intact groups* of subjects (e.g., students in classroom A versus classroom B, morning clinic patients versus afternoon clinic patients, workers on early shift versus late shift, mothers giving birth at hospital A versus hospital B, and so on). Schematically, it is identical to the randomized version discussed earlier (except for the absence of randomization). If pretesting reveals that the two groups do not differ significantly on the variable(s) of interest, threats to internal and external validity surrounding this design are essentially identical to those of its true experimental counterpart. If pretesting shows the groups *are* different at the start, however, attributing change measured at posttest strictly to the intervention becomes more difficult.

The counterbalanced design. Thus far, the designs that we have discussed, while increasingly more complex, are still relatively simple ones. The counterbalanced design exposes each group to *all* interventions, however many there are, but in a different order. This plan is illustrated on the next page.

Intervention Variations

Replication:	X_a	X_b	X_c	X_d
1	A	B	C	D
2	B	D	A	C
3	C	A	D	B
4	D	C	B	A

Column means:

In the counterbalanced design, groups are designated A - D, and intervention variations are designated X_a - X_d. Each group receives a different X at a given time, and each X precedes and follows each other variation of X an equal number of times. To interpret the

Test Performance (Score) as Related to Method and Time

	Method		
	Lecture	Discussion	Mean
Time			
60'	46	38	42
75'	40	32	36
Mean	43	35	

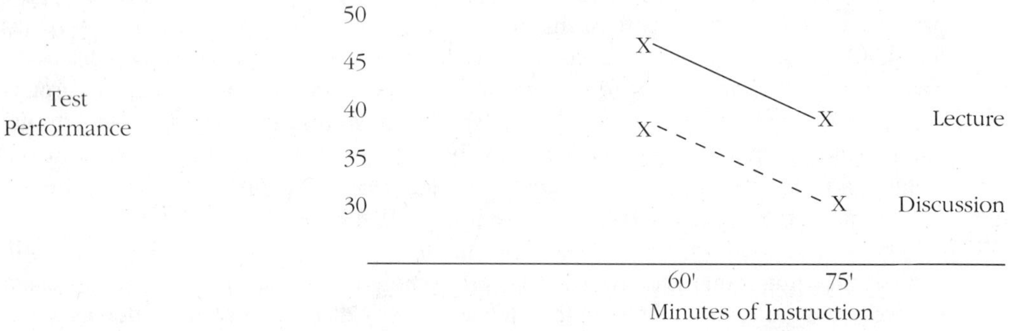

Test Performance

50
45
40
35
30

60'   75'
Minutes of Instruction

Lecture
Discussion

Figure 10.1 A 2 x 2 Factorial Design without the Presence of an Interaction Effect

effectiveness of each intervention, investigators compare the mean scores for all groups on the posttest for each intervention. That is, the mean posttest score for X_a can be compared with the mean posttest score for all groups for X_b, X_c, and X_d. This design controls for the possibility that intact groups of subjects are not equivalent prior to intervention (a concern inherent with the previously discussed design). On the down side, this design is vulnerable to certain interaction effects, e.g., selection-maturation (Isaac & Michael, 1971) and to multiple-treatment interference (Fraenkel & Wallen, 1990). In multiple-treatment interference, the effects of one X carry over and combine with measurements on the next X. Where the assumption of no carry-over effect cannot be made, the utility of the counterbalanced design is diminished.

Factorial designs. Classical experimental designs examine the variation of a single variable at a time, and hold all other relevant conditions constant. The factorial design extends the number of relationships that can be examined in a single study. It has two chief advantages according to Fraenkel and Wallen (1990). First, it is a modification of the posttest-only control group design or the pretest-posttest control group design (with or without randomization) that permits exploration of additional independent variables. Second, the factorial design allows an investigator to examine whether an independent variable has any interaction effect with one or more other variables. A simple 2 x 2 factorial design is illustrated in Figure 10.1 *without* an interaction effect present, and in Figure 10.2 *with* an interaction effect.

In Figure 10.1, the lecture method is shown to be superior to the discussion method regardless of the time of instruction. Thus, no interaction effect is present, as seen by examination of the tabled data, as well as by inspection of the diagram. In Figure 10.2, test performance was better in the instructional period of shorter duration, regardless of method. However, persons in 60' instructional periods performed better when taught by lecture, while persons in the 75' sessions performed better when taught by a discussion method. Therefore, even though persons did better when exposed to shorter instructional periods, how well they did was dependent on which method was used. The investigator is not able to conclude that lecture is better than discussion, or vice versa, since time of instruction interacts to affect test performance.

Factorial designs more complex than the 2 x 2 are employed. A 2 x 3 design might have gender (male or female) as one variable and smoking cessation method (cognitive restructuring, stimulus control, contingency contracting) as another. Designs such as 3 x 3 or 2 x 2 x 2 are also possible, but go beyond the intended scope of this text.

Time-series designs. A time-series design involves repeated measurements or observations over time, including times before and after the intervention. A basic time-series design is illustrated below.

Pretest				Intervention			Posttest	
O1	O2	O3	O4	X	O5	O6	O7	O8

Test Performance (Score) as Related to Method and Time

Time	Method		Mean
	Lecture	Discussion	
60'	48	42	45
75'	32	38	35
Mean	40	40	

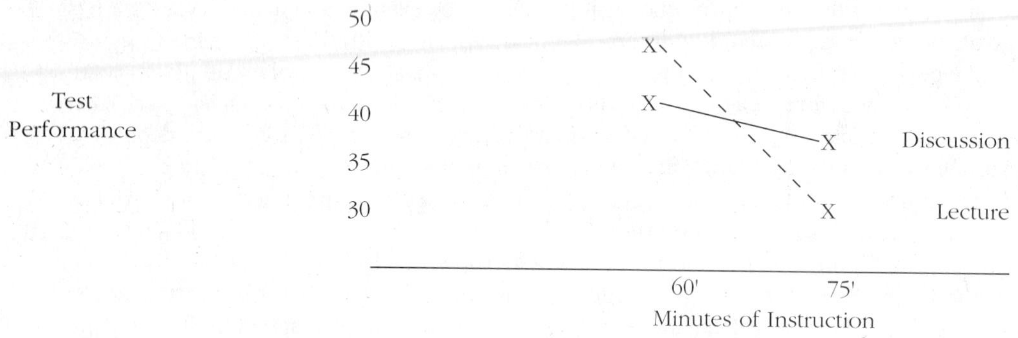

Test Performance (50, 45, 40, 35, 30) plotted against Minutes of Instruction (60', 75') showing Discussion and Lecture lines.

Figure 10.2 A 2 x 2 Factorial Design with the Presence of an Interaction Effect

This design is like the one-shot case study except that several measures are taken before and after the introduction of the intervention, thus providing more control over threats to internal validity. For instance, if there is no significant difference in the four pretest scores, the difference between O_4 and O_5 cannot be attributed to maturation, the effects of testing, or regression toward the mean. Moreover, the effects of selection and mortality can be controlled or accounted for. The chief limiting threat is contemporary history, if an event occurred between O_4 and O_5 that could magnify or diminish the apparent true effects of X. History can be controlled for, too, if the investigator is able to add a control group that receives everything that the intervention group receives *except* the intervention.

Summary

Program evaluators have many ways in which they can measure the effectiveness of an intervention by using quantitative approaches. Inherent in any evaluation approach are threats to internal validity that the investigator must try to control for or measure. Some threats are beyond the investigator's control, and always lurk about as confounding factors. Studies may be quantified using nonexperimental, true experimental, or quasi-experimental designs. The investigator's ability to manipulate the environment in which an evaluation is performed will dictate which set of methods and designs is appropriate. Solving design and methodological issues is one of the most basic challenges of being a researcher or program evaluator. It is also one of the most satisfying.

Case Study

Tucker, L.A., Martin, J.R., & Harris, K. (1997). Effects of a strength training program on the blood lipid levels of sedentary adult women. *American Journal of Health Behavior*, *21*(5), 323-332.

The authors report the effects of a 12-week strength training program on LDL and HDL cholesterol in a group of sedentary women (mean age = 42.8 years) versus women in a comparison group. A pretest, dual posttest experimental design with randomization was employed. What issues related to experimental design, internal validity, and external validity occur here? What sampling limitations are involved? What additional confounding factors were present or could have been present? Under more ideal circumstances, how could the design of this study have been improved to strengthen both internal and external validity?

Student Questions/Activities

1. What problem related to internal validity might occur if one wanted to measure the impact of a Wisconsin law eliminating cigarette vending machines on per capita tobacco sales, if Illinois and Minnesota (which have no such laws) were used as comparison states? Explain.

2. In a pretest-posttest control group design, how does one control for the confounding effects of subject mortality?

3. What ethical considerations are at play when one wishes to employ a true experimental design with an unexposed (i.e., untreated) control group? What are some possible solutions to these dilemmas?

4. A regular criticism of experimental designs among health educators is that they are difficult logistically to carry out in school settings, thereby reducing the possibility of getting good demonstrative data about the efficacy of school health education. Would you agree or disagree? Explain. To arrive at a more complete answer to this question, it might be interesting to meet with administrators from your local school district, and discuss the various obstacles and issues involved in doing health education research and evaluation in schools. Feedback from administrators, as well as inherent obstacles, are likely to vary from locale to locale.

5. For each of the following situations, which design or designs might be useful?
   a. A comparison of two ways of teaching senior citizens about using medications.

b. The effectiveness of six-month weight training program on grip strength and muscle mass in a group of college athletes.

c. The possible effects of gender, age, race, and socio-economic status on cigarette and smokeless "spit" tobacco use among 10th-grade students.

d. The effectiveness of reinforcement on smoking control in a group of individuals who have recently completed a smoking cessation program.

Recommended Readings

Ewart, C.K., Young, D.R., & Hagberg, J.M. (1998). Effects of school-based aerobic exercise on blood pressure in adolescent girls at risk for hypertension. *American Journal of Public Health, 88*(6), 949-951.

African American ninth-grade girls with blood pressures above the 67th percentile were randomly assigned to either a special aerobics class for one semester, or a standard physical education class. At the end of the study only those girls assigned to the aerobics class had increased their estimated cardiorespiratory fitness. Moreover, the aerobics group experienced a significantly greater decline in systolic blood pressure. After reading this article, consider the sources of measurement error and any threats to internal validity. How could this study have been improved methodologically? To what extent does this study illustrate the compromises that must be made in evaluation designs when working in applied settings such as schools? Explain.

Cousins, M., & McDowell, I, (1995). Use of medical care after a community-based health promotion program: A quasi-experimental study. *American Journal of Health Promotion, 10*(1), 47-54.

A community-based intervention to reduce ambulatory care visits, thereby reducing health care costs, was implemented. Volunteer participants (n=520) and 932 matched controls were assessed prior to and after the program. A quasi-experimental, nonequivalent comparison group design was used. The evidence collected did not show that the intervention group reduced visits. In fact, with respect to some measures, the intervention group had more primary care visits and services. How do you explain this phenomenon? To what extent do you think the findings are a result of a weak intervention? Weak measures? If you could repeat the study, what would you change?

Telljohann, S.K., Everett, S.A., & Price, J.H. (1997). Evaluation of a third grade sexual abuse curriculum. *Journal of School Health, 67*(4), 149-153.

A 24-item knowledge survey was administered to third grade students (n=236) exposed to a sexual abuse curriculum as well as to students not exposed (n=195). Both pretest and posttest measures were taken. Intervention subjects significantly increased their knowledge about sexual abuse between pretest and posttest. After reading this article, consider the timing of exposure (both pretest and posttest) to the instrument, and how timing might have affected the measured impact of the curriculum. The authors discuss several limitations to the study, but are there threats to internal validity present here that are not mentioned by the authors? How could you improve on the design of this study, including reducing measurement error? Explain.

References

Ary, D., Jacobs, L.C., & Razavieh, A. (1990). *Introduction to Research in Education*, 4th edition. Fort Worth, TX: Holt, Rinehart and Winston.

Best, J.W., & Kahn, J.V. (1989). *Research in Education*, 6th edition. Englewood Cliffs, NJ: Prentice Hall.

Campbell, D.T., & Stanley, J.C. (1966). *Experimental and Quasi-experimental Designs for Research*. Boston: Houghton Mifflin Company.

Cook, T.D., & Campbell, D.T. (1979). *Quasi-experimentation*. Boston: Houghton Mifflin Company.

Fink, A., & Kosecoff, J. (1978). *An Evaluation Primer*. Beverly Hills, CA: Sage Publications.

Fraenkel, J.R., & Wallen, N.E. (1990). *How To Design and Evaluate Research in Education*. New York: McGraw-Hill.

French, J.F., & Kaufman, N.J. (Eds.) (1981). *Handbook for Prevention Education*. Rockville, MD: National Institute on Drug Abuse, DHHS Publication No. (ADM)83-1145.

Green, L.W., & Gordon, N.P. (1982). Productive research designs for health education investigations. *Health Education, 13*(3), 4-10.

Isaac, S., & Michael, W.B. (1971). *Handbook in Research and Evaluation*. San Diego: EdITS.

Schofield, J.W., & Anderson, K.M. (1984). Combining quantitative and qualitative methods in research on ethnic identity and intergroup relations. Paper presented at the Society for Research on Child Development Study Group on Ethnic Socialization, Los Angeles.

Shortell, S.M., & Richardson, W.C. (1978). *Health Program Evaluation*. St. Louis: C.V. Mosby Company.

Worthen, B.R., & Sanders, J.R. (1987). *Educational Evaluation*. New York: Longman.

Wright, S.R. (1979). *Quantitative Methods and Statistics*. Beverly Hills, CA: Sage Publications.

Chapter 11

Qualitative Evaluation: Methods and Designs

Chapter Objectives

After completing this chapter, you should be able to:

1. Identify several contexts in which using qualitative evaluation strategies is desirable and appropriate.
2. Distinguish between the salient features of qualitative evaluation methods versus quantitative evaluation methods.
3. Describe several qualitative data collection methods, and illustrate each with an application to the evaluation of health education and promotion programs.
4. Synthesize potential situations where quantitative and qualitative strategies in program evaluation can be combined.

Key Terms

formative evaluation

graffiti

observer bias

observer effect

triangulation/triangulation of evidence

Introduction

In Chapter 10 we looked at quantitative paradigms for conducting evaluation of health education programs. Powerful as they are, quantitative techniques do not tell us everything that we would like to know about the *how's* and *why's* of program operation and delivery. Fortunately, there are *qualitative* evaluation models and techniques that can assist us in addressing the types of questions that quantitative techniques do not answer adequately. This chapter addresses qualitative evaluation methods, and explores circumstances where their implementation is both useful and appropriate. Some specific applications of qualitative methods in health education settings are discussed.

Qualitative Evaluation in Perspective

In *quantitative* evaluation (see Chapter 10), the investigator seeks answers to questions concerning "how well" or "to what extent" a program achieves its objectives, "how much" learning or behavior change occurs, and the degree to which program dimensions can be linked to a particular set of outcomes. At times, an evaluator also might wish to gain a more complete understanding of how the program functions. Consider the presentation of a lesson about AIDS in a high school classroom setting. How do teachers present the lesson? What kinds of activities support the lesson? Are there particular teacher characteristics (good or bad) that enhance or detract from the lesson? How do the teachers perceive their task, as compared to how the students perceive it? If learning occurs in an effective manner, why is this? Or, if learning does not occur, what is it about the teacher, the students, the material, the environment, or the interaction of these factors that interferes with the educational process?

These types of issues are ones dealing with the quality of the program under investigation. Studies that address the quality of relationships, activities, situations, or materials are referred to as *qualitative evaluations* (Fraenkel & Wallen, 1990). Whether one speaks of evaluative or basic research, qualitative methods differ from quantitative approaches in that there is greater emphasis placed on holistic descriptions of various phenomena. That is, qualitative investigators examine the minute details of what goes on with respect to a given activity or a given environment. One might say that qualitative evaluation tells us what really makes a program "tick" or "not tick."

While qualitative approaches may be quite variable, Bogdan and Biklen (1982) have identified five characteristics that these methods have in common. First, they involve a naturalistic setting in which the context of activities is integral to the evaluation. That is, they involve the investigator spending time observing the routines and rituals of the persons around whom the evaluation is centered. Consequently, if the evaluation is of a worksite health promotion program, the evaluator is likely to observe people during and after work, meet formally or informally with workers to gain insights concerning their impressions of the program, and compare these impressions to those held by persons responsible for program delivery, program managers, and other personnel. The evaluator may use nothing except a notebook to record observations and comments. Or, the evaluator may use audio or video equipment to make a more permanent record of the data.

A second commonality of qualitative approaches is that they do not ordinarily involve the reduction of data into numbers. Therefore, the data *are* the transcripts of interviews, the diaries, the personal field notes, the photographs, or the tape recordings that help to convey meaning about the settings and places under study. As Fraenkel and Wallen (1990) point out:

Gestures, jokes, conversational gambits, artwork or other decorations in a room -- all are noted by qualitative researchers. To a qualitative researcher, no data are trivial or unworthy of notice (p.368).

Thirdly, qualitative evaluation is concerned with *process* as well as *product*. Whereas *quantitative* evaluation seeks to explain *what* happens, *qualitative* evaluations try to identify *how* and *why*. Thus, a qualitative evaluation of a successful group smoking cessation program might consist of examination of how the participants interacted with each other and with the group leader (i.e., group dynamics), how the words and recommendations of behavior change specialists, education specialists, pulmonary disease or coronary disease specialists, and other program speakers were translated into action by the participants. It is not an uncommon occurrence for a program to function well in one setting under the direction of a particular individual, but to perform poorly (or at least less well) in another setting, under the leadership of a different person. Why do such discrepancies occur? Is it the facilitator? Is it the setting? Is it the people who make up the participant group? Such questions are best addressed through qualitative methods. In the implementation stages of a program, even one that has goals and objectives that eventually will be evaluated by quantitative measures, qualitative methods can be extremely useful in providing early feedback about program performance and program dynamics. Such feedback is an essential component of **formative evaluation** (see Chapter 1). Based on this kind of feedback, structural changes can be made in a program that ultimately will result in improved effectiveness or efficiency. Without the benefit of such feedback, a potentially good program might flounder or fail to live up to the needs of the people it was designed to serve.

A fourth characteristic of qualitative approaches is that they tend to involve *inductive* rather than *deductive* reasoning. A *quantitative* investigation is likely to begin with a hypothesis or research question. A *qualitative* study is one in which the data collection is done first, only after which the investigator begins deciding what the important or relevant questions to consider are. In fact, an important application of qualitative studies may be in generating research questions or hypotheses. Therefore, qualitative studies can be antecedents of quantitative investigations.

A fifth common thread with qualitative methods is the investigator's keen interest in understanding the people who are under study. Capturing the motives and reasons for people's behaviors, and the values that underlie these behaviors are of genuine concern. Investigators want to be able to understand other people's perspectives, not just their best interpretation of others' perspectives. Accurate portrayal of perceptions is a critical priority of the qualitative evaluator. In Table 11.1, some of the conditions under which qualitative evaluation may be especially useful are identified.

Table 11.1 Circumstances under which Qualitative Evaluation Should be Considered

Whenever:

- individualized client/student/patient outcomes are being emphasized
- decision makers desire to understand the dynamics and processes of how a program works
- in-depth information is desired about particular clients, cases, or program sites
- the unique aspects of a program are being assessed
- how clients experience the program is of interest
- formative evaluation is being stressed
- unobtrusive or less obtrusive data collection is needed
- case-specific quality assurance is an issue
- an evaluation especially responsive and tailored to the individualized interests of stakeholders is required
- program goals are vague or as yet undetermined
- quantitative measures fail to measure outcomes determined to be important
- evaluation is still exploratory
- the evaluability of a program is unknown, and the type of appropriate summative procedures is unclear
- there is a need to add depth, detail, and context to statistical data and other quantitative measures
- new measurement perspectives are desired

Adapted from: Patton, M.Q. (1987). *How to Use Qualitative Methods in Evaluation.* Newbury Park, CA: Sage Publications, pp.40-42.

Qualitative Methods

Having briefly examined some fundamentals of qualitative evaluation, it is time to look at specific methods. Qualitative researchers and evaluators have a wide array of methods available to them. We will examine some of the more commonly employed strategies in the remainder of this chapter. The reader should keep in mind that the list of descriptions provided is not an exhaustive one. Moreover, the approaches that are identified are not necessarily mutually exclusive. The distinctiveness of one approach versus another one to which it bears similarity may be due primarily to the context in which it is employed. Furthermore, one's evaluation purpose, available resources, and concurrent use of other evaluative techniques will play a role in the choice and utilization of specific methods.

Naturalistic Observations

This technique involves observation of individuals in so-called natural settings, i.e., non-laboratory settings where people congregate to perform typical or routine activities. Examples of the use of this strategy to examine behavior might include studying the interactions of preschool children on a playground, studying the waiting room activities of patients in a clinic, studying the handwashing behavior of persons in a restroom, studying teacher-pupil interactions in a classroom, studying the social interactions of persons in a singles bar, and so on. The evaluator's aim is to capture a "slice of life" without manipulating any of the variables under investigation. A certain amount of **observer effect** may not be avoidable, however. The known or suspected presence of an observer may cause people to alter their behavior, and hence, influence the conclusions drawn. **Observer bias** is also a potential problem. Regardless of how hard one may try to be impartial, one is limited to what is noticed, what is judged to be important, and what one expects to see in the first place.

Participant-observer Studies

Sometimes the investigator can get a better look at what is being observed by becoming a participant as well as an observer. To study what it means to be homeless and without a job, there is nothing quite as effective in learning the dynamics of homelessness as spending several days as a "street person." In the 1960s, John Howard Griffin, a Caucasian and author of the book *Black Like Me*, had his skin color changed chemically. He subsequently observed first hand what it was like to move about in some areas where racial prejudice was strong. Clearly, the strength of the participant-observer procedure is the first hand experience it can provide the investigator. When other persons know that observations are being made, the shortcomings of observational studies noted earlier surface, and confound the investigator's ability to make accurate interpretations of what is seen.

Ethnographic Studies

Ethnography employs participant observation, other observational techniques, interviews, and formal and informal interactions with people to obtain a global impression of a given society, group, institution, setting, or set of circumstances. According to Fraenkel and Wallen (1990), the emphasis is on "documenting or portraying the everyday experiences of individuals by observing and interviewing them and relevant others" (p.374).

An example of a question that might be addressed using ethnographic techniques is: *What is it like to be an unmarried, pregnant adolescent?* The investigator's objective would be to document the daily experiences of girls in this situation, and to assess the girls' interactions with such persons as parents, siblings, teachers, friends, health care providers, including physicians, social workers, and others. Pregnant adolescents, once identified and recruited into a study, would be observed over a period of time (perhaps the duration of pregnancy and early parenthood). The investigator's concluding evaluative document would portray the experiences of these girls as completely and fully as possible, perhaps using exact quotations and other evidence to "capture" the affect of the situation of interest. Ethnographic interviewing might be employed to answer other questions that do not lend themselves well to conventional data collection methods: (1) Why do some people fail to take precautions regarding sexual activity, and thus, expose themselves to the risk of acquiring HIV or other sexually transmissible infections? (2) In a given culture, why are certain pregnancy prevention approaches acceptable, but others are not? (3) How do young people become recruited into the "drug culture" to use or sell drugs to other youngsters?

A special type of ethnographic study is known as *street ethnography*, because the study is focused on a particular site -- a street corner, a park, a playground, or so on. If one is to understand the street culture of the drug addict, the prostitute, or the gang member, the best way to achieve this end is to "hit the streets." Street ethnographers encounter the problem of entry to the community of people to be studied -- at least the problem of *safe* entry. Proponents of street ethnography point to the failure of traditional fact finding strategies, such as surveys, to gather adequate data about street cultures, deviant groups, or rare cultures (Marshall & Rossman, 1995).

In-depth Interviewing

This strategy has been described by Kahn and Cannell (1957) as "a conversation with a purpose" (p.149). Interview style may vary from brief, casual conversation to formal and lengthy interactions. The in-depth interview differs from the heavily structured interview in that it unfolds more like normal conversation (Marshall & Rossman, 1995). The interviewee's perspective is allowed to be revealed as the conversation proceeds. The outcome can be rich data and understanding of the participant's view of the world, or at least that part of it in which the investigator has interest.

All interviewing requires skill and practice. Poor interviewing skills, poor phrasing of questions, or inadequate knowledge of the subject's culture or frame of reference may result in little data being obtained. A further weakness of the technique is the assumption that subjects who are interviewed are truthful in their responses. There must be a strong element of trust between the subject and the interviewer for high quality data to be obtained. The interviewer must be comfortable with other people, as well as be a skilled listener.

Elite Interviewing

An elite interview is specialized in that it focuses on a certain type of respondent. Such respondents are usually influential, prominent, and well-informed people who can provide a unique perspective on the issue being addressed in the qualitative study. The social, political, financial, or administrative position of the interviewees may give them access to information not otherwise obtainable. A person seeking to evaluate the perspective of CEOs with respect to the efficacy of company health promotion programs might use the elite interview approach. Getting to elite individuals can be difficult, though, because such people often are well insulated, have serious time commitments and constraints, and therefore, have limited availability. Thus, the investigator may need strong sponsorship, special introductions, and other help to make contact with elite individuals.

Focus Group Interviewing

"The focus group interview or discussion is a qualitative approach to learning about population subgroups with respect to conscious, semi-conscious and unconscious psychological and sociocultural characteristics and processes" (Basch, 1987, p.411). Focus groups have been used primarily in the past for market research -- finding out what people seek in certain products, where people shop and why, how they evaluate a product, and so on. Their utility has been summarized by Bellenger, Bernhardt, and Goldstucker (1976):

- Generation of hypotheses that can be tested quantitatively at a future time.
- Generation of information helpful in constructing a consumer questionnaire.
- Providing background information about a product or line of products.
- Collecting impressions about new products where there is little existing information.
- Stimulating new ideas about existing products.
- Generating ideas for creative concepts.
- Interpreting quantitative data that have been obtained previously.

Simmons (1985) has identified three additional uses of the focus group interview: to carry out formative evaluation of program planning; to assess the design of message strategies; and to conduct needs assessment.

The focus group interview approach has been used to study health and health education issues with selected groups such as high school students for developing a nutrition education video (James, Rienzo & Frazee, 1997), women and health care practitioners to obtain their views on barriers to effective family planning (McDermott, Bryant, Westhoff, Marty, Holcomb, Kroetsch, Lopez & Kent, 1996), college students to identify salient issues related to campus alcohol abuse (Emery, Ritter-Randolph, Strozier & McDermott, 1993), women responsible for family food purchases (Shepherd, Sims, Cronin, Shaw & Davis, 1989), senior citizens (Keller, Sliepcevich, Vitello, Lacey & Wright, 1987), pregnant teenagers (Kisker, 1985), and persons with hypertension (National Heart, Lung, and Blood Institute, 1979). Identification of what is wanted or what is acceptable provides not only *feedback* on existing resources, but also *feedforward* concerning the creation of new materials.

The group moderator will recruit participants on the basis of some important trait or characteristic that they possess that is pertinent to the investigation. The moderator will prepare a list of topics or general questions and issues that will be discussed, and distribute these to group participants. Although actual group size may vary, a composition of eight to twelve members often is ideal. The purpose of the focus group, as well as the homogeneity or heterogeneity of the membership, may determine the most suitable size. The role of the moderator is a critical one, because it is important that one or two persons not be allowed to dominate the discussion, or express their views so forcefully that other persons in the group are intimidated, frustrated, or bored. All opinions and beliefs expressed in the focus group are legitimate, and the facilitator must avoid being judgmental. A non-threatening environment (physical as well as psychological) is needed for successful participation and elicitation of responses. Persons acting as moderators must undergo interviewer training and practice before leading a group. For optimal effectiveness, the moderator may have a colleague present to take notes or to record observations, so as to be able to concentrate on leading the group, following up on ideas, and making smooth transitions from issue to issue. Excellent sources for more in-depth information about conducting focus groups include those by Krueger (1988), Morgan (1988), Stewart and Shamdasani (1990), and Morgan and Krueger (1998).

Historical Analysis

A historical analysis is an account of events that occurred in the past, and may include an interpretation of the impact such events have on current attitudes, values, and practices. Historical data may come from a variety of sources, including records of all types, reports, newspaper accounts, diaries and memoirs, archival documents, folklore, fiction, songs, poetry, and art (Marshall & Rossman, 1995). Historical analysis might be an effective technique for evaluating such issues as: (1) the factors that gave rise to the adoption of legislation that created programs like Medicare and Medicaid; (2) the persons, events, and social movements that have prevented the development of a comprehensive national health plan in the United States; and (3) the reasons why the United States, despite superior technology, lags behind many other countries in the world in terms of key indices of health status. Means (1975) illustrates the use of historical approaches to ascertain explanations of current school health practices in his classic work, *Historical Perspectives on School Health*. Persons using historical analysis must forever be cautious of introducing bias to studies resulting from the imposition of current thoughts and values on problems of previous eras. The accuracy and authenticity of some historical accounts may always leave some doubt as one attempts to reconstruct events as they actually occurred (as any American historian who has ever tried to evaluate the events at the Alamo, the Little Big Horn, the JFK assassination scene, or the Watergate break-in would no doubt confirm). Furthermore, the ability of the investigator to interpret historical documents and relics is a constant limitation. Nevertheless, historical analysis allows the evaluator a great deal of freedom to speculate and bring new perspective to important issues.

Content Analysis

Content analysis has been defined as "any technique for making inferences by objectively and systematically identifying specified characteristics of messages" (Holsti, 1969, p.14). Krippendorff (1980) states that "content analysis is a research technique for making replicable and valid inferences from data to their context" (p.21). Let us simply say here that content analysis is a strategy for studying the content of messages that has applications in both program planning and evaluation.

As an evaluation and research tool, content analysis has had an interesting history. In 18th century Sweden, the procedure was used by officials of the Lutheran church (the state church of Sweden) to count and to judge the words used in religious sermons and hymns to prove or to disprove the introduction of heresy. Heresy was considered a crime, the conviction of which could result in life imprisonment or execution. Because of the seriousness of the crime, this analysis technique was used by people on both sides of the controversy (Dovring, 1973; Holsti, 1969; Krippendorff, 1980; Rosengren, 1981). Holsti (1969) estimates that during World War II, 25 percent of the use of content analysis was "political research using propaganda materials" (p.21).

Many creative studies are now being done in diverse areas such as art, literature, and music (Paisely, 1984), cartoons and comic strips (Ehrle & Johnson, 1961; Chavez, 1985; Sofalvi & Drolet, 1986), antidepressant drug advertisements (Goldman & Montagne, 1986) and the content of suicide notes (Leenaars, 1986; Leenaars & Balance, 1981). Other uses of the technique in the health area have included content analysis of statistics reported in the *New England Journal of Medicine* (Emerson & Colditz, 1983), the *Journal of Educational Psychology* (Goodwin & Goodwin, 1985), and the *Journal of School Health* (Rudolph, McDermott & Gold, 1985), health-related articles found in women's magazines (Miller, Sliepcevich & Vitello, 1981), and health subjects addressed in *Health Education* (Sliepcevich, Keller & Sondag, 1986-87).

Content analysis requires careful planning, including performance of at least the following steps: (1) establishing specific objectives to be achieved or questions to be answered; (2) locating the sources of data from which questions will be answered; (3) describing a method or data collection scheme that will yield a representative sample or range of data; (4) identifying a data coding or classification protocol; and (5) making a decision concerning the summarization or data analysis procedure to be employed. More information about specific methods and application of content analysis can be obtained in a book by Weber (1985).

Case Studies

The case study is a qualitative evaluation approach in which the investigator attempts to organize social data for the purpose of viewing what Best and Kahn (1989) call the "social reality" (p.92). The case study examines a social unit, such as a person, a family or household, a worksite setting, a community, or almost any kind of institution as a whole. The unit of analysis, thus, may be a single subject. To collect and organize information, the investigator may employ in-depth interviewing, observation, records, reports, or virtually any other type of method or source of data discussed elsewhere in this chapter.

The case study has been made famous in fields like psychiatry by persons such as Sigmund Freud. Information obtained through a single case may not be generalizable to other settings and times, but it may allow the investigator to understand the dynamics of relationships, and other important variables that lead to decisions, attitudes, behaviors, and other relevant measures of program performance. An in-depth case study analysis of the design, implementation, growth, and permanent establishment of a single worksite health education and promotion program, including key personnel, may not guarantee the success of a program implemented elsewhere. However, it might provide considerable guidance to persons initiating a worksite health program idea. If compared to another case study of a program that failed, relevant variables might surface that indicate critical features that distinguish programs that succeed from ones that fail.

Films, Photographs, and Videotape Recording

This combination of data collection and recording procedures is identified by Marshall and Rossman (1995) as *visual anthropology* or *film ethnography*. They are used to capture the significant daily events, routines, or lifestyles of a particular group under study. They can be preserved to provide a permanent visual image of people and events, and when accompanied by a descriptive narrative, provide a rich source of data. Since the images are visual, such supplementary data as body postures, facial expressions, and other nonverbal communication signals are available for study and interpretation (see *Kinesics* later in this chapter). Film ethnography may be particularly effective as a means of recording, and subsequently studying in detail, the reaction of children to an activity, a learning exercise, or a particular assigned task. By means of film or videotape, social interactions, levels of leadership and group participation, activity level, and involvement can be viewed and measured. The recording of audience and actors participating in a skit with a race-prejudice theme might provide unique insights about the effectiveness of skits to engage children in the relevant issues.

Marshall and Rossman (1995) identify several weaknesses of the film ethnography approach. They caution the prospective user that bias (planned or unplanned) in filming can "manipulate reality." Moreover, the ethics of filming, as well as other intrusive aspects of the activity must be taken into consideration. Finally, the costs and technical expertise required to produce a quality end product may be prohibitively high.

Kinesics

Speech effectively conveys meaning, but nonverbal cues, signs, and signals can be quite effective, too (as any motor vehicle operator who has just cut off another vehicle can attest if the other driver responds with what has become a popular gesture on roadways). Kinesics is the study of body communication. Motions ranging from the nod of the head, to one's overall body posture, hand position, or arm gesture may reveal important evaluative information to supplement verbal feedback and cues. It is possible that certain kinesics could even be taught to people (e.g., adolescents) as devices for responding to challenging situations, such as being offered tobacco, alcohol, or other drugs. A shrug, a facial grimace, or a look of disgust following the offer of drugs may be a nonverbal countermeasure that could be evaluated for effectiveness.

Kinesic analysis is limited by the lack of universal meaning attached to certain gestures, and the cultural specificity of other nonverbal responses. For example, in one culture, direct eye contact may signify caring, concern, and empathetic intimacy; in a different culture, the identical kinesic activity might be interpreted as rude, invasive, threatening, or destructive. Good kinesic interpretation can only be made by experts. Nevertheless, kinesics provides a qualitative tool that has potential in the health education arena that has gone largely unexplored at this point in time.

Nominal Group Process

The nominal group process is a "structured meeting that attempts to provide an orderly procedure for obtaining qualitative information from target groups who are most closely associated with a problem area" (Fink, Kosecoff, Chassin & Brook, 1984, p.980). In an organization such as a public health department, someone might use the nominal group process as a means of prioritizing health problems to be addressed educationally in the community during the coming year. A group size of five to eight well chosen individuals is ideal (Van de Ven & Delbecq, 1972). In application, the process might proceed in the following sequence:

- Identify and bring together a panel of people whose expert judgments and opinions are valuable.
- Instruct each panel member to develop a written list of health problems to be addressed. This step is performed without consultation or discussion.
- When this task is completed, individuals present in turn the items on their respective lists. This process is carried out until all of the items on each of the lists are exhausted. The items are recorded so that all panel members can view them (e.g., on a flip-chart or chalkboard).
- A structured discussion ensues involving the items on the composite list. Each idea is evaluated separately, and any individual may express a view in defense or criticism of the merit of a particular item. Clarifications are made as necessary. Discussion proceeds until everyone who has a thought to express is permitted to do so.
- Each individual proceeds to evaluate the priorities, and to develop a revised and prioritized list based on the discussion that occurred.
- The panel's collective views are assessed to arrive at a consensus decision.

The nominal group process may be used for whatever creative purpose that the organizer can establish. For instance, the process may be used to identify content of items on a written survey or interview schedule which must be highly targeted, yet limited in scope. Van de Van and Delbecq (1972) provide a more in-depth presentation of the organization and delivery of the nominal group activity for exploratory health studies.

Delphi Technique

The Delphi technique is another technique whose aim is to use expert opinion to arrive at consensus about planning or problem-solving issues. It has been employed to study a wide range of issues from population growth to warfare and weapon systems (Brown, 1968). In the health education and promotion arena, it has been used to examine perceptions of the meanings assigned to the construct of "wellness" (Mullen, 1983), and to determine the nature of the spiritual dimension of health (Banks, Poehler & Russell, 1984).

With the Delphi technique, expert participants are polled, usually by means of a mailed, self-administered questionnaire. The procedure may have evolved out of criticism of the nominal group process, in which an outspoken, forceful, or highly persuasive individual can influence the outcome of the group's activity. The advent of electronic mail (i.e., e-mail) has facilitated the use of the Delphi technique by reducing cost and expediting feedback and dissemination.

The Delphi technique conventionally proceeds through three or four rounds, after each of which the results are tabulated and shared with the participants. After examining group feedback, individuals may modify their opinions, rankings, priorities, and so on in response to new information, modification of thought, or other reasons and events. The process typically is declared to be over when one of two events occurs: (1) a convergence of opinion is apparent, i.e., a level of consensus that may have been established at the onset of the process; or (2) a point of diminishing returns is reached (i.e., no further changes in group opinion, or significantly reduced response rate from participants).

Unlike the nominal group process, the Delphi technique permits participants to express views confidentially and impersonally -- thereby minimizing the overt influence that any one or two individuals can have on the group's overall opinion. Moreover, since e-mail or conventional mail is the mechanism for providing input and feedback, the use of experts is not limited to a particular region or geographic area. Furthermore, the number of rounds of activity used is open-ended, and restricted only by participants' lack of willingness to respond indefinitely. Reliability of the Delphi strategy increases with the number of rounds used as well as with the size of the participant group.

The Delphi technique does have limitations. The number of expert panelists, while initially large, may decline with the number of rounds used. Panelists lose interest, become fatigued, or develop other interests and demands that do not permit time for further response. The coordination of a large number of panelists may be an arduous task. The Delphi technique does not permit discussion among the panelists, so is not useful if personal contact is necessary or desired. Finally, there is debate over the means and criteria by which "experts" are chosen, and thus, some warranted concern about the validity of the process (Sackman, 1975).

Quality Circles

The quality circle is a strategy originally developed in the United States, but used widely in Japanese industry and in several European countries (Schillemans, De Grande & Remmen, 1989). The aim of the quality circle is to increase an organization's macro level problem-solving capacity by involving as much as possible, the individuals who are most directly involved with the delivery and receipt of services. A quality circle, then, is a group of people who meet at regular intervals to discuss problems and to identify possible solutions. One of the basic premises of the quality circle approach is that responsibility for quality control is moved from the top to the bottom of the decision making hierarchy.

The quality circle concept can be used to make evaluation an integral aspect of the program intervention process, and not simply a separate assessment activity (Schillemans, et al., 1989). Suppose we were faced with the task of evaluating a volunteer health agency-based smoking cessation program targeted for delivery to groups. Quality circles might be comprised of the following individuals: program clients, health educators, physicians, psychologists, other health professionals, and agency personnel. Numerous quality circles may exist simultaneously, each having a slightly different focus. In the present illustration, quality circle tasks may focus on client retention, adaptation to lifestyle change, responding to and coping with withdrawal symptoms, social support, barriers to permanent change, self-efficacy, skill development, logistical concerns, and other issues. Schillemans, et al. (1989) describe the process of the quality circle as follows:

Each circle follows six basic principles in its operation. First, the circle is small and meets at regular intervals for a certain period of time. Second, everyone involved in the production process participates. Third, participants behave in the quality circle as equals; all comments and suggestions are equally valid. Fourth, the discussion focuses on things that the group can actually influence. Fifth, the members of the circle provide any material (for example, literature, experience) that will be used during the process. Sixth, the circle is led by a circle leader who has the skills needed to lead a group; he or she should not outrank the other participants (pp.21-22).

The utility of quality circles in evaluation is that service recipients are intimately involved, and thus, able to offer a perspective not otherwise readily apparent to service providers. The use of quality circles is time-consuming, and critics of the approach point out that direct payoffs for individual clients/patients or providers are few. More detailed explanations and critiques of the approach are described by Schillemans, et al. (1989) and Galli and Corry (1986).

Unobtrusive Techniques

Unobtrusive techniques are data collection methods that do not require the direct participation or cooperation of human subjects. The most common of the unobtrusive techniques can be divided into the following general descriptive categories: (1) physical traces; (2) archival data; and (3) unobtrusive observation.

Physical evidence can be an important source of data, as any investigator who has examined the scene of an unwitnessed traffic accident can attest. Skid marks, for instance, provide evidence that can help the investigator reconstruct the accident, and make inferences about vehicle direction, speed, attempt to take evasive action, and other important details. The use of physical evidence can help us to evaluate programs in creative ways. For instance, one measure of the popularity of an innovative reading program to expand reader options might be based on the wear and tear on selected library books. Similarly, the popularity of jogging along a particular route after a promotional campaign might be evaluated, in part, by assessing the amount of grass along the trail before and after the campaign, the increased grooving of the dirt surface over time, and related indirect measures. With the establishment and growth of technology, the popularity of computer-based websites, homepages, and so on can be evaluated by electronically recording the number of "hits" a site receives, and thus, a trail of physical evidence becomes established. The use of physical evidence alone may not always be adequate for thorough and decisive evaluation. However, in conjunction with other qualitative or quantitative measures, unobtrusive measures may play an important corroborative role. The use of more than one means of measuring or evaluating a particular phenomenon is known as **triangulation** (or **triangulation of evidence**), and helps the evaluator to construct a more complete descriptive or predictive picture of a given event or relationship (Strauss & Corbin, 1990).

Archival data also may be useful for making inferences. Consider our reading improvement program again. A change in the pattern of library book withdrawals would support the notion that the program was altering previous reading habits. One interesting aspect of archival information is **graffiti**. It seems that groups who differ by generation or culture may have distinct ways of expressing graffiti -- on the exterior walls of public buildings, on the tops of school desks, in the pages of library books, and on the walls and surfaces of restrooms. Changes in political thought, sexual mores, and other sociological phenomena can be evaluated, in part, by the study of this unusual source of archival data. The use of graffiti in evaluation is not conceptually new. Cave art, depictions, and scribbles, which might be defined as prehistoric graffiti, have long provided the anthropologist or archeologist with useful data on which to base a prediction of the important elements of a primitive culture.

The use of various observational approaches has been discussed earlier in this chapter, and so, will not be repeated in detail here. Unobtrusive (i.e., undetected) observation aims to minimize stimulus factors, such as observer effect, to which subjects might react. Variables of possible importance to the investigator, such as subjects' expressive behavior, physical activity, language behavior, may be studied in this manner. The recent ethical issues surrounding the use of human subjects not given the opportunity to provide informed consent to be studied (see Chapter 3) somewhat limits the circumstances under which this approach should be authorized.

Summary

Evaluators of health education and health promotion programs have had to become increasingly adaptable in their approaches to providing explanations of program events and outcomes. Part of the adaptation has been in learning to incorporate qualitative models, measures, data collection techniques, and designs into their overall evaluative planning and thinking. The use of qualitative methods helps to promote interdisciplinary research and evaluation between health educators and other social scientists. Use of qualitative strategies, singularly or in combination, provides the evaluator with greater flexibility in solving problems not readily addressed by traditional quantitative tools. Moreover, the present and future possibilities of combining quantitative and qualitative methods presents evaluators with rich and powerful strategies for arriving at answers to questions that will strengthen the delivery and outcomes associated with health education and promotion programs.

Case Study

Mahloch, J., Thompson, B., & Taylor, V.M. (1998). Use of qualitative methods to develop a motivational video. *Journal of Health Education*, *29*(2), 84-88.

The authors used a focus group and other interview methods to develop and evaluate a video designed to motivate women to have regular mammograms. What were the selection criteria for participation in the focus group? In this instance was a single focus group adequate? What factors might have suggested the use of multiple focus groups and the designation of particular participation criteria? To what extent could this type of information have been ascertained using quantitative data collection and evaluation methods? If you were to replicate this study, what changes would you make to bolster generalizability, and why would you make these specific alterations? Describe a contemporary area of interest to health education professionals in which the focus group approach would be useful in obtaining feedback about the appropriateness of educational materials, or in providing "feedforward" concerning the development of new materials? What additional qualitative techniques, besides the focus group approach, might help guide your evaluation strategy?

Student Questions/Activities

1. Imagine that you and some fellow students are part of a team that is evaluating your own academic unit. What criteria will you use in your evaluation? Explain which qualitative measures and data collection lend themselves to this type of study. Be as specific as possible.
2. Identify a health education program in your community that could be improved through evaluation. Use a nominal group process to determine which aspects of the program will be evaluated, and which methods will be employed in the evaluation.
3. What could the qualitative evaluator who uses ethnography, observation, and interview techniques do to enhance validity and reliability, and minimize investigator bias in data collection and reporting? Explain.
4. Locate an individual who is involved in focus group interviewing. See if you can become a participant or a recorder. Identify an issue in health education which

could become illuminated through focus group interviewing. Recruit subjects for your focus groups, develop a list of topics to be addressed, work through practice sessions, and if possible, actually gather appropriate data that could be used to make recommendations about the issue you chose.

Recommended Readings

Ellis, C., & Bochner, A.P. (eds.). (1996). *Composing Ethnography.* Walnut Creek, CA: AltaMira Press.

This unique edited work helps to establish the interface of social science and humanities through a presentation of alternative forms of qualitative writing. Contents of this volume includes autoethnography, sociopoetics, and reflexive ethnography. It will introduce you to methods of research that are relatively unexplored in the health education and promotion arena.

Marshall, C., & Rossman, G.B. (1995). *Designing Qualitative Research,* 2nd edition. Newbury Park, CA: Sage.

This book describes the intellectual, political, and technological reasons for the advent and growth of qualitative methods in program evaluation and basic research. It represents a real "how to" book that will be of use to novices and senior analysts alike.

Morgan, D.L., & Krueger, R.A. (1998). *The Focus Group Kit.* Thousand Oaks, CA: Sage.

This six-volume work was composed by two of the premiere scholars on the use of focus groups in the U.S. today. Beginning with an explanation of the utility of focus groups, this collection explores focus group planning, question development, moderating guidelines, involving community members in focus groups, and analyzing, interpreting, and reporting results of focus groups. This series of books has a very practical design to it that makes it useful to novices, as well as to more experienced focus group interviewers.

References

Banks, R.L., Poehler, D.L., & Russell, R.D. (1984). Spirit and human-spiritual interaction as a factor in health and in health education. *Health Education*, *15*(5), 16-19.

Basch, C.E. (1987). Focus group interview: An underutilized research technique for improving theory and practice in health education. *Health Education Quarterly*, *14*, 411-448.

Bellenger, D.N., Bernhardt, K.L., & Goldstucker, J.L. (1976). *Qualitative Marketing Research*. Chicago: American Marketing Association.

Best, J.W., & Kahn, J.V. (1989). *Research in Education*, 6th edition. Englewood Cliffs, NJ: Prentice-Hall, Inc.

Bogdan, R.C., & Biklen, S.K. (1982). *Qualitative Research for Education: An Introduction to Theory and Methods*. Boston: Allyn & Bacon.

Brown, B.B. (1968). *Delphi Method: A Methodology for the Elicitation of the Opinion of Experts*. Los Angeles: Rand Corporation.

Chavez, D. (1985). Perpetuation of gender inequality: A content analysis of comic strips. *Sex Roles, 13*, 93-102.

Dovring, K. (1973). Communication, dissenters and popular culture in eighteenth century Europe. *Journal of Popular Culture, 7*, 559-568.

Ehrle, B.J., & Johnson, B.G. (1961). Psychologists and cartoonists. *American Psychologist, 16*, 693-695.

Emerson, J.D., & Colditz, G.A. (1983). Use of statistical analysis in the *New England Journal of Medicine. New England Journal of Medicine, 309*, 709-713.

Emery, E.M., Ritter-Randolph, G.P., Strozier, A.L., & McDermott, R.J. (1993). The use of focus group interviews for identifying salient issues concerning college students' alcohol abuse. *Journal of American College Health, 41*(3), 195-198.

Fink, A., Kosecoff, J., Chassin, M., & Brook, R.H. (1984). Consensus methods: Characteristics and guidelines for use. *American Journal of Public Health, 74*, 979-983.

Fraenkel, J.R., & Wallen, N.E. (1990). *How to Design and Evaluate Research in Education*. New York: McGraw-Hill.

Galli, N., & Corry, J.M. (1986). Quality circles and health promotion planning. *Health Education, 17*(1), 13-16.

Goldman, R., & Montagne, M. (1986). Marketing "mind mechanics:" Decoding antidepressant drug advertisements. *Social Science & Medicine, 22*, 1047-1058.

Goodwin, L.D., & Goodwin, W.L. (1985). An analysis of statistical techniques used in the *Journal of Educational Psychology,* 1979-1983. *Educational Psychologist, 20*, 13-21.

Holsti, O.R. (1969). *Content Analysis for the Social Sciences and the Humanities*. Reading, MA: Addison-Wesley Publishing Company.

James, D.C.S., Rienzo, B.A., & Frazee, C. (1997). Using focus groups to develop a nutrition education video for high school students. *Journal of School Health, 67*(9), 376-379.

Kahn, R., & Cannell, C. (1957). *The Dynamics of Interviewing*. New York: John Wiley.

Keller, K.L., Sliepcevich, E.M., Vitello, E.M., Lacey, E.P., & Wright, W.R. (1987). Assessing beliefs about and needs of senior citizens using the focus group interview: A qualitative approach. *Health Education, 18*(1), 44-49.

Kisker, E.E. (1985). Teenagers talk about sex, pregnancy and contraception. *Family Planning Perspectives, 17*, 83-90.

Krippendorff, K. (1980). *Content Analysis: An Introduction to its Methodology*. Beverly Hills, CA: Sage Publications.

Krueger, R.A. (1988). *Focus Groups: A Practical Guide for Applied Research.* Newbury Park, CA: Sage Publications.

Leenaars, A.A. (1986). Brief note on latent content in suicide notes. *Psychological Reports, 59,* 640-642.

Leenaars, A.A., & Balance W.D.G. (1981). A predictive approach to the study of manifest content in suicide notes. *Journal of Clinical Psychology,* 37, 50-60.

Marshall, C., & Rossman, G.B. (1995). *Designing Qualitative Research,* 2nd edition. Newbury Park, CA: Sage.

McDermott, R.J., Bryant, C.A. Westhoff, W.W., Marty, P.J., Holcomb, D.R., Kroetsch, M.A., Lopez, G.E., & Kent, E.B. (1996). Birth control and family planning: research findings for a social marketing plan. *Florida Journal of Public Health, 8*(1), 33-38.

Means, R.K. (1975). *Historical Perspectives on School Health.* Thorofare, NJ: Charles B. Slack, Inc.

Miller A.E., Sliepcevich, E.M., & Vitello, E.M. (1981). Health related articles in the six leading women's magazines: Content, coverage, and readership profile. *Health Values, 5*(9), 254-264.

Morgan, D.L. (1988). *Focus Groups as Qualitative Research.* Newbury Park, CA: Sage Publications.

Morgan, D.L., & Krueger, R.A. (1998). *The Focus Group Kit.* Thousand Oaks, CA: Sage.

Mullen, K.D. (1983). *Wellness Constructs: A Decision Theoretic Study.* Unpublished Doctoral Dissertation, Southern Illinois University at Carbondale.

National Heart, Lung, and Blood Institute, National High Blood Pressure Education Program. (1979). *Focus group study among aware hypertensives and social supporters, conducted July 10-13, 1979.* U.S. Department of Health, Education and Welfare, Public Health Service, National Institutes of Health.

Paisely, W.J. (1964). Identifying the unknown communicators in painting, literature, and music: The significance of minor encoding habits. *Journal of Communication, 14,* 219-237.

Patton, M.Q. (1987). *How to Use Qualitative Methods in Evaluation.* Newbury Park, CA: Sage Publications.

Rosengren, K.E. (ed.) (1981). *Advances in Content Analysis.* Beverly Hills, CA: Sage Publications.

Rudolph, A., McDermott, R.J., & Gold, R.S. (1985). Use of statistics in the *Journal of School Health* 1979-1983: A content analysis. *Journal of School Health, 55,* 230-233.

Sackman, H. (1975). *Delphi Critique.* Lexington, MA: D.C. Heath.

Schillemans, L., De Grande, L., & Remmen, R. (1989). Using quality circles to evaluate the efficacy of primary health care. In R.F. Conner & M. Hendricks (eds.). *International Innovations in Evaluation Methodology.* New Directions for Program Evaluation, no. 42. San Francisco: Jossey-Bass.

Shepherd, S.K., Sims, L.S., Cronin, F.J., Shaw, A., & Davis, C.A. (1989). Use of focus groups to explore consumers' preferences for content and graphic design of nutrition publications. *Journal of the American Dietetic Association, 89,* 1612-1614.

Simmons, J. (1985). *Comparison of marketing focus group and health education small group process*. Paper presentation at the annual meeting of the Society for Public Health Education, Washington, D.C.

Sliepcevich, E.M., Keller, K.L., & Sondag, K.A. (1986-87). RAPP: Content analysis of *Health Education*, 1984 and 1985. *Health Education, 17*(6), 16-21.

Sofalvi, A.J., & Drolet, J.C. (1986). Health-related content of selected Sunday comic strips. *Journal of School Health, 56*, 184-186.

Stewart, D.W., & Shamdasani, P.N. (1990). *Focus Groups: Theory and Practice*. Newbury Park, CA: Sage Publications.

Strauss, A., & Corbin, J. (1990). *Basics of Qualitative Research*. Newbury Park, CA: Sage Publications.

Van de Ven, A.H., & Delbecq, A.L. (1972). The nominal group as a research instrument for exploratory health studies. *American Journal of Public Health, 62*, 337-342.

Weber, R.P. (1985). *Basic Content Analysis*. Beverly Hills, CA: Sage Publications.

Chapter
12

Survey Methods and Evaluation

Chapter Objectives

After completing this chapter, you should be able to:

1. Explain how and why surveys are used to collect information.
2. Discuss the advantages and disadvantages of conducting surveys.
3. Identify questions and issues pertinent to the selection of a survey instrument.
4. Compare mail surveys, group administered surveys, electronic mail surveys, telephone interviews, and face-to-face (one-on-one and group) interviews as data collection methods.
5. Describe a systematic process for conducting a mailed survey.

Key Terms

behavioral data

central location intercept interview

cover letter

descriptive data

focus group interview

group interview

home delivery interview/drop-off survey

method effect

preferential data

presurvey letter

scheduled interview

Introduction

Before beginning any study, it is wise to define the questions to which answers are needed. Perhaps the best way to begin the formulation of these questions is to review the theoretical perspectives and previous research in the area under consideration. Without questions to answer, the investigator will find it difficult to specify the study objectives that ordinarily provide a road map of the project to be undertaken. For the remainder of this chapter, we will assume that you already have determined that collecting data by using a survey is the most appropriate method for the questions of interest to be answered.

Why Surveys Are Used

Surveys began gaining broad acceptance in 1935 when George Gallup conducted weekly polls on national political and consumer issues for private and public sector clients. Since Gallup was operating the American Institute of Public Opinion for profit, he was concerned about cost and time factors. Gallup polls remain today as tools in politics, as well as in other endeavors where decisions need to be driven by data about popular opinion.

Surveys have become more complex and sophisticated with the advancement of technology. Still, the survey is the best method for social scientists to describe, explain, or explore a population that is too large to observe directly.

Using proper sampling methods (see Chapter 13), surveys permit investigators to reveal the characteristics of a school, worksite, patient care setting, or community by studying individuals who represent these entities, and to do so in a relatively unbiased and scientifically rigorous manner. Investigators may generalize about an entire population by drawing inferences based on data drawn from a small portion of the entire population. Surveys used in health education and health promotion not only examine health topics related to individuals, schools, worksites, communities, and other entities, but also may include social, political, economic, cultural, and environmental issues as well.

As with most data collection techniques, surveys offer advantages as well as disadvantages. The major advantages of surveys are that they employ a standardized method of data collection which can be administered to a large sample relatively fast. In addition, data analysis is uniform and does not usually require subjective interpretation in the way that analysis of qualitative data does.

A primary disadvantage of surveys is the possible low response rate. Whether the survey is mailed or distributed in a group setting, only those respondents motivated to complete and return the survey become sources of data, regardless of how sophisticated the method used for obtaining the sample was. Surveys only tap persons who are available to participate and amenable to doing so. In self-administered surveys, the investigator is not present to probe, clarify and motivate the respondent to complete the survey, and therefore, loses control of the response pattern, and even whether or not the questions get answered by someone other than the selected respondent (Frey & Oishi, 1995). Table 12.1 summarizes several of the commonly cited advantages and disadvantages of using surveys in evaluation and related endeavors.

Table 12.1 Advantages and Disadvantages of Various Survey Data Collection Methods

Method	Advantages	Disadvantages
Face-to-face	high flexibility greater complexity possible diverse populations reached high response rate validity of instructions	high cost interviewer-induced bias subject reluctance stressful endeavor interviewer safety concerns anonymity not guaranteed
Telephone	rapid data collection less costly than face-to-face increases anonymity large scale accessibility validity of instructions high flexibility	less control less credibility no visual cues not everyone has a phone call screening is popular
Self-administered	lowest cost rapid response validity of instructions high flexibility	may not be generalizable self-selection few open-ended questions
Traditional mail	low cost convenience anonymity no interviewer bias	risk of low response rate slow data collection self-selection few open-ended questions low flexibility
Electronic mail	low cost ease and convenience almost instantaneous	must have e-mail access self-selection lacks anonymity risk of being "purged" lack of "cueing" must be short noninvasive items only

Selecting a Survey Instrument

A thorough review of the literature can tell the investigator whether a previously used instrument is appropriate, or, if the creation of a new instrument is desirable or necessary. Either decision has subsequent payoffs and potential compromises. With a well-developed and previously used instrument, the investigator has the opportunity to confirm or refute previously identified results. On the other hand, a well-established instrument may not be specific enough to the needs of the current investigation. If a new instrument is developed, the investigator assumes the burden of establishing its reliability and validity (see Chapter 7). Whether the investigator chooses an existing instrument or develops a new one, the following questions should be considered before proceeding with a pilot study:

- What is the purpose of the survey? Will the data generated from the survey answer the research questions?
- Who are the survey respondents? Will the type of respondents needed be able, available and willing to answer this survey in a timely manner? What are the incentives (as well as possible disincentives) for responding to the survey?
- How will the survey be administered? What logistical issues need to be addressed before the survey can be administered? How much time is required to complete the survey?
- What procedures has the investigator initiated to keep the responses confidential or anonymous? How will codes be used to replace confidential information such as the respondent's name, address, or social security number?
- What is the method of analysis? Does the investigator have the personnel and resources to enter and analyze the data?

Types of Data Generated from Surveys

Surveys allow the investigator to collect descriptive, behavioral, and preferential data (Rea & Parker, 1997). **Descriptive data** characterize the respondent's income, age, education, ethnicity, household size, zip code, health, employment, socioeconomic or marital status, religion and a variety of other demographic variables. Such demographic information enhances the investigator's ability to describe and understand the respondents and how the sample represents the larger population. Not all demographic variables will be useful in every situation.

Behavioral data examine activity patterns of individuals, so that the investigator can generalize to the behavior of the larger population. This information is useful when planning the implementation of a health behavior change program. Since many health education programs involve behavioral change, it is important to know the current behavior before attempting to implement a change. It may be important to collect relevant demographic data along with the behavioral data so as to be able to make inferences about the smaller, more unique segments of the population. For example, if the desired outcome is to increase mammography participation through a media campaign, it is useful to know the preventive health care behaviors as well as demographic information for the eligible women intended to respond favorably to the campaign. Lastly, **preferential data** are used to seek public opinions on a variety of topics such as political issues or social conditions. Unlike descriptive and behavioral data, preferential data are predictive and future oriented.

Even though there are three distinctive types of data generated from surveys, actual data collection incorporates some aspects of each type to explore the complex relationships among demographics and survey items themselves. For instance, in studying teenage pregnancy, it is important to know not only the demographic characteristics of the pregnant females, but also the factors related to family members and male partners. Results may be enhanced if the survey asks a respondent about whether her mother or older siblings were teen mothers, the age of the father of the baby, the number of other household members, the pregnant teen's relationship to the other household members, family history of domestic violence or substance abuse, and other possible associated factors. Although such variables are not the usual type of demographic information sought in surveys, these demographic data probably allow the investigator to give a broader and richer explanation of results.

Survey Strategies

Two common survey methods are interviews and self-administered paper-and-pencil surveys. Interviews may be performed with groups or with individuals. They may be done face-to-face or they may be performed by telephone. Self-administered surveys may be mailed to potential respondents, be provided to individuals to complete, as in health care settings, or may be administered in group settings such as in schools, university classes, other educational settings (e.g., prenatal classes, smoking cessation classes, and so on), worksites, or at conferences. It is becoming increasingly common to use the Internet and electronic mail to collect survey data.

Following a brief description of each type of survey design, the remainder of this chapter focuses on a detailed discussion of how to conduct a mailed survey. The reader is *alerted* here to the fact that the creation, administration, and analysis of surveys is a subject of greater complexity than often believed. Therefore, further reading from sources such as those listed at the end of this chapter is recommended to gain a more comprehensive understanding.

Face-to-Face Interviews

There are two commonly used categories of interviews: face-to-face administered and telephone administered. Although conducting interviews is a labor intensive exercise for the interviewer as well as the interviewee, the payoff often is in the richness of the understanding that emanates from data obtained in this manner.

The face-to-face interview may be conducted in either individual or group format, and has the advantage of providing the interviewer with visual and auditory cues from the participant, as well as the norms of conversational and interpersonal interaction. These cues allow the investigator to provide an explanation of the question, or to probe deeper into an area of concern. Face-to-face data collection is said to have "high flexibility" because it can be adapted to suit the needs of both the interviewer and subject. If directions need clarification, or definitions of terms need to be given, or an explanation of a question needs to be made, the format is flexible enough to accommodate such requirements. However, the advantage of greater in-depth knowledge comes at the price of possible interviewer bias. As illustrated in Table 12.1, each strategy has pros and cons. The investigator must decide which survey design is most likely to yield the data needed, given the budgetary constraints under which the study is to take place.

If you choose to conduct individual interviews, there are three options: scheduled, central location intercept, and home delivery (also known as door-to-door interviews). **Scheduled interviews** take place at a scheduled time in the respondent"s home, school, workplace or other agreed upon setting. Though this format potentially allows the interviewee to be in a familiar and comfortable location, it is met with increasing reluctance since the respondent has to allow strangers in the home, or meet someone unknown to them at some other setting. In addition, unless the investigator is hired to conduct the interviews, it is difficult to gain permission from employers to interrupt work time for to conduct the interviews.

Central location intercept interviews often are conducted in shopping malls and parking lots. The idea is to "intercept" potential respondents as they avail themselves for an unrelated activity. The technique is used primarily for conducting marketing surveys, though its use is getting expanded to include other purposes as well. More about this method is described in Chapter 8 and Chapter 11.

Home delivery interviews (door-to-door surveys) allow the investigator to give the survey to only specific individuals living within a designated geographic area. The investigator may wish to have the survey completed only by couples with children under five years of age. Instead of mailing the survey to a sample of every household in a specific zip code of interest, interviewers knock on doors, and inquire if the residents meet the study criteria before administering the survey. With this type of design, there are several options for retrieving the survey, the investigator may wait for the respondent to complete the survey, return later the same day or the following day to obtain the completed survey, leave a self-addressed, postage-paid envelope for the respondent to return the completed survey, or mail the survey to specific households followed by the investigator walking through the neighborhood collecting the completed surveys within a few days. Research shows that when the investigator either delivers the survey, picks it up, or both, the completion rate is higher than with straightforward mail surveys (Babbie, 1990). This technique of data collection is also referred to as the **drop-off survey** (Salant & Dillman, 1994).

Group interviews are used extensively in marketing research to solicit the opinions of targeted subsets of potential customers for a new product or marketing strategy (Frey & Fontana, 1991). Group interviews are more efficient and economical than one-on-one interviews, and they have the positive aspect of being able to get people to come to a consensus of opinion about a particular issue. Furthermore, persons who may be rather withdrawn in a single interview, may feel more at ease or participatory when they get to hear and digest the opinions of others in a group. On the other hand, groups can be intimidating and actually suppress the comments of less confident people. Groups, though they may seem to be reaching consensus, could in fact just be reaching a state of conformity without real in-depth analysis of the issue at hand. In some instances, if group members are polarized over an issue, the group process can actually intensify the polarity rather than bring people to agreement. It can also be the case than one or two aggressive, gregariously talkative, or manipulative group members can sway opinion without any "real discussion" taking place.

A specific type of group interview is the **focus group interview** which consists of eight to twelve individuals who share their views or opinions on a specific topic of interest. Besides being conducted for market research, focus groups are used in all stages of instrument design. Before an instrument is developed, a focus group of participants who identify with the issue might be asked to give opinions on the topics of interest. For example, a focus group comprised of HIV+ individuals may be asked their opinion on how to improve quality of care. Later, after an instrument is developed, but before the data are collected, a focus group interview might help to establish the relevance and clarity of the items covered in the instrument. Lastly, focus groups may explain, confirm or refute findings of instrument data. Elsewhere in this text, you can find information about use of focus groups for pilot testing (Chapter 8), and for other qualitative evaluation (Chapter 11). Since focus groups involve specialized skills and practice, you also are advised to read further on the topic from the list of recommended readings supplied at the end of this chapter.

Telephone Interviews

This approach has gained popularity because of several advantages over other interviewing methods. The increasing number of individuals with telephones permits access to more potential respondents, and accomplishes this fete with less intrusiveness than the door-to-door strategy. In addition, the availability of random digit dialing provides access to unlisted and new telephone numbers (Waksberg, 1978). Telephone surveying also is more cost-efficient and faster than door-to-door interviews, and is designed to reduce interviewer error. The use of toll-free 1-800 or 1-888 numbers permits a wide calling area at relatively low cost. Moreover, the use of the telephone for surveying permits an unlimited number of callbacks. If the caller is informed that the call may be monitored to improve quality, special equipment may be used which allows the investigator to monitor quality as operators conduct the interviews. In addition, large commercial interviewing companies utilize computer-assisted telephone interviewing systems to script and cue interviewers concerning responses, record the data electronically on computer as responses are provided, and thus, increase quality control. Whether the data are being collected by a commercial enterprise or by a few interviewers in a small office, each telephone interview has a set of standardized questions and an accompanying script which clarifies how to motivate the respondent to continue with the interview while maintaining a conversational tone (Frey & Oishi, 1995). Successful telephone interviewing depends on the auditory signals, the quality of communication between the interviewer and the respondent, and whether a question is likely to be understood if read exactly as it is written (Aday, 1996).

Though telephone interviewing can be a quick and efficient means of collecting data, there are notable shortcomings associated with this technique. Persons receiving calls at home have become increasingly suspicious of a caller's intention. The recipient of the call may fear that the caller is about to make a carefully disguised sales pitch or ask for a donation -- two things that make many individuals feel awkward. The call recipient may abruptly terminate the call without hearing the real intention. Some people receiving a telephone call from a stranger may fear that the purpose of the call is for "screening" potential victims of home burglaries, assaults, or other possible crimes. More and more telephone owners have invested in answering machines to screen calls, and thus, "weed out" low priority calls, which may include persons performing legitimate telephone surveys.

The success of telephone surveying is also thwarted by the many "busys" and "no answers" that fail to produce results and add to the tedium of the exercise. The caller has to be a person who is well prepared for this kind of activity, and one who is patient and diplomatic enough to speak with persons who will be annoyed that they have had their favorite TV program interrupted, have had to abandon their dinner guests, or thanks to their attention to your interview attempt, have to go undo the mischief their children have gotten into.

Finally, the time of day associated with calling can be crucial to getting a representative sample. Calls restricted to daytime may provide access primarily to people who do not work outside of the home, children, or babysitters. Calls limited to the evening are likely to be confronted with some of the screening obstacles identified above. A letter that comes to a person's home or place of business a few days prior to the initiation of the telephone call may prepare that individual in advance. Thus, the recipient of the call may experience some reduction in suspicion or reluctance to participate if forewarned that a "legitimate" call will be coming.

While the obstacles to telephone surveying may be many, the strategy is used widely and with success. The Behavioral Risk Factor Surveillance Survey (BRFSS), one of the major ways in which the U.S. Centers for Disease Control and Prevention monitor health risk behavior in the adult population, has been administered traditionally by means of telephone with relatively few design problems (Gentry, Kalsbeek, Hogelin, et al, 1985; Siegel, Brackbill, Frazier, et al., 1991). Recently, some states have adopted the telephone survey strategy to conduct more localized BRFSS data collection for needs assessment, feedback on current interventions, and future program planning (Brownson, Schmid, King, et al., 1998).

Self-Administered and Mailed Surveys

Whether a self-administered or mailed survey is used, investigators rely on accompanying instructions and visual appeal to motivate the potential respondent into completing the survey. In both situations, the respondent must understand the question without needing extensive clarification.

Self-administered surveys may be conducted with individuals or groups. Individual or one-on-one survey completion allows the interviewer to answer questions which may arise as the survey is completed, and produces results about which data analysts can have confidence. On the other hand, this option is expensive and time-consuming. However, administering surveys to groups is relatively low in cost, fast, and may be supervised or unsupervised. A supervised format is preferred because it allows for consistent instructions, simultaneous administration, availability to answer questions, and the monitoring of completion. Unsupervised surveys may yield more representative samples, but fail in providing a consistent motivational stimulus to all respondents (Bourque & Fielder, 1995).

The mailed survey is the most common self-administered variety of survey. As with other types of data collection strategies, there are several advantages and disadvantages. Although mailed surveys are often perceived as being faster, and, being among the less complex methods, they require a substantial amount of planning and preparation. A primary shortcoming of the mailed survey is the risk of a low response rate. To overcome this potential hazard, investigators have developed a number of ways to increase the likelihood of the survey being completed and returned. Among other suggestions, Torabi (1991) advises that mailed surveys be relatively short, be written clearly, offer concise directions, and keep open-ended questions to a minimum. Additional strategies for promoting more optimal response rates are discussed below.

Conducting a Mailed Survey

As with any type of research study, it is essential to conduct a pilot test prior to initiating the actual study (see Chapter 8). After pilot test results are examined, any changes are incorporated into the survey or study design. Also, pilot testing allows the investigator to estimate the cost of the study in terms of time and money, as well as numerous other logistical issues (Bourque & Fielder, 1995). A pilot test is especially important when conducting a mailed survey because the potential respondents do not have the advantage of communicating with the investigator to ask questions, seek advice, or clarify instructions for completion. The investigator should allocate enough time to follow each of the steps identified, and to conduct the pilot test with the same exact criteria as the actual study.

Step 1: Determine the Sample Size

The first decision to be made related to cost is the size of the sample. Any mailed survey will involve personnel expenses and direct costs, such as postage, envelopes, and printing. Actual costs will change over time and may vary to some extent by geographic region. A sample needs to be only as large as is required to make the inferences desired. Having a sample that is too small will limit the extent to which inferences can be made. Having a sample that is larger than necessary is wasteful of resources. Methods for determining sample size are described in Chapter 13 and more detailed references are provided.

Step 2: Select the Instrument

From a practical standpoint, it is recommended that the investigator consider the cost of the instrument. Some instruments are available only through specific vendors and require the investigator to purchase the questions, answer key, and interpretation guidelines. On the other hand, many instruments are available at no cost from the author or are available in books which provide detailed information for administration, reliability and validity data, and methods of analysis.

Step 3: Obtain Mailing Lists of Names and Addresses

There are two common ways to obtain names and addresses. First, if a professional organization represents the type of desired respondents, membership mailing lists may be purchased from the appropriate organization. Second, if the sample is drawn from the general population for a specific geographical area, it is possible to purchase a mailing list. Check the local yellow pages of the telephone book for appropriate listings under the heading of "Mailing Lists." It is necessary to inquire about the available format, because some lists are on preprinted labels, while other lists are on computer diskette or paper. Often retyping a large list is more time-consuming and costly than paying additional cost for preprinted labels. But, if four or five sets of labels are needed, it may be cheaper to retype the list and print the labels yourself.

Step 4: Develop A Coding and Tracking System

After the address labels are obtained, and prior to mailing the surveys, one needs to develop a detailed plan for coding and tracking the surveys. Without a systematic way of knowing to whom surveys were sent, the investigator has no way of knowing who responded and who needs to be sent a second packet. Also, the tracking systems allow the investigator to record the date when each survey was returned, and the type of individual who responded after the first mailing, after the reminder/thank you postcard, and after a second or third mailing. For example, it may be useful to know that nurses responded before physicians, or that individuals living in a rural area responded before those in an urban setting. Careful tracking provides data on those individuals who never returned the survey. This non-response data is useful when attempting later to generalize results to a larger population.

In addition to the obvious advantages of tracking the exact date on which each survey was returned, there is another advantage that is important, but often ignored. Suppose the investigator sends out a large survey to women over the age of 50 to determine their knowledge, attitudes and beliefs about breast cancer. After the first mailing, a famous woman is diagnosed with breast cancer and makes a public plea for all women to obtain a mammogram. As the investigator, it is essential to know which surveys were returned before the national event and which were returned after the media intervention. Without a careful tracking system in place, the results of the survey might be erroneous. (For further explanation, see the discussion of *contemporary history* in Chapter 10).

Step 5: Format the Survey

Appearance. The mailed survey must be appealing at first glance to encourage the potential respondent to continue reading. Visual appeal and clear audience salience is considered a part of face validity (see Chapter 7). Survey designers find that mailed surveys presented in a booklet format are most appealing.

Along with the instrument format, the investigator needs to determine if the survey will be presented in a computer scanning format. An advantage of using computer-read optical scan forms is the cheaper and faster method of data entry that is provided. Data entry by hand can be slower, as well as more expensive and labor intensive. Although computer scanning is faster and cheaper, a chief disadvantage is that it makes use of the booklet format more difficult since forms cannot be folded. In addition, respondents may not darken the desired spaces completely, which leads to erroneous or missing data. Furthermore, the investigator must supply the correct type of pencil to facilitate completion of the optical scan sheets.

Size of paper. If the double-sided survey is printed on 8½" x 14" paper and folded in half, it fits into a 7" x 9" envelope after trimming. Since this size envelope is unusual, the potential respondent is more likely to open it. If the envelope is never opened, the survey has no chance of being completed and returned.

It is worth the time to experiment with alternating the size of the paper and the envelope to decrease postage costs. For instance, it may be cost effective to pay a few cents extra per page to have the paper trimmed after the copies are printed, to decrease the weight and save a few cents per survey on the postage (Dillman, 1978; Dillman, 1983).

Color of paper. Since printing customized colored envelopes is costly, white envelopes are acceptable. However, the survey may be printed on an easy-to-read, light pastel paper (Torabi, 1991), a point which may help to decrease the chance of the survey booklet being lost among the pile of white paper on the potential respondent's desk or countertop.

Font. The survey booklet is printed in a 10-point or 12-point font with adequate margins and white space to avoid eye strain. Some survey designers suggest using upper and lower case fonts for the questions, and only upper case fonts for the responses. This technique allows the potential respondents to identify the choices quickly (Dillman, 1978; Dillman, 1983).

Literacy level and cultural sensitivity. If the survey is mailed to the general population, it is important to conduct a readability test. An 8th-grade readability level is considered acceptable for the general population. For special populations (e.g., persons known to be low literacy, some Medicaid recipients, persons for whom English is a second language) a 6th-grade reading level is more desirable. Of course if literacy is a serious issue, face-to-face interviews or another format other than a paper-and-pencil survey method may be preferred. For older adult groups, a method other than a written survey may yield a better return. Moreover, it is important to verify with a pretest the meaning of words across various cultures. If the meaning of a particular word or phrase is not understood, the respondent is likely to guess or mark an inappropriate response. If the survey is aimed at low literacy respondents, the investigator should avoid the all-caps response format mentioned previously, because there is evidence that use of all upper case letters may be more difficult to read for low literacy individuals (Doak, Doak & Root, 1985).

Matsumoto (1994) points out that cross-cultural or cross-lingual comparisons using translated surveys may be more difficult to accomplish than commonly believed. Even if the written or spoken words used in translation are the same, there is no guarantee that the words have identical meanings and idiomatic interpretation across languages or cultures. A technique known as *cultural tailoring* (Pasick, D'Onofrio & Otero-Sabogal, 1996) of items may require the special assistance of linguists, cultural anthropologists, and other experts. Pilot testing (Chapter 8) is an important part of matching literacy and *cultural sensitivity*.

Booklet cover. The survey booklet is simple and includes a small graphic design with the name of the institution conducting the project to lend credibility. The investigator's name should not be on the cover. Respondents are more likely to respond to an institution or agency than to an individual (Torabi, 1991) unless the sponsoring agency is one of negative notoriety or one mired in controversy.

First page. The inside of the cover page remains blank to provide an uncluttered appearance. The first inside page of the booklet states a question that is related to the topic and which can be answered easily. For example, *How would you rate your health today?* with response anchors such as: (a) excellent, (b) very good, (c) good, (d) fair, (e) poor. This first question serves as a "hook" to get the survey recipient to turn the page and complete the remaining portion of the survey. The data collected from this first question are not necessarily used in the data analysis.

Arrange the questions. After selecting the instruments to be used in the survey, it is necessary to determine a logical order for the questions to appear in the booklet. For instance, if there are three instruments, and two of them have a Likert scale format, the two similar formats are grouped together.

As for the placement of the demographic questions, most researchers agree that the demographic questions should be placed at the end of the survey. If the demographic questions are at the beginning, the potential respondent may find the questions boring or too personal, and thus, be less likely to complete the remaining questions. When the demographic questions are at the end, the respondent has already invested time in completing the survey, and therefore, is more likely to answer the demographic questions and return the survey (Bourque & Fielder, 1995; Dillman, 1978; Dillman, 1983).

Last page of booklet. It is best to keep the back cover blank with an invitation for the respondent to write-in any further comments related to the survey design or the topic. Although these comments may or may not be useful in the data analysis, such qualitative data may be beneficial in the development of future research. If there are specific questions that are printed intentionally on the last page of the booklet, they may be overlooked by the respondent, or presumed to be something other than part of the intended survey.

Step 6: Write the Presurvey Letter and Cover Letter

About one week before mailing the survey, some researchers suggest mailing a **presurvey letter** to each potential respondent. This presurvey letter also describes the purpose of the survey that will arrive within a few days, the purpose of the study, the reason their opinion and participation is important, the name of the institution and person conducting the research, and an invitation to call if more information is desired. This presurvey letter adds to the overall cost of conducting the survey, but has been shown to increase the response rate in some instances (Bourque & Fielder, 1995).

The **cover letter** is enclosed with each survey booklet, and states the purpose of the research and encourages participation. The institution, along with the investigator's name, address and telephone number are also provided so that the potential respondent may call if more information is desired. The cover letter confirms that the research has been approved by the institutional review board (see Chapter 3), how data are to be used, and how the identity of the respondents will be protected.

The investigator should sign each presurvey letter and cover letter in a colored ink with a ballpoint pen. This personal touch illustrates to the potential respondent that the investigator cares enough about the research to sign each letter by hand. Photocopied form letters are less labor intensive, but may seem too impersonal to the addressee, and therefore, decrease the likelihood of obtaining a response.

Step 7: Select the Envelope and Postage Option

Envelopes. As previously discussed, the survey should be mailed in a 7" x 9" envelope. The envelope should contain the cover letter, the survey, and the self-addressed, stamped return envelope (SASE). The return envelope should be the same size and folded in half, so the potential respondent does not have to fold the survey to fit it into another size of envelope. Some researchers design questionnaires in such a way that they can be refolded so that the stamp and return address appear on the outside. This technique is most appropriate for short, one-page surveys. The advantage to this technique is that the survey will not be separated from the envelope, and possibly, not get returned. However, the disadvantage is that the folding procedure may be confusing and must include a glue strip in compliance with regulations for use of first class postage (Babbie, 1990). Moreover, the additional cost of the folding design must be weighed against the cost of using the SASE design.

Postage. Once the survey is printed and the envelopes are purchased, it is advisable to take the complete template to the post office, and discuss the cost and time factors associated with using postage stamps versus bulk rate mailing or business-reply envelopes for mailing the surveys, as well as for the SASE for the returned surveys. Although using postage stamps is more convenient, if the survey yields a low response rate, a financial loss is incurred on the lost postage. If the bulk rate option is chosen, the investigator must check with the local post office for rates and the specific zip code sorting procedures. Bulk rate postage is generally the cheapest option. However, the less predictable delivery schedule may not outweigh the cost savings. In addition, if potential respondents notice the bulk rate postage, they may be less likely to evaluate the survey as important and worthy of their time.

The business-reply postage option saves money because postage is billed only for returned surveys. This option does require the establishment of an account with the local post office, payment of an additional surcharge for each returned envelope, and printing the business-reply graphic on the envelopes. This option is cheaper if a low response rate is anticipated. Since there is no way to predict the response rate, the surcharge fee and additional envelope printing charge may decrease the postage savings. Figure 12.1 gives cost estimates for printing, instrument, envelope and postage costs.

Step 8: Determine When to Mail the Survey

In addition to the appearance of the mailed surveys, it is important to consider the time of year in which the survey is mailed. Since the entire process may take up to five or six weeks, not including the pilot test phase, it is advisable to consider what events may compete for the potential respondent's time and attention. For instance, if the survey arrives in December, it may be viewed as holiday "junk mail" and discarded without being opened. If the survey arrives in the summer, it may lay unopened while the respondent is on vacation. Another time to avoid is the week prior to April 15th, since the high volume of tax returns being handled by the U.S. Postal Service may increase the chances of the survey being delayed or lost.

More specifically, if the survey is sent to the potential respondent's place of employment, it is best to have it arrive toward the end of the work week, since the beginning of the work week usually has greater competing demands.

Item of Purchase	Cost per 500	
Printing:		
presurvey letter	500 @ $ .08 =	$ 40
cover letter	500 @ $ .08 =	$ 40
reminder/thank you		
postcard	500 @ $ .08 =	$ 40
4 pages duplexed on		
8"x14" pastel paper	500 @ $ .10 x 8 =	$ 400
Instrument:		
Existing (purchase/user fee)	500 @ $1.00 =	$ 500
or self-created (no cost)		$ 0

Figure 12.1 Eastimating the Cost of Mailing 500 Surveys

Envelopes:

500 presurvey	500 @ $ .01 =	$ 5
500 1st mailing	500 @ $ .08 =	$ 40
500 1st mailing SASE	500 @ $ .08 =	$ 40
450 2nd mailing	450 @ $ .08 =	$ 36
450 2nd mailing SASE	450 @ $ .08 =	$ 36
300 3rd mailing	300 @ $ .08 =	$ 24
300 3rd mailing SASE	300 @ $ .08 =	$ 24

Postage:

500 presurvey	500 @ 1 oz. x $ .32 =	$ 160
500 1st mailing	500 @ 2 oz. x ($ .32 + $ .23) =	$ 275
500 1st mailing SASE	500 @ 1 oz. x $ .32 =	$ 160
500 postcards	500 @ $ .20 =	$ 100
450 2nd mailing	450 @ 2 oz. x ($ .32 + $ .23) =	$ 248
450 2nd mailing SASE	450 @ 1 oz. x $ .32 =	$ 144
300 3rd mailing	300 @ 2 oz. x ($ .32 + $ .23) =	$ 165
300 3rd mailing	300 @ 1 oz. x $ .32 =	$ 96

Total estimated cost: $2073 to $2573

Figure 12.1 Continued

Step 9: Prepare the Reminder/Thank You Postcard

Seven days after the first survey packet is mailed, a reminder/thank you postcard should be sent to the entire sample. This postcard thanks those respondents who have returned the survey and reminds those who have not yet done so that it is not too late to participate. Again, each postcard is signed with a ballpoint pen to add the personal touch. Torabi (1991) concludes that a follow-up reminder could increase the response rate as much as 25%. Isaac and Michael (1990) found that one reminder boosted response rate by over 20% and a second follow-up increased response by an additional 12%. Text for a sample reminder/thank you postcard is shown in Figure 12.2.

Step 10: Prepare for the Second Mailing

The second mailing occurs approximately 2 to 3 weeks after the initial survey packet and includes a slightly revised cover letter, another copy of the survey, and a self-addressed, stamped return envelope. The new cover letter conveys the message that a response is important and that this letter is the second attempt to obtain participation. This cover letter also should thank persons if a response has already been sent, since there is a chance that this mailing crossed the response in the mail.

Today's Date

Dear Respondent,

About one week ago, you received a survey about breast cancer screening. Your name was randomly selected from a list of women over the age of 50 years in your area to participate in this survey.

If you have already returned the survey, please accept our sincere thanks. If not, please complete it today. Since the survey was sent to only a small number of women, we need *your* response if the results are to accurately represent the opinion and experiences of women.

If you did not receive the survey, or if it has been misplaced, please call me at 1-800-555-6700 and I will send you another one immediately.

Sincerely,

Your Name
Your Organization or Institution
Your Address

Figure 12.2 Sample Text for Reminder/Thank You Postcard

Step 11: Determine an Acceptable Response Rate

For mailed surveys, a response rate of at least 50% is *adequate*. A response rate of at least 60% is considered to be *good*, and a rate of 70% or higher is assessed as *very good* (Babbie, 1990; Fox, Crask & Jonghoon, 1988). If the suggested guidelines are followed, a return rate of approximately 40% can be expected from the first mailing, a 20% return from the postcard and second mailing, and a 10% return from the third mailing. The actual return rate after each mailing will determine how aggressive the investigator chooses to be in conducting subsequent follow-up mailings.

Step 12: Decide on the Need for a Third Mailing

Two to three weeks after the second mailing, a third survey packet is sent as one last attempt to obtain a response. If the highest possible response rate is important and if there are adequate resources, the third mailing can be sent by certified mail. This technique confirms to the non-respondent that a response is highly valued. If funding is not available for certified postage, a third mailing with first class postage may gain a few more of the reluctant-to-respond individuals. In at least one instance (Isaac & Michael, 1990), a third mailing resulted in only a negligible increase in response rate, so the return on one's investment must be weighed carefully.

Electronic-mail: How Useful in Conducting Surveys?

The use of electronic-mail (i.e., e-mail) for data collection is largely an unexplored concept (Kittleson, 1995; Kittleson, 1997). There are, however, numerous reasons to believe that e-mail will be a major channel for survey data generation in the near future. According to Kittleson (1997):

E-mail has several advantages over the U.S. Postal Service. It is relatively easy to use, can be transmitted and received almost instantaneously, and in many instances, is cost free to the user. With budgets being cut, postal rates continually on the rise, and more individuals having access to the Internet, the use of e-mail as a communication mechanism is gaining in popularity. (p.193).

In a study comparing response rates of an e-mail survey and one sent using the U.S. Postal Service, Kittleson (1995) found that the majority of e-mail users responded within three days of receiving the survey. In a later study to determine the optimal number of effective follow-ups to an e-mail survey, Kittleson (1997) found that up to four follow-ups provided over a 12-day interval yielded only a 47.5% overall response rate. Though this response rate might be deemed "adequate" if regular mail survey standards are applied, several possible explanations for a lower than expected return deserve consideration. According to Kittleson (1997):

First, e-mail messages sent to a person typically enter a "zone" that can be described as a "waiting phase." While in that zone, an individual can look at the message and decide whether to save or discard it. To avoid an overflow of messages, many computer systems will purge messages after a certain period of time. Occasional users of e-mail (i.e., those who review their messages less than once a week) may have their messages purged automatically even before they have an opportunity to view them (p.195).

A person who receives a survey in the mail, and does not discard it immediately, may receive a regular reminder of its presence because it occupies space on top of a desk and is in frequent view. An infrequent or unskilled e-mail user, on the other hand, may not receive such a cue, and therefore, forget that there is a survey to which a response has been requested. As Kittleson (1997) puts it: "The old adage, *out of sight, out of mind,* may be especially relevant to e-mail messages" (p.195).

Without question, one of the present limiting factors with e-mail surveys is the "anonymity factor." E-mail informs the receiver from whom the message has been sent. Thus, for all but the most mundane of subjects, a user may not want an identity revealed to the person conducting the survey.

What suggestions can be offered about use of e-mail for carrying out a survey? Absolute recommendations may have to come in the future since e-mail itself is still in a relative period of infancy. For now, Kittleson (1997) advises that a minimum of one follow-up memo be sent 4 to 7 days after the original e-mail. A second reminder may not add significantly to the response rate, but it probably will do no harm. Constant or ongoing reminders may discourage response by annoying survey recipients (Kittleson, 1997; Rucker, 1984). E-mail surveys should be short in length to avoid the tedious and bothersome task of scrolling back and forth on the computer monitor. Finally, until the anonymity issue is resolved, items appearing on e-mail surveys should be impersonal or contain only "noninvasive" items.

The Method Effect

With surveys performed by face-to-face or telephone methods, the interviewer controls the pace of data collection and the sequence in which questions are asked (Salant & Dillman, 1994). With self-administered, paper-and-pencil surveys, the subject controls both of these phenomena. Moreover, the greater anonymity permitted by self-administered methods may influence the nature of the data that are reported and used to draw conclusions. It should come as no surprise that the method used to collect data can profoundly influence the range, quality, and validity of the information gathered. This phenomenon has been labeled as the **method effect**. It is a source of measurement error about which the evaluator must be keenly aware. The complete elimination of measurement error when conducting surveys is probably not a realistic goal. However, paying careful and close attention to the steps of survey purpose, questionnaire development, pilot testing and related issues will minimize the influence of method. Salant and Dillman (1994) conclude:

It is critical to recognize that self-administered questionnaires are written for people to read, whereas interview questionnaires are written for people to hear. In mail surveys, our goal is to design a visually appealing questionnaire that encourages people to respond, thereby reducing the potential for nonresponse error. In interview surveys, our goal is a questionnaire that communicates effectively to the interviewer and sounds good when read to the respondent. Again, the result is a higher response rate. In both cases, a well-designed questionnaire helps ensure that people's answers are as accurate as possible (p.135).

Summary

This chapter examined various methods and strategies for developing and conducting surveys. Each approach has accompanying advantages and disadvantages that must be weighed carefully before initiating any survey project. The mail survey continues to be the most widely used survey method, but it is possible that technology will spawn new and more cost-effective techniques. Decisions about which method to use revolve around cost, but also around such issues as time, the literacy of potential respondents, the evaluator's ability to standardize items and questions, how much flexibility is required in the data collection process, one's concerns about social pressure and response bias, and how such things as validity (construct, internal, external, etc.) are affected by choice of method. The task of survey development and administration is an arduous one, and one whose sophistication should never be underestimated. Beyond the overview that we have provided in this chapter, there are numerous resources whose only focus is examining the strengths and pitfalls of survey methods. We advise the liberal consultation of the recommended readings and references identified at the end of this chapter to magnify your chance of producing good survey data.

Case Study

Brownson, R.C., Schmid, T.L., King, A.C., et al. (1998). Support for policy interventions to increase physical activity in rural Missouri. *American Journal of Health Promotion*, *12*(4), 263-266.

This study reports on the results of a random-digit dialing telephone interview performed on residents of a rural part of Missouri following the implementation of a project aimed at increasing physical activity in the population. How were data used for (1) needs assessment; (2) estimation of program penetration; and (3) future program planning? How do you suppose the study and its results might have been different if a method other than telephone interviews was used for data collection? What limitations does this study have?

Student Questions/Activities

1. As described in this chapter, the use of e-mail to conduct surveys has been explored only recently. If you are a member of an Internet users' group or listserv, construct a survey following the instructions in this chapter. Experiment with format, length, question types, and follow-up reminders.
2. Using the step-by-step procedure outlined in this chapter, construct a survey on a topic of interest to the students or the administration in your department or college.
3. Interview faculty concerning the use of surveys in their evaluation and research. Ask them to describe their experiences with various survey strategies.
4. Locate a commonly used survey that is prepared in English. Write a short essay concerning what difficulties might arise if the survey were to be translated to another language for use in a different country.

Recommended Readings

Aday, L.A. (1996). *Designing and Conducting Health Surveys: A Comprehensive Guide*, 2nd edition. San Francisco: Jossey-Bass Publishers.

The author provides criteria for evaluating the accuracy and reliability of survey questions, as well as guidelines for developing both objective and subjective types of items. Real examples from notable health surveys are used.

Dillman, D.A. (1978). *Mail and Telephone Surveys: The Total Design Method.* New York: John Wiley.

This book is one of the true handbooks for creators and users of surveys. Dillman introduces his "total design method," the basis for many of the suggestions contained in the chapter you have just completed.

Fink, A. (Ed.). (1997). *The Survey Kit.* Thousand Oaks, CA: Sage.

This nine-volume work was composed by premiere survey research experts. The first volume is a survey researcher's handbook, and is followed by volumes addressing question development, carrying out self-administered and mailed surveys, conducting telephone and in-person interviews, designing surveys, sampling, measuring reliability and validity, analyzing data, and reporting results. This series can be useful to novices, as well as to more experienced survey researchers.

References

Aday, L.A. (1996). *Designing and Conducting Health Surveys: A Comprehensive Guide.* San Francisco: Jossey-Bass Publishers.

Babbie, E. (1990). *Survey Research Methods*, 2nd edition. Belmont, CA: Wadsworth.

Bourque, L.B. & Fielder, E.P. (1995). *How to Conduct Self-administered and Mail Surveys.* Thousand Oaks, CA: Sage.

Brownson, R.C., Schmid, T.L., King, A.C., et al. (1998). Support for policy interventions to increase physical activity in rural Missouri. *American Journal of Health Promotion, 12*(4), 263-266.

Dillman, D.A. (1978). *Mail and Telephone Surveys: The Total Design Method.* New York: John Wiley.

Dillman, D.A. (1983). Mail and other self-administered questionnaires. In P.H. Rossi, J.D. Wright, & A.B. Anderson (Eds.), *Handbook of Survey Research.* San Diego, CA: Academic Press.

Doak, C.C., Doak, L.G. & Root, J.H. (1985). *Teaching Patients with Low Literacy Skills.* Philadelphia, PA: Lippincott.

Fox, R.J., Crask, M.R., & Jonghoon, K. (1988). Mail survey response rates. *Public Opinion Quarterly, 52,* 467-491.

Frey, J.H. & Fontana, A. (1991). The group interview in social research. *Social Science Journal, 28,* 175-187.

Frey, J.H. & Oishi, S.M. (1995). *How to Conduct Interviews by Telephone and in Person.* Thousand Oaks, CA: Sage.

Gentry, E.M., Kalsbeek, W.D., Hogelin, G.C., et al. (1985). The Behavioral Risk Factor Surveys: Design, methods, and estimates from combined state data. *American Journal of Preventive Medicine, 1,* 9-14.

Isaac, S., & Michael, W.B. (1990). *Handbook in Research and Evaluation for Educational and the Behavioral Sciences*, 2nd edition. San Diego, CA: EdITS Publishers.

Kittleson, M.J. (1995). Comparison of the response rate between e-mail and postcards. *Health Values*, *19*(2), 27-29.

Kittleson, M.J. (1997). Determining effective follow-up of e-mail surveys. *American Journal of Health Behavior*, *21*(3), 193-196.

Matsumoto, D. (1994). *Cultural Influences on Research Methods and Statistics*. Pacific Grove, CA: Brooks/Cole.

Pasick, R.J., D'Onofrio, C.N., & Otero-Sabogal, R. (1996). Similarities and differences across cultures: Questions to inform a third generation of health promotion research. *Health Education Quarterly*, *23*(Supplement), S142-S161.

Rea, L.M. & Parker, R.A. (1997). *Designing and Conducting Survey Research*. San Francisco: Jossey-Bass.

Rucker, M. (1984). Personalization of mail surveys: Too much of a good thing? *Educational and Psychological Measurement*, *44*(4), 893-905.

Salant, P., & Dillman, D.A. (1994). *How To Conduct Your Own Survey*. New York: John Wiley.

Siegel, P.Z., Brackbill, R.M., Frazier, E.L., et al. (1991). Behavioral risk factor surveillance. *Morbidity and Mortality Weekly Report*, *40*(SS-4), 1-23.

Torabi, M.R. (1991). Factors affecting response rate in mail survey questionnaires. *Health Values*, 15(5), 57-59.

Waksberg, J. (1978). Sampling methods for random digit dialing. *Journal of the American Statistical Association*, *73*, 40-46.

Chapter
13

Methods and Strategies for Sampling

Chapter Objectives

After completing this chapter, you should be able to:

1. Explain the role of sampling in research and evaluation studies.
2. List and explain the components of a sampling design.
3. Distinguish between probability and nonprobability sampling.
4. Compare and contrast strengths and weaknesses of various nonprobability sampling methods presented.
5. Compare and contrast strengths and weaknesses of various probability sampling methods presented.
6. Identify sources of bias that occur in sampling.
7. Apply methods of estimating sampling error.
8. List and explain various criteria for estimating desirable sample size.
9. Discuss the limitations of making inferences to groups beyond the sample studied.

Key Terms

confidence interval

confidence limits

generalizability

intact group

nonprobability sample

nonresponse bias

oversample

probability sample

sampling error

selection bias

table of random numbers

Introduction

Since it is not usually feasible to study every subject or person possessing a particular population characteristic or trait, it is necessary to define and limit the scope of our effort in carrying out a study. This task is accomplished through a process known as sampling. While the concept of sampling is a relatively easy one to understand, the sophistication of some sampling techniques is frequently underestimated. Because of a tendency that less experienced investigators have to ignore the importance of selecting samples in appropriate ways, many investigations do not tell us as much as they otherwise could. This chapter will examine the most common approaches to selecting samples, and describe the benefits and liabilities associated with each approach.

What is Sampling?

One of the primary purposes of conducting investigations is to make observations and identify principles that have universal application or **generalizability** (Best & Kahn, 1989). In carrying out research and evaluation activities in health education, it is common to want to know some characteristics of the group of people to whom we wish to make inferences. Suppose, for instance, we want to know something about the tobacco use status of eighth-grade students in a particular community. How do we go about collecting this information? One way would be to ask, perhaps by means of an anonymous questionnaire, how frequently one smokes cigarettes, dips snuff, chews tobacco, or uses other tobacco products, and how much of each of these products is used. But whom would we ask, and how would we decide whether the students surveyed were representative of all eighth-graders in our community?

Clearly, if we were able to survey all eighth-graders (and assume that they told us the truth), we would be able to determine with virtual certainty that the group represented the tobacco use habits of eighth-graders in the community. The task of having our results be generalizable with respect to the eighth-grade class in the community would not be a difficult one. If our community were sufficiently small, it might indeed be feasible to conduct just such a survey that *did* involve all members of the eighth-grade class. However, it often is impractical to examine the entire *population* of individuals about whom we wish to make inferences. If the population of interest consisted of all eighth-graders in New York City, or all eighth-graders in the United States, the assignment would be most formidable. To conduct a study of this magnitude would require much effort and money. Thus, it almost goes without saying that some populations are so large that their characteristics cannot be measured readily. Therefore, we must scale down our effort, and examine a *sample* of that population. Sampling allows one to make valid generalizations after careful measurement of the variables of interest in a relatively small segment of the population. A measured value from a sample is called a *statistic*, and the population value inferred is known as a *parameter*.

The accuracy with which research and evaluation questions can be answered depends on the adequacy of the sampling design. A sampling design requires thoughtful planning and preparation. According to some authorities (Salant & Dillman, 1994; Smith & Glass, 1987), the sampling design should consist of the following steps:

- Careful definition of the population.
- Selection of a sample from the population.
- Observation or measurement of the variable in the sample.
- Estimation of the variable in the population based on measurements taken in the sample.
- Statement of the accuracy of the estimates.

Though sampling is a procedure frequently and routinely employed by investigators, it is by no means one that should be done without considerable thought. There are at least two distinct categories of procedures from which one can address the issue of sampling: the **probability sample** and the **nonprobability sample**. We will begin our formal review of sampling strategies by examining the traits and varieties of these two approaches to sample selection.

Nonprobability Samples

Nonprobability samples are ones that take advantage of subjects who are available and accessible to the investigator. In fact, "availability," "accessibility," or "willingness to participate" may be the only criteria for inclusion in a particular investigation. Not everyone within a given population has an equal chance of being selected for the sample to be studied. There are several common ways by which nonprobability samples are chosen.

Samples of Convenience

Perhaps the most frequently employed strategy is known as the *sample of convenience*, or as it is also known, the *sample of opportunity*, the *accidental sample* (Popham, 1988), or the *haphazard sample* (Green & Lewis, 1986). Perhaps you have been a participant in a study that employed this technique. This method is the least complex form of sampling, and the one that provides the investigator with the least amount of ability to make defensible generalizations. It is, perhaps, unfortunate that this sampling technique is often employed by a large number of health educators conducting studies. Health educators are not alone in their use of this low-level sampling approach, as any undergraduate college student who has taken Psychology 101 will attest. Since it is common for psychology students to be participants in surveys and other investigative activities of college professors and their graduate student assistants, it is facetiously said that the science of psychology could be defined as *the study of rats, pigeons, and college freshmen*. However, freshmen psychology students are not representative of all students at that same institution, and certainly are not representative of college students everywhere. If all freshmen have to take psychology, it might be argued that these students could be representative of the freshmen class, but one still would not be on solid ground in professing such a relationship. Would all academic majors be represented? Would race and gender distributions be equitable? If it is an eight-o'clock class in the morning, would it be representative of those students who sleep late and take afternoon or evening classes? One cannot automatically respond affirmatively to these questions.

Samples of convenience frequently allow the investigator the advantage of using **intact groups** of subjects (i.e., students in a classroom, workers in factory, patients at a health care setting, etc.). They also are able to permit an investigator to collect a large amount of information, from a large number of people, and in a relatively small amount of time. The opportunity sample can be useful for such things as generation of hypotheses, refinement of research questions, or exploration of issues not previously examined. Therefore, this sampling technique is not altogether without value.

In the study of eighth-graders that was pondered earlier, consider what erroneous conclusions the investigator might draw about the prevalence of tobacco use if the school or group chosen to "sample" was one that had adopted a strong religious or moral posture with respect to cigarettes and other tobacco products. On the other hand, what might be the result if the sample was selected from a rural area of the country that specialized in cultivation of tobacco products? It should be obvious that this approach to sampling does not permit generalizable conclusions to be drawn, since representativeness cannot be assumed.

Because of several pragmatic considerations, administrative limitations, and other factors, health education program evaluators may have no other choice but to use the sample of opportunity. It is a fact of life that health educators, like many other persons who are asked to perform research and evaluation studies, must function in the real world of what is practical to do, rather than in an ideal world that allows the easy manipulation of people and variables. Manipulation of variables is not so difficult in the laboratory world of test tubes, beakers, white rats, and experimental hybrid corn plants. It is more difficult to arrange people in so orderly of a fashion. The underlying message is a simple one: *If a sample of opportunity is all that is available, you need to be cautious about unwarranted generalizations. If it is practical to employ higher level probability sampling techniques such as those presented later in this chapter, samples of opportunity ought to be used to a minimal extent.*

Volunteer Samples

In some survey research, investigators use what is called *volunteer sampling* (Smith & Glass, 1987). You are probably asking yourself why a particular method is singled out and called a volunteer sample. After all, isn't any sampling of people where there is a choice to participate or not participate, in essence, a volunteer sample? In one respect the answer is clearly "yes." However, in volunteer sampling as we mean it here, a person plays an active role in becoming part of a sample. You see volunteer sampling in action almost every day. Television stations or networks often take polls where one actively, and completely voluntarily, calls a special number to record a vote or point of view (and is usually charged somewhere between $.50 and $1.00). Popular magazines such as

Psychology Today have conducted numerous polls that required readers to complete a questionnaire, tear it out of the magazine, and mail it in (usually at their own expense) to become part of a large data set. Some popular magazines conduct reader surveys about sensitive or controversial topics (e.g., attitudes and practices related to extramarital sex). The results of such surveys make interesting reading while we are getting our hair cut, or while we are waiting for our semi-annual dental examination, but to what extent do they represent the population, or even the usual readership of the magazine that initiates the survey? Can the readerships of these periodicals be characterized in some way? What type of individual is motivated enough to complete and return a published survey questionnaire? How do these people compare in attitudes and practices to persons who read the magazines, but who are not motivated to return a survey, or to those people who never even look at these magazines? Some surveys, like the one described above, result in thousands of completed questionnaires from a volunteer sample. Obviously, if the topic under investigation is one of great audience salience, the likelihood of recruiting numerous volunteers is good. This possibility is the biggest asset of volunteer sampling. However, generalizability is still problematic.

Grab Samples

Another example of nonprobability sampling is selection of subjects using the *grab sampling method* or the *central location intercept method*. The term is practically descriptive of the means by which subjects are chosen for participation in a study - i.e., they almost are literally grabbed. You may have seen this type of sampling done in places such as shopping malls, busy intersections, athletic stadiums, college campus student centers, or other similar locations where large numbers of people congregate. The technique has two chief advantages: (1) acquiring a large sample in a relatively short period of time, and (2) getting at hard-to-reach target audiences in a cost-effective way (National Cancer Institute, 1992). Potential respondents are stopped and asked whether they will participate. Specific screening questions are usually asked to see if the person meets a particular criterion for inclusion in a survey (e.g., being married, being a nonsmoker, or possessing whatever the criterion trait of interest happens to be).

This method has been used by the National Cancer Institute (NCI) to sample people's reactions to alternative written communications about skin cancer that have not yet been released for mass distribution. As intercepts, the NCI workers used construction sites and heavily populated beaches to interview persons who were exposed excessively to the sun (National Cancer Institute, 1992). Properly phrased questions can be of assistance in pilot testing (i.e., audience testing) materials before they are disseminated to the general population (see Chapter 8). The technique can help one to assess a person's comprehension of the materials, individual reaction, personal relevance, credibility, and recall of information. The central location intercept interview is commonly used in market research. The sample you get, though, becomes one comprised of volunteers -- those who are willing to be distracted long enough from their intended activities to be interviewed, or to answer a brief paper-and-pencil questionnaire. Major segments or sub-groups may not be represented when the central location intercept method is employed, as can be seen from the following example.

Suppose you wished to use the central location intercept interview to collect data from high school students about marijuana and alcohol use. Assuming that you went through a proper approval process with the institutional review board (see Chapter 3), the plan might be to station yourself outside the school's main exit at the end of the school day with the intention of stopping students and asking for their cooperation. Think for a moment about what problems might arise in arriving at representativeness? First, you would miss any student who left by any exit other than the main one. Second, any student who was involved in varsity sports, intramural sports, clubs and activities, or any student who was on detention for misbehavior might not be available for hours. Third, all students who had to catch one of the school buses probably would have to head straight for his or her respective bus to avoid being left behind. These are just some of the problems that one would encounter. These problems are not insurmountable, but they are not readily addressed either. It is easy to see why representativeness is difficult with this particular sampling method. Although respondents may not be representative of the general population, or even a particular target population, a large number of people still can be accessed in a relatively short period of time. As with opportunity sampling, if you use this sampling method, you need to be alerted to its limitations.

Homogeneous Samples

Green and Lewis (1986) discuss a broad category of sampling known as *homogeneous sampling* which consists of three illustrative scenarios with relevance for health education evaluators and researchers: the *extreme case*; the *rare element* or *deviant case*; and, the *strategic informant*. In the first of these, the extreme case sample, only persons with an extreme value of the variable under study are included. Thus, persons with severe hypertension, with morbid obesity, or extreme anorexia nervosa might qualify for inclusion in a given sample. In the second instance, people having a low frequency trait or special condition, such as cigarette smoking, HIV/AIDS, albinism, or transsexualism might comprise a unique sample. Finally, strategic informants are those individuals, who because of their key position, special expertise, or high level of training in a narrow area or discipline are recruited to participate in a study (e.g., an expert panel to predict the major health issues in the first two decades of the 21st century). Strategic informants can play an important role in helping to develop consensus around an important issue or set of issues.

Judgmental Samples

On occasion, you may have cause to use what is called *judgmental* or *purposive sampling*. In application, the investigator attempts to select subjects on the basis of whatever he or she thinks is a "typical" student, worker, drinker, smoker, marijuana user, or whatever group is the target of the study. Already you should be asking yourself -- who are these "typical" people, and what constitutes their being "typical"? More often than not, the meaning of "typical" is in the mind of the beholder, and is purely a judgment. This is not to say that the technique is without some merit. The purpose of a study may be to explore behaviors and practices that are unique to a few individuals, or at least, to a distinct segment of the population. Sampling individuals possessing a particular trait can be a useful exercise. Selecting purposive samples of former smokers, recovering alcoholics, sex offenders, individuals who have overcome great personal obstacles to go on to success, and other groups with special traits, may ultimately illuminate the solution to a problem, or guide the design of a responsive intervention. As with other nonprobability sampling methods, generation of research questions and hypotheses are important outcomes associated with the use of judgmental or purposive samples.

Snowball Samples

According to Babbie (1982) sometimes the only way to locate people appropriate for a study is through a referral process. Suppose you wanted to study the people who participated in a gay and lesbian rights rally. Chances are that there would be no list available from which to select a sample. If you knew a few individuals who attended the rally, you could ask them to identify others whom they knew participated in the demonstration. You could then seek out those persons, interview them, and ask them to name additional people who attended. This strategy goes on and on until the investigator gets no new names, or until the objective of the study is met. The technique described here is known as *snowball sampling*. As with other nonprobability sampling strategies, the generalizability of the snowball sample is in doubt. In the example above, the persons most likely to be identified are the ones who were the most visible or the most active during the rally. The extent to which these individuals represented other participants could not be determined with any certainty. While far from being a perfect sampling technique, Babbie (1982) perhaps sums up its value best when he writes: "The choice may be one of learning something of questionable generalizability or learning nothing at all" (p.126).

Quota Samples

A frequently used form of nonprobability sampling is quota sampling. In this approach, the evaluator relies on insight with respect to key demographic variables such as gender, race and ethnicity, religious affiliation, income, and so on. Quota sampling calls for the assignment of proportions (or quotas) when seeking information about knowledge, attitudes, beliefs, or practices in a given population. Therefore, a comparison of attitudes toward family planning options might employ quotas of sex, race, religion, and income to examine the impact of each of these traits taken separately, and in combination, on acceptability of certain birth control options. If the population parameters of these demographic variables are known, the proportions selected for inclusion in the study can reflect these parameters. That is, for example, if it is known that the racial mix of a population is 77% Caucasian, 13% African American, 7% Hispanic, 2% Asian American,

Table 13.1 Summary of Nonprobability Sampling Procedures

Sampling Procedure	Primary Descriptive Element
Convenience	Includes any available subject meeting some minimum criterion usually being part of an accessible intact group.
Volunteer	Includes any subject motivated enough to self-select for a study.
Grab	Includes whomever the investigators can access through direct contact, usually for interviews.
Homogeneous	Includes individuals chosen because of a unique trait or factor they possess.
Judgmental	Includes subjects whom the investigator judges to be "typical" of individuals possessing a given trait.
Snowball	Includes subjects identified by the investigator, and any other persons referred by initial subjects.
Quota	Includes subjects chosen in approximate proportion to the population traits they are to represent.

and 1% Native American, you could select a sample on the basis of these proportions. If you had decided that it was only feasible to have 100 subjects in the study, the proportions would be $77 + 13 + 7 + 2 + 1 = 100$. Of course, there is a problem with this method. To what extent will the seven Hispanics, two Asian Americans, and the lone

Native American reflect the actual population parameters of their respective groups? To overcome this deficit, persons who perform quota sampling often choose to **oversample** minorities to help ensure that a reasonable range of group traits gets represented. Thus, if the size of the group to be studied still is limited to 100 individuals, the respective proportions may be more on the order of 45 : 20 : 15 : 10 : 10. As you can see, some of the diversity in the Caucasian group might be missed, as the magnitudes of the other proportions are increased. Thus, there is something of a trade-off when oversampling is performed without increasing the total sample size. In addition, as more and more key demographic traits are factored into selection of a sample, the complexity of the process increases. Thus, even nonprobability sampling techniques can become quite sophisticated.

We have spent a great deal of time talking about, and giving examples of nonprobability samples. Despite the fact that much criticism is leveled against these techniques by sampling "purists," who advocate use of probability samples only, they serve important functions, as we have pointed out. The quantity of space we allocate to their discussion is defensible, since most health education specialists are forced by circumstances to use them much of the time. It is important, therefore, to understand their utility, and their limitations, equally well. A summary of the major characteristics of nonprobability sampling methods is provided in Table 13.1. Green and Lewis (1986) give their justification for using nonprobability sampling methods:

- When a complete listing of elements comprising the population is neither currently nor potentially identifiable.
- When sensitive information is available from a nonprobability sample, but only superficial data could be obtained from a probability sample.
- When resources are too limited to recruit subjects using probability methods, and the choice is collecting data that may not be generalizable, or collecting none at all.
- When the desire is to make inferences only about the sample, and not a larger population, as in the case of an agency that prepares progress reports on the status of its own program participants.
- When the integrity of a random sample may become compromised by field workers and data gatherers who do not appreciate design sophistication, deviate from the sampling plan, and introduce a bias that cannot be estimated.

Probability Samples

A basic principle of probability sampling is that a sample will tend to be representative of the population from which it is chosen, if every member of the population has a mathematically equal chance of being included in the sample. Representativeness means that the sample accurately embodies the characteristics of the population that are relevant to the study. If we have our population of eighth-grade students to consider again, we can examine the concept of representativeness a little more closely. If we determine that the relevant characteristics of this population are: (1) their current status as a user or nonuser of tobacco products, and (2) their attitudes about tobacco products and tobacco users, then a representative sample drawn from this population should reflect the tobacco use status of students as well as their attitudes toward use and users.

A *simple random sample* is a sample in which each eighth-grader in the entire population of eighth-graders has an equal chance of being studied. Because each student has an equal likelihood of being selected, random sampling reduces the chance of getting a nonrepresentative group to study. There are several ways of choosing a sample randomly. The most popular has been through the use of a **table of random numbers**, such as that likely to be found in the appendix of many statistics books. The table is likely to consist of a series of five-digit random numbers such as the ones shown in Table 13.2.

To see how to employ a series of random numbers to select a sample, pretend that of 1500 eighth-grade students, you want to sample a total of 300 of them. You would begin by numbering the students in the population consecutively from 1 to 1500. Then, entering the table of random numbers, you would go through selection of the first 300 four-digit numbers that fell between 1 and 1500. In the abbreviated table above, you would select the following 15 numbers initially: 1232, 147, 1305, 1134, 1129, 1432, 987, 1496, 1243, 1098, 1027, 26, 343, 1, 667. Students corresponding to these 15 selected numbers would be included in your sample. You would go on using the random number table until 300 unique numbers had been selected.

Table 13.2 Abbreviated Table of Random Numbers

12326	90170	14326	98768
01475	11297	09875	00014
13054	82379	14961	06678
11343	42321	12433	65654
30653	62125	10983	31231
72655	72145	10276	88765
72846	62869	00267	80982
72147	62081	03433	32541

The advent of personal computers has made the generation of random numbers even easier than using a table of random numbers. An investigator who wishes to create random numbers can do so by writing a simple number generating program, and printing out the numbers.

The result would be 300 randomly generated integers (whole numbers) between 1 and 1500. Of course, the easiest way of all to perform this task is to have the student names on a computerized list, and have a computer program randomly generate actual names, rather than have to match names with numbers. Some computers have "built-in" programs that perform this function with the simple administration of a keyboard or mouse command. In any case, computer technology has assisted the process of choosing a sample.

In the example we have been considering, the probability of a particular individual named Joe Mize (#1232) being selected first is 1 in 1500. If we return Joe's number to the original pool after he is selected, the second person also has a 1/1500 chance of being selected. Putting numbers that already have been selected back in the original pool of numbers is known as *random sampling with replacement*. If Joe's number had not been returned to the pool of possible selections, the next person would have had a 1/1499 chance of being drawn. If we continued in that matter of nonreplacement, the last person picked would have had a 1/1201 chance of being picked, somewhat different odds than those Joe Mize had. This latter technique is known as *random sampling without replacement*. Replacing numbers that already have been used is a technicality in sampling, and for most persons, one that has minimal practical significance.

Random sampling eliminates as much of the investigator's **selection bias** as possible. With random sampling, there is greater probability that the true population parameters of interest will be included in the sample that is drawn. There is no way, however, to guarantee that true representativeness is achieved. The extent to which the sample represents the population is primarily a function of sample size. Any difference between the statistic measured in the sample and the actual parameter of the population from which the statistic has been calculated is known as **sampling error**. Babbie (1982) suggests the guidelines shown in Table 13.3 for estimating sampling error when simple random sampling has been the strategy used. Additional easy-to-understand reading about sampling error can be found in Fowler (1993).

Table 13.3 Estimate of Sampling Error Based Upon Sample Size

Sample size:	Accurate within:
100	10.00 percentage points
400	5.00 percentage points
1600	2.50 percentage points
6400	1.25 percentage points

Use the data in Table 13.3 when considering the following illustration of sampling error. If 55% of the eighth-graders in a community are girls, and a random probability sample of 400 is selected, the percentage of girls in the sample is likely to fall within 5 percentage points of the actual population mean. Thus, in a given sample of 400 students, it is likely that the actual percentage of girls will be between 50% and 60% (5 percentage points either side of the population parameter). Theoretically, if we were to choose sample after sample of 400 students using a totally random procedure, 95 out of 100 times the percentage of girls in the sample would fall between 50% and 60%. This theoretical distribution of girls in the sample is known as the 95% **confidence interval**, the standard most often used in reference to sampling error (Babbie, 1982). *The 95% confidence interval is equal to plus or minus 1.96 times the calculated sampling error.* If you pay attention to public opinion polls, or polls on voting preference taken prior to an election, you will hear pollsters speak of their estimate "accurate within X percentage points." It is this sampling error to which they refer.

How does one go about estimating sampling error? Even at the sake of being redundant, let us restate a point: Sampling error is based primarily on sample *size*, not on the *proportion* of the total population which it represents. For example, the sample size necessary to estimate the actual male-to-female ratio in the United States (population > 260,000,000) within 2.5 percentage points would be 1600 (see Table 13.3). To estimate the same ratio with the same degree of accuracy in the city of Tampa, Florida (population > 290,000) also would require a sample size of 1600. Why the same number? Babbie (1982) offers the following explanation:

The proportions are irrelevant because the probability theories upon which sampling is based assume that the populations are infinitely large; hence all sample sizes would represent 0 percent of the population. Only when the sample represents 5 percent or more of the total population do researchers take account of the proportion selected (p.110).

Sampling error is sometimes also known as the *standard error*. It also can be estimated in the following way (Smith & Glass, 1987). An estimate of sampling error in probability sampling is calculated by the square root of $P \times Q / n$, where P is equal to some proportion (e.g., females), Q is equal to $1 - P$, and n represents the sample size.

Suppose a simple random sample of n = 1600 is drawn from a population, and that 55% of the subjects are female (P), and 45% are male (1 - P). Perform the following computations:

1. .55 x .45 = .2475.
2. This decimal divided by 1600 gives a dividend of .0001546.
3. The square root of this dividend is approximately equal to .01245, and represents the percentage points (1.245) of sampling error.

The 95% confidence interval can be calculated by first multiplying 1.96 by the sampling error (1.96 x 1.245 = 2.440). Then, this calculated value is added to, and subtracted from, the known sample proportion of females (55%). Theoretically speaking, if simple random sampling continued to be carried out in the same manner, 95 out of 100 times the proportion of females selected will be between 52.56% and 57.44% (55 ± 2.440). These "boundaries" are known as the 95% **confidence limits**. Thus, we could estimate that the population value for the true proportion of females lies somewhere between 52.56% and 57.44%. We would be correct 95% of the time in making such statements using this method. The larger the sample that we draw, the narrower we can define the confidence limits. Small sample sizes allow us to calculate sampling error and confidence limits, but the confidence interval is likely to be quite large, and therefore, give us less informative results with respect to the population parameter of interest.

Additional Methods of Probability Sampling

The simple random sampling method is by no means the only method of probability sampling available to the investigator. Other methods of probability sampling can, in fact, get extremely sophisticated. The method one chooses depends to a large extent on how much time, money, and other resources are present. Although some probability sampling strategies are quite cleverly devised, they are not necessarily difficult to understand or use. Let us consider some variations of simple random sampling that are practiced routinely in evaluations.

"Fish Bowl" Samples

You are probably already familiar with the notion of drawing slips of paper or ticket stubs containing names or numbers from a fish bowl, or drawing them out of a hat. Anyone who has attended a party or banquet where door prizes are presented has probably seen this method of "randomness" in action. The contents of the container are shaken up vigorously, and either the person doing the drawing is blindfolded, or has the fish bowl (or hat) placed above the head so that names and numbers cannot be read before being selected. This method describes *fish bowl sampling*. Is this method truly a random one? Many sampling experts would argue that it is not. How do we know that every person has an equal chance of being selected? Suppose the tendency of the person doing the choosing is to select only from the top of the bowl. The people whose ticket stubs are in the middle or at the bottom may have zero chance of being selected. Suppose some of the pieces of paper are folded, thus obscuring them from being drawn, and others are not. Will the person simply pick out the first piece of paper that is encountered? You should begin to see by now that this method, although approximating simple random sampling, is somewhat less "scientific" than having a sample generated by a computer. Nevertheless, it is an acceptable sampling method if time and convenience are overriding factors.

Systematic Samples

If it is possible to list or identify everyone who makes up a particular population, another type of sampling procedure, known as *systematic sampling*, is possible. Best and Kahn (1989) indicate that this procedure often can approximate a random sample. In systematic sampling, the investigator selects each *n*th name from a list. In the sample of eighth-graders we have been talking about, if our sample of 300 were to be selected from a school district's roster of students, we would select the first name randomly, and then every 10th name (or 20th, or 30th) thereafter, until 300 names were picked. Thus, after the first person is chosen, the locations of all other persons to be in the sample are determined rather automatically. A chief drawback of systematic sampling is that some important portions of the population that are grouped together on the list might be omitted from being considered (Sowell & Casey, 1982).

Because lists of names are readily available, the systematic sampling approach is easy. Depending on the particular needs and objectives of a study, one could call upon many different types of lists. In addition to a roll call roster of students, one might select postal patrons with addresses in a particular zip code area or census tract, registered voters in a given precinct, persons listed in a telephone or city directory, drivers whose motor vehicles are registered with the licensing bureau, civil service workers in government offices, members of a particular trade union, participants in a health maintenance organization, discharge lists from local hospitals, and so on. Westhoff, McDermott and Harokopos (1996) used systematic random sampling to identify health compromising and health enhancing behaviors among middle school youth in a Florida school district. The accessibility of a list of all the middle school students in the district (and the cooperation of school officials) facilitated the process. The choice of this sampling method also permitted the investigators to draw a sample that was proportionately consistent with the racial and ethnic make-up of the school district.

Lists have their limitations as well, since not everyone is registered to vote, not all people have telephones or allow their name and number to be published, not all people register their motor vehicles, and so on. However, as a means of identifying and accessing large groups, lists that can be employed for systematic sampling are quite useful.

According to Popham (1988) systematic sampling can be used instead of random sampling when the investigator is certain their is no *periodicity* in the list being used. That is, when there is no reason to believe that every *n*th person (the interval being used) has a characteristic not shared by others on the list. Periodicity can occur unexpectedly, as in the example described below by Babbie (1973):

In one study of soldiers during World War II, the researchers selected a systematic sample from unit rosters. Every tenth soldier on the list was selected for the study. The rosters, however, were arranged in a table of organization: sergeants first, then corporals and privates -- squad by squad and each squad had ten members. As a result, every tenth person on the roster was a squad sergeant. The systematic sample selected contained only sergeants. It could, of course, have been the case that no sergeants were selected for the same reason (p.93).

Anyone who was ever in the army would tell you that, unless you were seeking a purposive sample, you probably would not want to study a group comprised entirely of sergeants. Fortunately, periodicity is a rare phenomenon, but one needs to be alerted to the possibility of it.

Stratified Random Samples

A variation of simple random sampling is *stratified random sampling*. With this particular strategy, the population is divided into categories, called *strata*, prior to sample selection. Each *stratum* is comprised of a population characteristic believed to be important in the study being undertaken. In our sample of eighth-graders, suppose we wished to evaluate the effects of a health education unit about tobacco on student knowledge, attitudes, and behaviors. What would be the relevant strata? One cannot say for sure, but it is possible that if 100% of students ride a bus to school, and come from several areas, strata might be constructed on the basis of whether the kids come from urban or rural settings. Perhaps socioeconomic status, sex, race, class standing or grade point average might comprise the bases for other *stratification* of the sample. While simple random sampling can provide the evaluator with a representative sample, further representativeness can be achieved through stratification - i.e., using supplementary information known about the population to organize or direct the selection of the sample by various relevant strata (Popham, 1988). Strata should be used *only* if there is evidence to suggest that these dimensions are relevant to the problem under study. Therefore, do not automatically subdivide a population on the basis of age, race, sex, or some other factor unless there *is* good justification for doing so (Popham, 1988).

On the basis of a literature review, previous studies, or an insightful hunch, an investigator might decide that residency (urban/suburban vs. rural) could have an impact on student response to the tobacco education curriculum. Such a hunch or hypothesis might be drawn especially if the study were being done in North Carolina, Virginia, Kentucky, or some other state where tobacco is a major cash crop, and persons who are raised around tobacco may be more inclined to disdain allegations about ill health effects, and use tobacco freely from an early age. Stratified random sampling might be in order in this instance. The evaluator performs two tasks: (1) operationally defines what constitutes urban, suburban, and rural residency for the purpose of this study; and (2) checks bus ridership to see which students come from which areas. Upon completing these activities, the evaluator determines that 33% of the students come from urban/suburban settings and 67% come from rural settings. In selecting a 300-student stratified random sample of the district's 1500 eighth-graders, the evaluator sees to it that 100 students (33%) are randomly selected from among the urban/suburban dwellers and 200 students are chosen from among the residents of the rural part of the school district. This stratified random sample will be more representative of the population with respect to residency than would a simple random sample. What is described here is a *proportionate stratified random sample*, because the proportions in the sample are the actual proportions of the population. When a particular trait (e.g., demographic characteristic, attitude, behavior, disease state) in a population occurs infrequently, but is of potential importance, one might chose to use a slightly different stratification approach. It involves the use of *disproportionate sampling*, where a sample is selected that purposely examines a larger proportion of individuals with a particular trait than what exists in the population. That is, the segment of the population with the characteristic under study is *oversampled*. To represent the low frequency trait more thoroughly, sample proportions equal in size to those persons with the trait and those without it, may even be selected. This special case of disproportionate sampling produces what is called a *fixed* or *constant stratified random sample*. A weighting procedure can be employed to estimate actual population characteristics.

Since sampling experts agree that stratified random sampling is able to guarantee representativeness better than simple random sampling, with respect to certain traits of the population, it is usually viewed as being a more refined method of sampling (Popham, 1988). Moreover, with stratification, sampling error is decreased, as is the magnitude of the confidence interval (Smith & Glass, 1987). It is possible to add other strata to the sampling design if it becomes evident that they are desirable. As the sampling design increases in complexity, the value of having a sampling expert on the evaluation team becomes a wise consideration.

Cluster Samples

Many times, it is not possible to select individuals at random, but it *is* possible to select schools, classrooms, communities, apartment complexes, churches, businesses, fraternities, or census tracts at random. When the sampling unit becomes groups instead of individuals, one is engaging in *cluster sampling*. Groups are drawn by random selection as in simple random sampling. In cluster sampling, all individuals who comprise the group (or cluster) are subjects for participation in the study. In the study of our eighth-graders, each school could be considered a cluster. If our hypothetical community has ten junior high or middle schools, and each school has approximately 150-200 eighth-graders, randomly selecting two clusters from among the ten available should give us the sample size of 300 that we are seeking.

Perhaps the two schools we chose were unique in some way. That is, because of their location in the community, they overrepresented some types of students and underrepresented others, thus, leaving us with an undesirable sampling situation. How could we modify our cluster sampling design to achieve a more favorable representativeness? One way would be to establish a two-step process for sample selection. In the first stage, we would choose a larger number of schools at random from our pool of ten, (five schools, for instance). In the second stage, we would randomly select eighth-grade classrooms from each of our five schools. Suppose each of the five schools has five eighth-grade classrooms, and each classroom has approximately 30 students. We could then randomly select two classrooms from each of the five schools. A quick computation would show that this sampling method gives us our 300 students (5 schools x 2 classrooms/school x 30 students per classroom = 300 students). The procedure we have just followed here is known as *multistage cluster sampling* or *area probability sampling*. In this particular instance, there were two stages. However, if our original sampling unit had been communities, we might have randomly selected only some of those communities to study. Then, within each community we might have selected only a few schools to study. Finally, within each school, we might have sampled only selected classrooms. This procedure, then, would have involved three stages (see Figure 13.1). The CDC's Youth Risk Behavior Survey (Brener, Collins, Kann, Warren & Williams, 1995) is one example of the use of a multistage cluster sampling technique.

When a population is quite large, accessing groups instead of individuals may be easier and less costly. Such an advantage is important when time, money, personnel, and other resources are at a premium. Cluster sampling, therefore, is highly recommended because of its efficiency. Efficiency, however, comes at a price with respect to precision.

The use of intact groups increases the chance of having an atypical or nonrepresentative sample. At each stage of sampling, there is sampling error added. Thus, the greater the

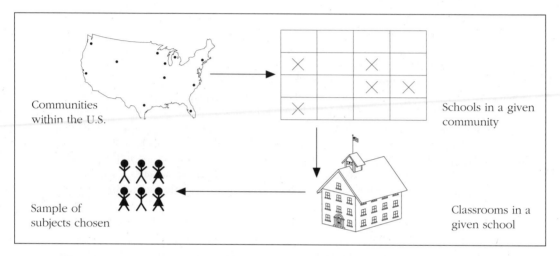

Figure 13.1 Schematic Diagram of Multistage Cluster Sampling

number of stages, the greater the sacrifice in sampling precision. Increasing the sample size and the homogeneity of the elements being sampled enhances representativeness (Babbie, 1973). A detailed description of all possible complexities of cluster samples is beyond the scope of this chapter. Suffice it to say, though, that cluster sampling also may involve a great deal of stratification. In our study of eighth-grade students, communities from which they are drawn could be stratified by region of the country, schools could be stratified by size, by urban versus rural location, and/or by public versus private sponsorship, and so on. Students could be stratified by gender, race, religion, and virtually any other conceivable demographic factor than would be deemed relevant to the study of interest. If you should ever find yourself requiring this level of sophistication, it would be wise to consult a sampling specialist.

Matrix Samples

Lord (1962) is credited with the development of a labor-saving procedure known as *matrix sampling*, that can be employed whenever one wants or needs to ask a large number of questions to a large number of people. Lord reasoned that if one only wished to make inferences about a group (as opposed to individuals), it was not necessary to ask every item to every person. This approach is quite relevant in testing situations where the performance of one group that received an educational intervention (experimental group) is being compared to the performance of a group that did not get the educational intervention (control group).

One begins with a population domain, say for instance, 1500 eighth-graders in a community school district. Assume that 1000 of these students were recipients of a tobacco education curriculum, and that the remaining 500 students did not receive this information. To test the efficacy of the educational intervention, each group is to take a 100-item objective test of knowledge.

The administration of 1500 examinations, together with their aggregate scoring and analysis, would be an arduous task for teachers or program evaluators. Moreover, students would require one or more hours to complete the examination. Of interest to the evaluator, however, is the group scores, not the performances of individual students. Consequently, the evaluator has some options as to how to proceed.

First, you could have all students take the 100-item test. As pointed out, this would be labor intensive for everyone. Second, you could select students from experimental and control groups by an appropriate probability sampling method, and give the 100-item test to just those students (*examinee sampling*). This action would save everyone some effort, but would still necessitate that some of the eighth-graders take the whole test, while others do not participate at all. Third, you could select items from the test by some probability sampling method, and give an abridged version of the test to all 1500 students (*item sampling*). This procedure would probably make the students a little happier, but the scope of the content on the examination might be compromised. Fourth, you could combine item sampling with examinee sampling, i.e., select a sample of questions and a sample of students. This method would reduce the evaluator's work some, but might compromise the item coverage, and it would still have some students taking a test while others do not. None of these solutions is very satisfactory. There is one other option, however, known as *multi-matrix sampling*, that solves the evaluator's dilemma.

According to Gold, Basch, and McDermott (1983): "Multi-matrix sampling combines the advantages of item and examinee sampling while still allowing the potential for greater scope of coverage and improved precision of measurement" (p.274). In the example above, the 100-item test can be randomly divided into 10 separate tests of 10 items each. Likewise, the experimental and control groups can be divided up randomly into groups of 25 students each (40 experimental and 20 control). The 10 tests can then be randomly assigned to the 60 samples of eighth-graders. Through multi-matrix sampling, one has complete population and item domain coverage. Furthermore, a 10-item test is much easier to administer by the teacher, to complete by the student, and to score and analyze by a computer, and to interpret by an evaluator. Some of the advantages of multi-matrix sampling include:

- Greater coverage of large item domains, especially when time is limited.
- Reduction in time required for testing.
- More acceptable to test-takers (especially children or others with short attention spans) and less threatening.
- Applicable to many item types, populations, and settings.

This approach also has noteworthy drawbacks, including:

- It is useful for group statistics only, not individual scores.
- Its logistics can be complex unless the level of cooperation is high among examinees and test administrators.
- The computations of group statistics require a computer.
- The context of the test-taking situation may produce response sets (a tendency to respond in a predictable way), or contribute to a sub-optimal performance by the examinee.

A summary of probability sampling methods appears in Table 13.4.

Table 13.4 Summary of Probability Sampling Procedures

Sampling Procedure	Primary Descriptive Element
Simple random	Each subject has an equal mathematical probability of being selected if random number generator is used.
Fish bowl	Approximates simple random sampling but has less precision.
Systematic	Uses a list to select subjects at a constant interval after first subject is picked at random.
Stratified random	Uses strata to ensure representation of key variables in the population.
Cluster	Samples groups at random instead of individuals.
Matrix	Simultaneously samples items comprising a test and persons comprising a group to make population estimates.

Adapted from: Babbie, E.R. (1982). *Social Research for Consumers*. Belmont, CA: Wadsworth, p.109.

Criteria for Evaluating Different Sampling Designs

Aday (1996) identifies four different criteria for evaluating various sampling designs. These criteria include precision, accuracy, complexity, and efficiency.

Precision refers to the extent to which the estimates derived from the sample reflect the population of interest. Thus, precision is a function of sampling error. The magnitude of the sampling error is related to sample size (smaller samples have more risk of error) and sample complexity (cluster samples have more risk of error than simple random samples).

Accuracy refers to the extent to which the estimates derived from the sample reflect systematic error or systematic bias. As identified elsewhere in this chapter, as well as in Chapter 12, bias occurs when some groups that are eligible for inclusion in the study are systematically excluded -- people without telephones are excluded from a telephone survey, women who work outside the home during the day are excluded from door-to-door surveys, school-aged youth who participate in extramural activities after school are excluded from central location intercept surveys performed on school grounds, and so on.

Complexity "refers to consideration of the amount of information that must be gathered in advance of doing the study, as well as the number of stages and steps that will be required to implement the design" (Aday, 1996, p.121). Thus, whereas simple random sampling is relatively straightforward, a multistage cluster sample introduces much greater complexity, as well as more labor intensity.

Efficiency refers to maximizing precision and accuracy to obtain sample estimates reflective of the population, and doing so at the least possible cost. Reading, consultation with experts, and experience lead to greater efficiency on the part of the evaluator.

Nonresponse - Then What?

You have planned your sampling procedure well and have decided on an appropriate method. With whatever complexity your resources, motivations, and other concerns allow for, you have chosen your sample. You have hired and trained telephone interviewers, developed valid and reliable instruments, printed questionnaires, or mailed surveys to your potential respondents. Everything went well except you did not get a very good rate of return. People turned you down on the street and over the phone. Mailed questionnaires never got farther than the recipients' circular files. Audience administered questionnaires came back to you blank or only partly completed -- some even with disparaging remarks about your ancestry. Where do you go from there?

Just because you toiled to select a representative sample does not necessarily mean that you will end up with one. Sampling error is greatly influenced by nonresponse. Writes Fowler (1993): "The effect of nonresponse on survey estimates depends on the percentage not responding, and the extent to which those not responding are biased - that is, systematically different from the whole population" (p.40). Any interpretation of results may be misleading, and causes what is known as **nonresponse bias**. What is an acceptable nonresponse rate? There is little agreement on this matter. Babbie (1990) indicates that a 50%-60% return on a mailed questionnaire is adequate to analyze. Smith and Glass (1987) suggest that nonresponse bias can be substantial even when the rate of return is as high as 80%.

What do you do about nonrespondents? Follow-up of nonrespondents is sometimes performed (e.g., postcard reminders, complete remail, telephone callback, etc.)

if time and other resources permit it. Even if follow-up increases the overall return rate, it may still bring in responses only from those people who are motivated (albeit less motivated or compulsive than the immediate respondents). It may be possible to test for the true representativeness of your respondents, however. If there are demographic or other relevant data available on the population from which the sample was taken, comparisons between respondents and the parent population may be made. If comparison reveals that the respondents are different, the extent to which one can make inferences is reduced. In the real world, one seldom gets a response rate as high as one would like. The best defense against low response rate is good planning and experience (see Chapter 12).

Statistical adjustments can sometimes be made to correct for nonresponse. Fowler (1993) cites the following example:

Suppose people 65 or older are known to constitute 20% of the adults in some population. Because of differential response, though, only 10% of the sample respondents are 65 or older. After the survey is done, a researcher could weight the answers of those 65 or older who responded so that they are the equivalent of 20% of the responses. To the extent that those 65 or older gave different survey answers from those who were younger, the resulting estimates might be better. This result, however, also depends on the over-65 respondents being similar to the over-65 nonrespondents, which may not be true (p.48).

A related type of statistical adjustment, involving the use of a weighting procedure, is illustrated later in this chapter (see Table 13.5).

There is still another possibility for the person wishing to address the problem of nonresponse. Suppose that a sample of 500 people is chosen to participate in a mailed survey, but responses are received from just 300 of the people. It is possible that some of the 200 nonrespondents would be willing to respond to a personal interview, perhaps by telephone. Even though this strategy is labor intensive and expensive, it may prove to be worthwhile if it substantially improves the overall response rate and decreases the amount of nonrespondent bias. and thus, reduces the sampling error. According to Fowler (1993): "Of course, the second round will also have nonresponse, and itself may still produce data that do not fully represent all nonrespondents" (p.48). If half of the original nonrespondents (100 of the 200 nonrespondents) are followed up on, any new respondents obtained through this phase of the study should be weighted by a factor of two if combined with the original data. If a fraction of the original nonrespondents other than half is used, a different, proportional weighting factor should be used. For the example above, an adjusted response rate (ARR) can be calculated as follows (Fowler, 1993):

ARR = Original Responses + (2x Responses from Nonresponse Sample) ÷ Original Total Eligible Sample

If the second round efforts result in obtaining 40 more respondents, the adjusted response rate becomes: ARR = 300 + (2x 40) ÷ 500 = .76 or 76%.

Sample Size: How Many Subjects Do I Need?

Another frequent dilemma of investigators is figuring out how large of a sample they need to select. There are several guidelines for determining an adequate sample size. Nachmias and Nachmias (1987) suggest that appropriate sample size is a function of the level of accuracy required or how large of a sampling error one is willing to accept. One needs a smaller sample if a 10% sampling error is acceptable, than if the required sampling error is 5% or less. If the population is fairly homogeneous with respect to the variable being studied, the sample size does not have to be particularly large. However, if the number of sub-groups one wishes to make inferences about is large, the sample size will have to increase in size. If stratified random sampling is used to enhance the probability of estimating population traits more precisely, sample size can be more moderate. In addition, descriptive survey studies should have larger samples than experimental studies (Best & Kahn, 1989). Finally, cost may be an overriding factor regardless of other criteria.

There is no wisdom in selecting a particular *sampling fraction* (sample size : population size) such as 5% or 10% (Fowler, 1993). Recall that it is primarily sample size, and not proportion (fraction), that determines sampling error. Specific formulas for calculating sample size for finding differences between means or proportions are available in Cochran (1963), Dillman (1978), Fowler, (1993), Gilbert (1976), Kish (1965), and Salant and Dillman (1994). In general, sample size is a function of the precision of estimate needed, the homogeneity of the variable within the population, the extent to which stratification and subclass analysis is required, whether the study is descriptive or experimental, and the cost of identifying or recruiting subjects.

Generalizing from Samples

There are two kinds of inferences that health education specialists want to make from studies of samples: *descriptive* and *explanatory*. Descriptive inferences occur when we describe the characteristics of a particular sample, and then, infer that this description would also hold true for the population. Such an inference is dependent on an appropriate probability sampling design, a high completion rate, and any additional checks of representativeness that can be done.

Even when a sample is found to be unrepresentative, meaningful descriptive and explanatory inferences can be made if weighting procedures are employed. An example of weighting is illustrated with respect to the data in Table 13.5. An investigator was interested in how the student body at her university felt about using condoms when having sex for the first time with a new dating partner. Despite observing probability sampling protocol, she got a sample that was not representative of the 50%-50% gender split that enrollment figures suggested existed at that school. Although such a sample would be unlikely in probability sampling, it is still possible. Women clearly were underrepresented. Upon inspection of the unweighted data, it appeared that slightly less than half of the students would use a condom during a first sexual episode.

The investigator then made a statistical adjustment to give women equal representation in the sample. By multiplying each woman's response by 2.33 (350/150), she created a hypothetical sample of 350 women to match the 350 men. Please note that when the weighting procedure is employed to compensate for misrepresentation, a majority of respondents now favors the use of a condom during a first sexual episode.

One certainly would have been misled about student attitudes if only the raw, unweighted data had been considered.

Table 13.5 Unweighted and Weighted Student Responses to the Question: "Would you use a condom if you were having sex for the first time with a new dating partner?"

		Men	Women	Total
Unweighted				
	YES	140	105	49.0%
	NO	210	45	51.0%
	TOTAL	350	150	100.0%
Weighted				
	YES	140	245	55.0%
	NO	210	105	45.0%
	TOTAL	350	350	100.0%

Unlike descriptive generalizations, explanatory inferences are not affected by the representativeness of the sample. The unweighted data in Table 13.5 clearly show that gender is an important factor in supporting the use of condoms during a first sexual episode. Women are far more likely to support their use (105/150 = 70%) than are men (140/350 = 40%). Thus, while having a nonrepresentative sample distorted overall student body opinion about condom use attitudes, it did not hide the strength of the association between gender and attitude.

Summary

Health educators who perform research or conduct evaluation studies that require knowledge of sampling have several strategies at their disposal. Whenever possible, probability sampling should be employed. Often, it is the case that probability sampling is neither more difficult, nor more expensive than opportunity sampling or other nonprobability methods. The sample design should fit the problem that is being investigated. When an evaluation calls for a sophisticated sampling design, a sampling expert should be employed or consulted. Sampling almost always requires some type of compromise on the part of the investigator. Whatever sampling design you use, you should be aware of its limitations as well as its strengths. You now should be able to read practically any research or evaluation report, make informed judgments about the appropriateness of the sampling technique used, and thus, be a better consumer of the literature and a more skilled practitioner of the activity.

Case Study

Jackson, C., Henriksen, L., & Foshee, V.A. (1998). The Authoritative Parenting Index: Predicting health risk behaviors among children and adolescents. *Health Education & Behavior, 25*(3), 319-337.

Jackson and her colleagues report on three separate studies involving the application of the Authoritative Parenting Index (API) scale with school-aged youth and the relationship between API scores and various health risk behaviors. Examine the samples and survey protocols for each of the three vignettes. What are the strengths of the sampling design? What are the weaknesses? How could this study be done in a way that would enhance representativeness? Explain.

Student Questions/Activities

1. On the evening news you hear that the results of a random telephone survey conducted by the Centers for Disease Control and Prevention estimate that 85% of Americans approve of mandatory drug testing of public school employees, and that this percentage is accurate within plus or minus 5 percentage points. Explain what this statement means in terms of sampling error and confidence limits. Is any confidence level stated or implied here?

2. Suppose that in the poll conducted in Question #1, 30% of the persons contacted refused to answer the question. In a general way, describe the effect that nonresponse might have on one's interpretation of the poll's results. Secondly, since public education is a large service industry in the country, it is likely that many of the persons called (whether or not they chose to respond) were education professionals. Does this possibility influence interpretations of the poll at all?

3. A person who is consulting with you on how to evaluate teachers' reactions to a recently implemented health education curriculum advises you to survey 20% of the 200 teachers who used the curriculum. Make a judgment about this advice and support your conclusion. Would the sampling method used influence your conclusion? Identify five approaches to choosing this sample.

Recommended Readings

Fink, A. (Ed.). (1997). *The Survey Kit*. Thousand Oaks, CA: Sage.

This nine-volume work was composed by premiere survey research experts. The first volume is a survey researcher's handbook, and is followed by volumes addressing question development, carrying out self-administered and mailed surveys, conducting telephone and in-person interviews, designing surveys, sampling, measuring reliability and validity, analyzing data, and reporting results. This series can be useful to novices, as well as to more experienced survey researchers.

Fowler, F.J. (1993). *Survey Research Methods*, 2nd edition. Newbury Park, CA: Sage.

This handy volume covers the "ins" and "outs" of surveys for research and evaluation. It addresses single-stage and multistage sampling, calculating sampling error, estimating needed sample size, implementing sampling designs, and correcting for nonresponse.

Salant, P., & Dillman, D.A. (1994). *How To Conduct Your Own Survey*. New York: John Wiley.

This textbook is recommended because of its extensive examples and integration of sampling and survey construction. It is useful in selecting the survey approach that is right for you, while avoiding common errors.

References

Aday, L. (1996). *Designing and Conducting Health Surveys*, 2nd edition. San Francisco: Jossey-Bass Publishers.

Babbie, E.R. (1973). *Survey Research Methods*. Belmont, CA: Wadsworth.

Babbie, E.R. (1982). *Social Research for Consumers*. Belmont, CA: Wadsworth.

Babbie, E.R. (1990). *Survey Research Methods*, 2nd edition. Belmont, CA: Wadsworth.

Best, J.W., & Kahn, J.V. (1989). *Research in Education*, 6th edition. Englewood Cliffs, NJ: Prentice-Hall.

Brener N.D., Collins J.L., Kann L., Warren C.W., Williams B.I. (1995). Reliability of the Youth Risk Behavior Survey questionnaire. *American Journal of Epidemiology, 141*, 575-580.

Cochran, W.G. (1963). *Sampling Techniques*, 2nd edition. New York: Wiley.

Dillman, D.A. (1978). *Mail and Telephone Surveys: The Total Design Method*. New York: Wiley.

Fowler, F.J. (1993). *Survey Research Methods*, 2nd edition. Newbury Park, CA: Sage.

Gilbert, N. (1976). *Statistics*. Philadelphia: W.B. Saunders.

Gold, R.S., Basch, C.E., & McDermott, R.J. (1983). Multi-matrix sampling: A valuable data collection method for health educators. *Journal of School Health*, *53*(4), 272-276.

Green, L.W., & Lewis, F.M. (1986). *Measurement and Evaluation in Health Education and Health Promotion*. Palo Alto, CA: Mayfield.

Kish, L. (1965). *Survey Sampling*. New York: Wiley.

Lord, F.M. (1962). Estimating norms by item sampling. *Educational and Psychological Measurement*, *23*, 259-267.

Nachmias, D., & Nachmias, C. (1987). *Research Methods in the Social Sciences*, 3rd edition. New York: St. Martin's Press.

National Cancer Institute. (1992). *Making Health Communication Programs Work: A Planner's Guide*. Washington, DC: USDHHS, NIH Publication #92-1493.

Popham, J.W. (1988). *Educational Evaluation*, 2nd edition. Englewood Cliffs, NJ: Prentice-Hall.

Salant, P., & Dillman, D.A. (1994). *How To Conduct Your Own Survey*. New York: John Wiley.

Smith, M., & Glass, G. (1987). *Research and Evaluation in Education and the Social Sciences*. Englewood Cliffs, NJ: Prentice-Hall.

Sowell, E.J., & Casey, R.J. (1982). *Analyzing Educational Research*. Belmont, CA: Wadsworth.

Westhoff, W.W., McDermott, R.J., & Harokopos, V. (1996). Acquisition of high-risk behavior by African-American, Latino, and Caucasian middle-school students. *Psychological Reports*, *79*, 787-795.

Chapter

14

Statistical Analysis of Data

Chapter Objectives

After completing this chapter, you should be able to:

1. Describe the uses of statistics in evaluation projects.
2. Organize a data set and develop a frequency distribution.
3. Calculate and interpret selected descriptive (univariate) statistics.
4. Describe the uses of bivariate statistical procedures.
5. Describe the uses of multivariate statistical procedures.
6. Define various terms applied to statistical analysis.

Key Terms

analysis of variance (ANOVA)
chi-square test
confidence interval
correlation
cross-tabulation
dependent variable
descriptive statistics
discriminant analysis
factor analysis
frequency distribution
geographic information systems (GIS)
incidence rate

independent variable
inferential statistics
mean
median
mode
multiple regression
odds ratio
prevalence rate
range
standard deviation
statistical significance
t-test

Introduction

We use statistics to organize and summarize data. We also use them to make inferences from a small group of observations (a sample) to the total group (a population). **Descriptive statistics** are used to organize and summarize data sets, and **inferential statistics** are used to generalize results from a sample to a larger population (Devore & Peck, 1993).

Descriptive statistics also are used to make sense of large data sets. For example, think of a personal health course with an enrollment of 100 students, where the students just took an exam. It would be difficult to make sense of how well any one student performed, compared to the others in the class, just by looking at the list of test scores. For this reason, teachers often provide the class average, or **mean**, when discussing test results with students. The teacher might also indicate the highest score (*maximum score*) and the lowest score (*minimum score*) for the test. In a 100-point test, the mean may have been an 85, the minimum score equal to 40, and the maximum score equal to 96. A student who received an 89 would know that the test score was "above average," yet not the highest score received on the test. In ways similar to this one, descriptive statistics are used in every day life.

Inferential statistics are used when one gathers data from a small group of people (preferably a group which was randomly sampled), but desires to make inferences about a larger population. We use sampling because it is often prohibitively expensive or impractical to study each person. Probability sampling procedures, as described in Chapter 13, allow us to estimate population values from the sample results. Surveys for political polls are good examples of how inferential statistics can be used. Various opinion polls often are reported on television. These polls estimate what percent of the population will vote for the Democratic candidate, what percent will vote for the Republican candidate, and so on. These results are not based on a survey of every person who will vote in the United States, but rather, on a sample of likely voters. The results, more often than not, are extremely accurate! Inferential statistics allow us to make generalizations from a sample to a population.

We also use statistical procedures to compare the effects of various interventions. For example, we might be interested in testing the effects of two drug education programs, to determine which one had the more positive impact on middle school youth. A quasi-experimental design (see Chapter 10) might be developed, where one group of youngsters receives program *A* and another group receives program *B*. At the conclusion of the study, we would collect data, and determine if one group had a greater increase in knowledge than the other, and, if one group showed a larger reduction in drug use. We could use a statistical technique called a *t-test* to see if one group had a higher mean score on the knowledge test. The results might show that group *A* had a statistically significantly higher score than group *B* at posttest time. These data would suggest that program *A* is more effective than program *B* in increasing drug education knowledge.

Another reason we might use statistics is to determine if there are relationships between different variables (Kachigan, 1986). Suppose we want to understand the relationship between cholesterol level and heart attack risk, or, the relationship between gender and alcohol use. Correlational statistical tests can examine if there is a statistically significant relationship between cholesterol level and heart attack, and chi-square tests can tell us whether males are more likely than females to be heavy drinkers.

In health education program evaluation, we use descriptive *and* inferential statistics to assess the degree to which an intervention program worked, to study how risk factors are related to diseases, and to describe information that comprises large data sets. In each case, we use the terms **dependent variable** and **independent variable** to describe the various treatments, interventions, risk factors, and outcomes studied. McKenzie and Smeltzer (1997) define independent variables as those variables controlled by the evaluator, whereas, dependent variables are the outcome variables being studied. For example, the types of drug education program being studied would be an independent variable, whereas, drug use behaviors, attitudes, and knowledge levels would be the dependent variables. Independent variables *affect* dependent variables. In the cholesterol example cited above, the independent variable is *cholesterol level*, while *heart attack risk* is the dependent variable. The independent variable causes a change in something. The dependent variable is the thing you are trying to predict. Independent variables are also known as *predictor variables*, and dependent variables are sometimes called *criterion variables*.

This chapter introduces you to some of the more commonly used statistical tools of health education program evaluation. Emphasis is placed on univariate procedures. However, we also will discuss bivariate and multivariate procedures.

Univariate Procedures

When you analyze a single variable, you use univariate statistical procedures. If you administered a classroom test to a group of students, you would usually describe that test in terms of univariate procedures. As discussed earlier, you might calculate a mean score (the class average), as well as identify the high and low scores. These statistics, along with several others, are commonly used to describe variables. In this section, we talk about raw scores, frequency distributions, measures of central tendency, measures of dispersion, and rates.

Raw Scores. The simplest way to describe a variable is to present all the scores for that variable in a table. In Table 14.1, you will find test scores of 111 students for a 20-point test. As you can see, a table of raw scores generally does not provide the reader with much information. The scores must be arranged or analyzed in some way to be more meaningful. One way of arranging scores is to use frequency distributions.

Frequency Distributions. **Frequency distributions** are rank-ordered sets of raw scores, from highest to lowest, or lowest to highest. Frequency distributions can present data in a number of ways, including frequency of raw scores, percentages, and cumulative percentages. Table 14.2 shows the frequency distribution for a set of scores. A review of the table indicates that there was one person who received one point on the test, and one person who scored a perfect 20 out of 20. Six people scored a 15.

Measures of Central Tendency. Three measures of central tendency are the **mean**, **median**, and **mode**. We use measures of central tendency, rather than raw scores

Table 14.1 Table of Raw Scores

1	3	4	4	6	6	8	8	8	8
2	4	5	7	7	9	11	11	11	11
2	4	5	6	6	6	10	10	10	10
3	5	6	7	7	9	11	11	11	11
3	5	5	7	7	7	8	8	8	8
9	9	9	9	9	9	9	11	12	12
10	15	10	15	10	14	10	13	10	13
17	16	17	18	16	19	15	12	14	12
13	17	13	16	13	17	13	15	13	15
16	14	16	14	19	14	15	14	18	14
20	12	11	12	11	12	12	10	12	13
18									

or frequency distributions, because they allow us to describe a set of data with one number. Along with measures of dispersion, they allow us to describe a data set in a succinct and understandable manner.

The mean is what the lay person calls the "average." The mean is calculated by adding up all the scores, and dividing that sum by the number of scores in the distribution. Statistically, the calculation of the mean is expressed as follows:

$$X_m = \sum_{i=1}^{n} X \div N$$

X_m = the mean of X
Σ = the Greek letter sigma which means to add up all numbers known as X (in our case, X is the set of test scores)
N = the number of scores analyzed (in our case, 111 scores)

The mean score may be the most frequently reported statistic in health education evaluation and measurement. The mean is an appropriate measure of central tendency for data which are interval and ratio in nature. In our sample data set, the mean score is 10.5.

The median is the "middle-most" score in the distribution. It is that score which equally divides the frequency distribution in half, with 50% of the scores being above the median, and 50% of the scores being below the median. The median is the appropriate measure of central tendency for ordinal data, and can also be calculated when using interval and ratio data. It is a useful statistic for ratio or interval data when the distribution of data is skewed. In these situations, reporting a median and mean is appropriate. The median score for our sample distribution is 11.

If in a test of 50 people, the most common score received was 15, then the mode would be 15 points. The mode is the most appropriate measure of central tendency for nominal data. It can also be used with ordinal, interval, or ratio data. Sometimes, in a

Table 14.2 Frequency Distribution of Scores

Score	Frequency	Percent	Cumulative Percent
1	1	0.9	0.9
2	2	1.8	2.7
3	3	2.7	5.4
4	4	3.6	9.0
5	5	4.5	13.5
6	6	5.4	18.9
7	7	6.3	25.2
8	8	7.2	32.4
9	9	8.1	40.5
10	10	9.0	49.5
11	11	9.9	59.5
12	9	8.1	67.6
13	8	7.2	74.8
14	7	6.3	81.1
15	6	5.4	86.5
16	5	4.5	91.0
17	4	3.6	94.6
18	3	2.7	97.3
19	2	1.8	99.1
20	1	0.9	100.0
Total	111	100.0	

Sample size	111	Maximum	20.0
Mean	10.5	Minimum	1.0
Median	11.0	Std Dev	4.3
Mode	11.0	Range	19

data set, there are two or more modes. In this situation, the distribution is said to be *bimodal*. We calculate the mode by simply counting up the most frequently occurring score in the distribution. In our example, the mode is 11.

When the data are *normally distributed*, i.e., in a bell-shaped curve, the mean, median, and mode are all the same number. When the data are skewed (do not form a normal distribution) these values are different. Figure 14.1 shows the relationships among three measures of central tendency when the data are normally distributed, positively skewed, and negatively skewed.

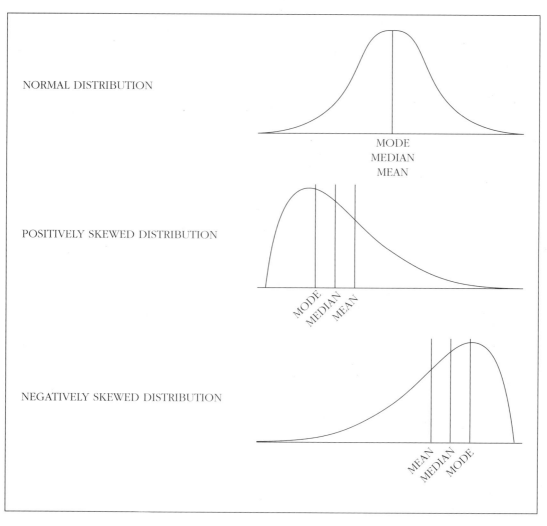

Figure 14.1 The Effects of Distribution on Measures of Central Tendency

Measures of Dispersion. Measures of dispersion describe the spread of scores in the distribution. Although measures of central tendency tell us a lot about the average, the middle-most score, and the most common score, they do not tell us how much the scores differ from each other. Knowing the class average on a test is 75 does not tell us what the highest and lowest score was, or where the greatest concentration or grouping of scores was. It is possible for three classes to have the same measures of central tendency, yet the spread of scores might vary widely. Figure 14.2 shows how we can have three distributions of scores with the same measures of central tendency but different measures of dispersion.

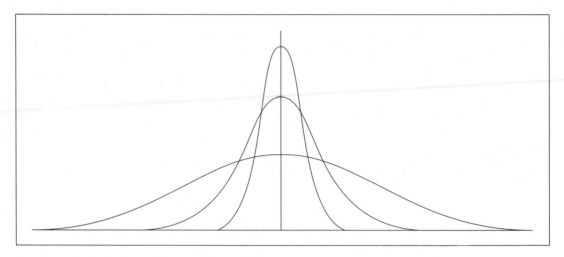

Figure 14.2   Three Distributions with the Same Measure of Central Tendency but Different Measures of Dispersion

The simplest measure of dispersion is the **range**. The range is calculated by subtracting the *minimum score* (e.g., lowest score received on the test) from the *maximum score* (e.g., highest score on the test). In our example, the minimum score was 1 and the maximum score was a 20, providing a range of scores of 19.

The **standard deviation** is a more sophisticated measure of variation. It tells us the variability of scores around the mean. Based on statistical theory, one standard deviation around the mean is where about 68% of the scores for the variable will fall. For example, if we had a test with a mean score of 75 and a standard deviation of 10, then we would know that about 68% of all test scores fell between the scores of 65 and 85. Standard deviations are used to describe where the highest concentration of scores are. In our sample data set, the standard deviation was 4.3. With a mean score of 10.5, we now know that approximately 68% of the scores on our sample test were between 6.2 and 14.8.

Standard deviations can be calculated in two ways, depending on whether a sample or population standard deviation is being estimated. They can be calculated as follows:

Standard deviation of a population

σ = the square root of $\Sigma(x_i-\mu)^2 \div N$

Σ = summation
$(x_i-\mu)^2$ = deviation of x from the population mean
N = number of cases in the population
σ = standard deviation

Sample estimate of the population standard deviation

s = the square root of $\Sigma(x_i-x_m)^2 \div n-1$

s = sample standard deviation
n = number in the sample
Σ = summation
$(x_i-x_m)^2$ = deviation of x from sample mean

Rates. In addition to measures of central tendency and dispersion, health education program evaluators often work with rates, especially rates focusing on disease, disability, death, and fertility. State and local health departments publish these vital statistics on an annual basis, and these data play an important role in measuring the health of the community or state. You have already been taught (see Chapter 9) the importance of vital statistics data in the needs assessment phase of program development.

Health educators use many different types of rates to describe health events. In reading an annual report from a local health department, you will undoubtedly come across terms such as *crude rates, age-adjusted rates, disease-specific rates, sex-adjusted rates, incidence rates,* and *prevalence rates.* Rates are essential for the comparison of health events from one group of people to another, from one geographic region to another, or from one time period to another. We cannot simply compare raw numbers of events, because populations differ in size from each other. Suppose county A has 45 alcohol-related highway fatalities, while county B has 145 such fatalities. Which county has a bigger problem? We cannot say for sure based on the information provided, because county B might have a huge population and one or more large cities, while county A is rural, and with few people. One-hundred forty-five fatalities around Chicago, Illinois might be a "blip" in the grand scheme of things, but 45 similar events around Monroe, Wisconsin would signal an epidemic! For this reason, when we make comparisons among populations, we must not only count the number of events (e.g., deaths, births, cases of illness), but must also count the total number of people (or population) in the region being studied. Rates are expressed in terms of a time period (usually a year), or in terms of population (often, per 100,000). So, we might hear that the rate of *Chlamydia trachomatis* is 800 cases per 100,000 population for 1999. We can compare the target population's rate to that of the state, the nation, and the year 2010 target rate. We would not be able to make those comparisons using only the actual numbers of cases.

A rate is calculated as follows:

$$\text{Rate} = \frac{\text{\# of events}}{\text{population in same area}} \text{ in a time period x } K \text{ (some constant)}$$

In 1995, there were 67,493 births in Wisconsin (population 5,119,240) according to Center for Health Statistics (1996a) data. The crude birth rate is calculated as follows:

$$\text{crude birth rate} = \frac{67,493 \text{ births}}{5,119,240 \text{ people}} = .01318 \text{ X } 1000$$

$$= 13.2 \text{ births per 1000 population}$$

There were 45,037 deaths in 1995 in Wisconsin (Center for Health Statistics, 1996b). The crude death rate is computed as follows:

$$\text{crude death rate} = \frac{45,037 \text{ deaths}}{5,119,240 \text{ people}} = .0879 \text{ x } 1000$$

$$= 8.8 \text{ deaths per 1000 population}$$

Rates can be expressed in a number of ways, including using percentages, or the number of events per 1000 people, per 10,000, per 100,000, or per 1,000,000 people. The less common the health event, the greater the number of people used in the denominator. For example, prevalence of smoking (relatively large number of smokers) often is expressed in percentages of population who smoke, whereas for rare types of cancers, the rate is described as the number of cases per 100,000 people (or, in some instances, per 1,000,000 people).

We frequently use *age-adjusted* and *disease specific* or *age-specific* rates when studying populations. In fact, age-adjusted or age-specific rates are the best ways to make comparisons, because populations vary by region with respect to age. Retirement communities in Florida and Arizona will naturally have higher rates of some chronic diseases than areas which have large concentrations of youth (e.g., college towns). On the other hand, college towns probably will have higher rates of certain diseases (e.g., sexually transmitted diseases) than retirement communities. One should never compare different types of rates with each other (i.e., crude rates from one locale and age-adjusted rates from another).

An **incidence rate** is a special type of rate which describes the number of new cases of a disease or other health event in a specific region during a given time period. A state with an incidence rate for *Chlamydia trachomatis* of 305/100,000 population experienced 305 new cases of the disease for every 100,000 people. If the state has a million people, how many new cases were identified for that year? Incidence is calculated as follows:

$$\text{Incidence} = \frac{\text{number of new cases of disease}}{\text{population at risk}} \text{ in a time period } \times K$$

The **prevalence rate** describes the number of new *and* existing cases of disease in a region for a period of time. A 1995 Wisconsin survey of 2210 adults revealed that 23% had been diagnosed with high blood pressure (Center for Health Statistics, 1996c). Thus, the prevalence rate of hypertension among adults is 23%. This rate would include people who have had hypertension for many years, as well as persons newly diagnosed. Prevalence is calculated as follows:

$$\text{Prevalence} = \frac{\text{total number of cases}}{\text{population at risk}} \text{ in a time period } \times K$$

Nelson and colleagues (1996) found that the prevalence of smokeless tobacco use for men was 6.5% in Indiana, 7.5% in Iowa, 14.4% in Montana, and 17.4% in West Virginia. These rates varied by age, education level, and place of residence (rural vs. urban). Their study shows how much variation is present by region, and allows federal health planners to concentrate prevention efforts in regions of highest risk.

For both incidence and prevalence rates, it is important to note that the population at risk is in the denominator of the ratio. If you were studying cervical cancer, only the number of women in the population of interest would comprise the denominator. For testicular cancer, only the number of men in the population would make up the denominator. This point also suggests that for infectious diseases (e.g., measles), persons who have already had the disease, as well as ones who have been immunized, should not be included in the denominator. In practice, such an adjustment may not happen, and can lead to flawed decisions.

It is becoming common practice in public health to report, not only the mean or percentage regarding the variable being studied (e.g., 17.4% of West Virginia men use smokeless tobacco), but the **confidence interval** as well. "A confidence interval for a population characteristic is an interval of plausible values for the characteristic. It is constructed so that, with a chosen degree of confidence, the value of the characteristic will be captured inside the interval" (Devore & Peck, 1993, p.391). Nelson, et al. (1996), found that 25.9% of the men in Montana between the ages of 25 and 34 used smokeless tobacco. The 95% confidence interval was 6.3%. What these data suggest then is that if we repeatedly sampled this population, 95% of the time, this confidence interval would capture the mean value (Devore & Peck, 1993)., Thus, the confidence limits (see Chapter 13) would be 19.6% and 32.2% (Kachigan, 1986).

Bivariate Procedures

Thus far, we have reviewed statistics which examine just a single variable. These univariate procedures are the most common statistical analyses used in evaluation studies. However, more sophisticated procedures are often needed to establish a relationship between variable x and variable y. When we study two variables simultaneously, bivariate procedures are used. Common procedures include cross-tabulations (with chi-square tests and odds ratios), t-tests, analysis of variance (ANOVA), and correlations.

Bivariate procedures are usually used to determine the presence of relationships or differences between groups. We might want to know if a greater proportion of boys, compared to girls, engage in aerobic physical activity, or, if intervention group A did better than control group B on a knowledge test. In these situations, we want to know if there is a real difference or real relationship present between the variables of interest. We are interested in determining whether or not the relationships studied are statistically significant. **Statistical significance** in experimental or quasi-experimental situations refers to whether the observed differences between the two or more groups are real or not, or, whether they are chance occurrences. Statistical significance from a correlational perspective asks the question of whether or not the observed (i.e., measured) relationship between two variables is *real* or not. Tests of statistical significance do not provide information concerning the size of the effect, or the strength of the relationship. They merely provide a probability statement that the observed relationship is real. Often, one can have a statistically significant result, but there may be little meaning or practical importance in the finding (Moore, 1992).

Before one begins testing a study's hypotheses, one usually establishes the statistical significance level that will be used to assess whether the observed relationship is real. By tradition, the significance level is usually set at .05 or .01. This criterion is referred to as the probability level or *alpha* level. A probability level of .05 would suggest that about 5 times out of 100 we would reject the hypothesis we are testing, when in fact, it is true. Thought of another way, it suggests that we are 95% confident that we have made the right decision (Spiegel, 1988). From still another perspective, an alpha level of .05 suggests that we are willing to be wrong 5% of the time in the decision we make based on the observed relationship. In general, the more critical the consequences of being wrong are, the more stringent we need to make the alpha level. Thus, for some biomedical tests or procedures that literally could be a matter of life or death, an alpha level of .001 or even .0001, would not be unusual.

Cross-tabulations allow evaluators to compare two nominal or ordinal variables to identify possible relationships between them. One might be interested in comparing 100 people with lung cancer, and 100 people without lung cancer, regarding previous smoking behavior. A cross-tabulation of data would look like Table 14.3.

Table 14.3 Comparison of Smokers and Nonsmokers Regarding Lung Cancer

Smoker?	Disease state		
	Lung cancer	No lung cancer	Total
Yes	90	20	110
No	10	80	90
Total	100	100	200

One can see that 90% of the people who had lung cancer were smokers. This figure compares to just 20% of the comparison population who were smokers. Is the relationship between smoking and lung cancer statistically significant? Two tests used to examine this relationship are the **chi-square test** and the **odds ratio**.

The chi-square value for this table is 98.99 (p < .001). This value indicates that these results would be expected to happen by chance less than once in 10,000 times. Thus, one can make the case that the relationship between smoking and lung cancer risk is probably quite real.

The odds ratio for this table is 36, with 95% confidence limits of 14.92 and 89.41. The odds ratio analysis suggests that smokers were 36 times more likely to have lung cancer than non-smokers. The odds ratio, combined with the chi-square test of significance, provides compelling evidence that smoking is strongly related to lung cancer. Although this case-control example is based on fictitious data, we know the health risks of smoking to be high. A review of the literature of 83 studies related to smoking suggests that the lowest relative risk of smoking related to lung cancer was 2.5 while the highest relative risk was 134.5 (van de Mheen & Gunning-Schepers, 1996).

Odds ratios are useful when studying risk for a particular disease or behavior. Schooler, Feighery and Flora (1996) used odds ratios to examine the risk of smoking among 7th-graders. Their data showed that youngsters whose parents smoked had more than twice the risk of being smokers themselves than peers with non-smoking parents.

Youth who had friends who smoked had 6.11 times the risk of smoking, as those whose friends did not smoke. With the aid of chi-square tests, they demonstrated that cigarette experimenters were more likely to have received promotional materials such as t-shirts, hats and lighters in the mail ($p<.001$). Odds ratios and chi-square tests are two ways in which we study the risk of disease, death, disability, or some behavior, when people are exposed to a factor or factors.

Whereas chi-square tests and odds ratios are used to study nominal data, the **t-test** and the **analysis of variance** (ANOVA) are used to study group differences, when the dependent variable is interval or ratio in nature. Suppose in the sample of test scores presented earlier (see Table 14.1), the class was actually delivered in two ways: through distance education and through traditional classroom style. We might be interested in assessing whether students in distance education did better, the same, or worse on a subsequent test. We could compare the mean scores of both groups using a t-test. Table 14.4 shows test performance data and descriptive statistics for both classes.

Table 14.4 Sample Test Performance Data for Distance Education and Traditional Classroom Students

	N	Mean	Standard Deviation
Distance education style	56	10.5	5.8
Traditional classroom style	55	10.5	1.6

The t-test results suggest that there was no significant difference between the two types of classes in terms of overall performance ($p = .991$). The mean scores were identical. However, note that the standard deviations for the groups are different. Are there still some differences between the performance of different people in these classes? If you have to think too long about this, go back in this chapter and read about methods of dispersion.

Because this class attracts a large number of part-time students, we might wonder if there are differences between students who take the class through distance education versus traditional learning, with respect to their full-time or part-time status. This analysis requires us to compare the mean scores of four groups. Such a comparison is easily done. Any time we compare three or more groups of mean scores, analysis of variance, or ANOVA, can be used. The data in Table 14.5 represent descriptive statistics from both classes by student status.

Table 14.5 Sample Data for Distance and Traditional Education Styles by Student Status

	N	Mean	Standard Deviation
Distance education style			
full time	27	9.1	0.8
part time	28	11.9	0.8
Traditional classroom style			
full time	28	16.0	1.8
part time	28	5.0	1.8

    The ANOVA results suggest a statistically significant difference among the four groups ($p < .001$). An examination of the mean scores shows that full-time students who used a traditional class format have the highest mean score (16.0), followed by part-time students in distance education (11.9), full-time students in distance education (9.1), and part-time students in traditional classes (5.0).

    So far we have talked about bivariate procedures which are used to determine if there are differences between groups. **Correlational** procedures are used to study the strength and direction of relationships between two variables, rather than differences. We speak in terms of correlations frequently in everyday life. When we say that height and weight tend to be correlated, we are suggesting that as people get taller, they have a tendency to weigh more, too.

    There are both positive and negative correlations. Being positive is not necessarily "better" than being negative. Rather, the notion of positive or negative merely describes the nature of the relationship. Positive correlations indicate that when one variable increases in value, so does the comparison variable. Height and weight, blood pressure and stroke risk, and cholesterol level and heart attack risk, are examples of positive correlations.

    In a negative correlation, when one variable increases in value, the other variable decreases. An example of negative correlation is risk of heart attack and exercise. The more a person exercises, the lower the heart attack risk. The more frequently one brushes his or her teeth, the lower the risk of getting a cavity. Figure 14.3 shows some examples of positive and negative correlations.

Correlations range in value from +1 to -1, with 0 indicating no relationship between the variables. The higher the value of the correlation coefficient is (regardless of direction), the stronger the relationship between the two variables.

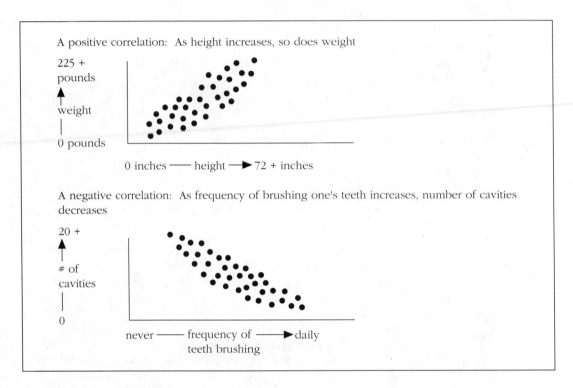

Figure 14.3 A Comparison of Hypothesized Positive and Negative Correlations

Copeland, Shope, and Waller (1996) studied factors related to adolescent drinking and driving among 3137 Michigan high school seniors, using correlational coefficients as part of their analysis. Drinking and driving were strongly correlated with a number of variables, including self-reported cigarette use (r=.32), as well as binge drinking (r=.64). Both of these correlates appear plausible. We know that, in general, adolescents who smoke are also more likely to drink. We also know that binge drinking is strongly related to drinking and driving. We can conclude from these correlational analyses that the results are plausible, and probably, accurate depictions of adolescent drinking and driving behavior.

It should be noted that there are many different types of correlation coefficients, such as Spearman's rho, Kendall's tau, and Pearson's r. The different types of coefficients are used situationally for different levels of data (e.g., ordinal, interval, or ratio).

Generally, Pearson's r is used for interval or ratio data, and Spearman's rho and Kendall's tau are used for ordinal data.

Multivariate Procedures

We use multivariate procedures to study more than two variables simultaneously. For example, we know that heart attack risk is related to several factors, including smoking, hypertension, exercise, nutrition, and heredity. When predicting complex behaviors or health events, it makes sense to use as many variables as possible in the analysis. Multivariate procedures allow us to do just that.

One of the most commonly used multivariate procedures is **multiple regression**. There are many types of multiple regression, including stepwise regression, logistic regression, and general linear regression. Although there are some differences among these models, they all seek to predict something (the criterion) using multiple predictors. One of the major assumptions of multiple regression is that we can predict something more accurately using several variables (multiple), than we can with only one variable.

In their drinking and driving study cited earlier, Copeland, et al. (1996) conducted multiple regression analyses. Their results suggest that:

offers of alcohol from friends, while strongly correlated with drinking/driving at the bivariate level, dropped out of the multivariate model entirely. Finally, the two high-risk behaviors of riding with a drinking driver and binge drinking had the most impact on the outcome variable, drinking/driving (p.258).

Their analysis shows an important feature of multivariate analyses. When some variables are analyzed in a bivariate manner, they are significantly related to the criterion. Those same variables, when put in an equation with many other variables, may not be statistically significant predictors. Multiple regression is a tool which enables evaluators to determine which variables, from among many, are the *best* predictors of the health event or issue of interest.

We use **discriminant analysis** when we are trying to classify people or objects into different categories, using several predictor variables. It is a procedure that can be used when trying to identify relationships between nominal level variables and ordinal, interval, or ratio level variables (Kachigan, 1986).

Sawyer and Beck (1989) used discriminant analysis to compare health concerns among current and former users of birth control pills. They found that concerns related to stroke, reduced sex drive, cervical and uterine cancer, expense, and vaginal infections were of much greater concern among those who used birth control pills than among former users. With these variables, they were able to classify correctly almost 80% of their subjects into either the user or former user groups. This example illustrates the primary classification value of discriminant analysis.

Factor analysis is used frequently in instrument development efforts, especially to study construct validity. Factor analysis is a data reduction technique which can be used to remove redundancy from a large set of correlated variables, and to identify a series of factors that are represented in the data set (Kachigan, 1986).

When developing instruments, one is often interested in identifying the different dimensions of the instrument. For example, we might develop a series of items related to behaviors, attitudes, and knowledge concerning low-fat diets. We might believe that we have designed an instrument based on these three factors. Confirmatory factor analyses can be run to see if we have indeed developed a three-factor instrument, or, if there are more than (or fewer than) three factors.

Gilmer, et al. (1996) studied the construct validity of a health survey for youth, using factor analysis. The study did not produce the expected results. Whereas they felt the physical activity scale would produce three unique levels of activity, it did not. They concluded that "the items did not represent the three levels of activity, or that the expectation that physical activities fall along a single dimension of activity from low to high MET is incorrect" (p.109). Thus, more developmental work to establish construct validity is needed.

Geographic Information Systems

We predict that there will be increasing use of **geographic information systems (GIS)** in health education evaluation studies in the future. GIS is particularly useful when trying to study geographic factors related to the health problem being studied. From a descriptive, epidemiologic perspective, geographic factors are known as "place factors" when disease occurrence is assessed. We know, for example, that certain diseases vary by region. One has a greater chance of acquiring frostbite in January, if in Winnipeg, Manitoba, than in Miami, Florida. On the other hand, one has a greater chance of developing skin cancer, if residing for years in Miami, than if living in Winnipeg. GIS can be used to study the distribution of diseases by regions of any dimension or size that is desired.

GIS can be used to study demographic trends in the population. A map showing the distribution of persons 65 years of age and older in a region can be used to plan for, or predict, needed or expected health services. Overlaying this map with roadways, health care facilities, and schools, enables planners to identify the best places to implement programs. Numerous additional prevention planning uses of "visual statistics" through GIS mapping are possible. Better interventions to address violent and other forms of crime, motor vehicle-related injuries, occurrences of low birth weight infants, needs of burgeoning population centers, identification of health and health care disparities, and a host of initiatives may be made more feasible thanks to GIS mapping strategies.

Summary

This chapter discussed the uses of statistics in health education program evaluation. Univariate procedures include frequency distributions, measures of central tendency, measures of dispersion, and rates. The use of confidence intervals was introduced. Next, common bivariate procedures, including cross-tabulations, chi-square tests, odds ratios, and correlation coefficients were presented. Tests of mean differences between groups include the t-test and ANOVA. The chapter concluded by introducing some multivariate procedures, and GIS applications in health education.

Case Study

Winkleby, M.A., Taylor, C.B., Jatulis, D., & Fortmann, S.P. (1996). The long-term effects of a cardiovascular disease prevention trial: The Stanford Five-City Project. *American Journal of Public Health*, *86*(12), 1773-1779.

Winkleby and colleagues describe a long-term follow-up of a community-based cardiovascular risk reduction program implemented in California. Their study suggested that community-based programs can maintain effects over a long time period. Which results did you find most interesting? Was the program equally effective for both males and females? Were the data presented in a manner which was understandable and reader friendly? If you were going to conduct a similar study, what would you do differently?

Student Questions/Activities

1. Create a frequency distribution using a set of baseball player batting averages (your favorite team, of course) printed in the Sunday sports page. What is the mean, median, mode, range, and standard deviation of the data set?
2. Identify some health-related examples where you would expect a positive correlation between two variables. Describe some examples of where a negative correlation would be present.
3. Propose a study which would use multivariate procedures in the analysis of the data. What would be your dependent and independent variables? What is the purpose of your study?
4. Select three health objectives from *Healthy People 2000*, or a more recent national or state document. Visit the local health department, and compare your county's performance on the specific objectives you selected. What do these data tell you? How can they be used for designing a health education program?

Recommended Readings

Gfroerer, J.C., Greenblatt, J.C., & Wright, D.A. (1997). Substance use in the US college-age population: Differences according to educational status and living arrangement. *American Journal of Public Health*, *87*(1), 62-65.

Gfroerer and associates, from the Office of Applied Studies at the Substance Abuse and Mental Health Services Administration, analyzed data from the National Household Survey on Drug Abuse. They concluded: "Substantial variation in substance use patterns within the college-age population suggests that overall rates of use for young adults should not be used to characterize specific subgroups of young adults" (p.62).

Office on Smoking and Health. (1996). Tobacco use and usual source of cigarettes among high school students - United States, 1995. *Journal of School Health, 66*(6), 222-224.

This paper presents data from the Youth Risk Behavior Survey. Using a three-stage sample design, data were collected from over 10,000 high school students throughout the 50 states and the District of Columbia. Data are presented on prevalence of tobacco use, characteristics of users, as well as source of cigarettes. All prevalence data are reported using both percentages and 95% confidence intervals.

Werch, C.E., Carlson, J.M., Pappas, D.M., & DiClemente, C.C. (1996). Brief nurse consultations for preventing alcohol use among urban school youth. *Journal of School Health, 66*(9), 335-338.

Werch and colleagues present results of an experiment designed to prevent alcohol use among inner-city youth. A comparison of pretest and posttest results, using a t-test, suggested that students who received the intervention showed a significant reduction in heavy drinking, while control subjects increased in their heavy drinking behavior.

References

Center for Health Statistics. (1996a). *Wisconsin Births and Infant Deaths, 1995.* Madison, WI: Department of Health and Family Services.

Center for Health Statistics. (1996b). *Wisconsin Deaths, 1995.* Madison, WI: Department of Health and Family Services.

Center for Health Statistics. (1996c). *Health Counts in Wisconsin.* Madison, WI: Department of Health and Social Services.

Copeland, L.A., Shope, J.T., & Waller, P.F. (1996). Factors in adolescent drinking/driving: Binge drinking, cigarette smoking, and gender. *Journal of School Health, 66*(7), 254-260.

Devore, J., & Peck, R. (1993). *Statistics: The Exploration and Analysis of Data,* 2nd edition. Belmont, CA: Wadsworth.

Gilmer, M.J., Seck, B.J., Bradley, C., Harrell, J.S., & Belyea, M. (1996). The youth health survey: Reliability and validity of an instrument for assessing cardiovascular health habits in adolescents. *Journal of School Health, 66*(3), 106-111.

Kachigan, S.K. (1986). *Statistical Analysis: An Interdisciplinary Introduction to Univariate and Multivariate Methods.* New York: Radius Press.

McKenzie, J.F., & Smeltzer, J.L. (1997). *Planning, Implementing, and Evaluating Health Promotion Programs*, 2nd edition. Boston: Allyn and Bacon.

Moore, D.S. (1992). What is statistics? In Hoaglin, D.C., & Moore, D.S. (Eds.). *Perspectives on Contemporary Statistics*. Mathematical Association of America, MAA Notes Number 21: Author.

Nelson, D.E., Tomar, S.L., Mowery, P., & Siegel, P.Z. (1996). Trends in smokeless tobacco use among men in four states, 1988 through 1993. *American Journal of Public Health*, *86*(9), 1300-1393.

Sawyer, R.G., & Beck, K.H. (1989). Oral contraception: A survey of college women's concerns and experiences. *Health Education*, *20*(3), 17-21.

Schooler, C., Feighery, E., Flora, J.A. (1996). Seventh graders' self-reported exposure to cigarette marketing and its relationship to their smoking behavior. *American Journal of Pubic Health*, *86*(9), 1216-1221.

Spiegel, M.R. (1988). *Theory and Problems of Statistics*, 2nd edition. New York: McGraw-Hill.

van de Mheen, P., & Gunning-Schepers, L. (1996). Differences between studies in reported relative risks associated with smoking: An overview. *Public Health Reports*, *111*(5), 420-426.

15

Assessing Program Costs and Effects

Chapter Objectives

After completing this chapter, you should be able to:

1. Describe the purposes of cost analysis.
2. Discuss ethical issues related to cost analysis.
3. List the different types of costs.
4. Compare and contrast cost-identification analysis, cost-effectiveness analysis, and cost-benefit analysis.
5. Describe a reference case.
6. Explain how perspective of analysis is a factor in assessing program costs.
7. Identify how sensitivity analysis is used in the decision-making process.
8. Describe methodological issues related to cost analyses.

Key Terms

cost-benefit analysis
cost-effectiveness analysis
cost-identification analysis
direct costs
distributive justice

indirect costs
perspective of analysis
quality adjusted life years (QALYs)
reference case
sensitivity analysis

Introduction

It is becoming increasingly important to be able to identify program costs as well as associated benefits, when proposing new health programs for organizations. Whether one works for a school, a county health department, a hospital or clinic, a fitness center, a worksite program, or any other settings, health educators are increasingly being called upon to justify new programs as well as existing ones.

Administrators of large health care organizations must make decisions concerning which programs will be implemented and "institutionalized" as a part of the organization. This administrative need not only means deciding which health education programs are to be implemented (e.g., which smoking cessation program is most effective *and* most cost-effective), but also deciding if a health education program is to be implemented at all. With finite resources, program administrators must rely upon cost analytic techniques to help them make informed decisions.

When conducting cost analyses, it is important to consider the notion of **perspective of analysis**. Perspective refers to the point of view from which the analysis is based. Is the analysis conducted from a patient perspective, from an insurance company or HMO perspective, from a physician perspective, or from a societal perspective? Each perspective has its unique viewpoint concerning program costs and benefits, and analysis of a program from one perspective might yield different results than if viewed from another. Russell, Gold, Siegel, Daniels, and Weinstein (1996) provide the following example. A person may become sick, and an HMO or other insurance provider might not worry at all about how long it takes a person to return to work....the loss of productivity might not figure into the cost analysis. For the employer, however, it may matter a great deal how long it takes to get an employee back to work. If the employer conducted the cost analysis, time spent away from work, disability payments, and other factors might be considered in the analysis. Thus, when cost analysis is performed, one must always be aware of the perspective of the analysis.

Perspective of analysis is related to Guba and Lincoln's (1989) idea of understanding different stakeholder needs when evaluating one or more programs. Stakeholders will have diverse viewpoints on what is considered acceptable, high quality, cost-effective, and so on. When conducting a cost analysis, it is important to state clearly the perspective from which the analysis is being conducted.

One must also be sure that the effects of the program are being assessed accurately. One may have very accurate cost data. However, if robust evaluation methods have not been used to evaluate program effectiveness, then cost analysis is certainly suspect, if not altogether useless. A "cheap" program that doesn't produce the desired results isn't much good to anyone.

A Conceptual Example

An example of a program which has received much scrutiny in recent years is the DARE (Drug Abuse Resistance Education) program. This program enjoys widespread support from law enforcement personnel, but receives widespread criticism from public health specialists, particularly drug and alcohol prevention experts. Ennett, Tobler, Ringwalt, and Flewelling (1994) describe a meta-analysis of the DARE program, comparing the results of rigorously evaluated DARE programs to the results of other types of drug education programs that have been similarly evaluated. They report that the DARE program effect size means were smaller than the effect size means of programs emphasizing social and general competencies, and those using interactive teaching strategies for all outcomes examined. In terms of short-term results, DARE was less effective than the other programs which were studied.

This analysis of the DARE program has several program cost implications. For example, some authorities argue that DARE is an expensive program. Many police departments employ one or more DARE program officers, just to run the program. Second, when school administrators, teachers, and parents implement the DARE program, they generally do not implement other drug education programs. Why should they? They already have one drug education program. This neglect of other competing programs means that dollars are allocated to a program of uncertain efficacy. Ennett, et al. (1994), therefore, provide a conceptual basis for evaluation that can be incorporated as part of a cost-effectiveness analysis. Take note, that when conducting these types of analyses, it is important to remember alternative points of view. For example, Gorman (1995) wrote a response to the Ennett, et al. study, disagreeing with the methods used to conduct the analysis. A good cost-effectiveness analysis will consider multiple viewpoints when examining program effects and their associated costs.

Program Costs

Cost analytic studies require the accurate determination of program costs. This task, known as **cost-identification analysis**, is a more difficult process than it first seems. At a minimum, the evaluator ought to be able to identify the different costs which are incurred as a result of implementing the program. An examination of program costs includes an inspection of various "ingredients" that are part of program implementation. Levin (1988) has described a three-pronged approach to identifying the costs of a program using the ingredient approach:

- Identify the ingredients.
- Determine the value or cost of ingredients and total costs of program.
- Analyze costs using an appropriate framework.

Identifying Ingredients

An evaluator must first identify all of the ingredients necessary for program implementation. These ingredients include personnel (full-time, part-time, volunteers), costs of facilities, equipment, and materials. One must be sure to account for both direct and indirect costs (see Chapter 4) when collecting these data. **Direct costs** are those costs that can be traced to a specific cost object, while indirect costs cannot be associated with a particular cost object. For example, a person who is working solely in the project of interest would contribute to the overall direct costs through salary and fringe benefits. **Indirect costs** are incurred when more than one unit receives benefit from the particular cost being analyzed. If several programs share one building, then the costs of rent and utilities would be considered indirect costs. If a supervisor oversees more than one unit, those costs would generally be considered indirect as well (Larson, Spoede, & Miller, 1994). The important message here is that one must be careful to measure all costs of the program. Often, costs are "hidden," and therefore, are not considered in the assessment of total program operating costs. This error will cause a serious problem leading to underestimation of overall costs of running the program.

Determining the Value of Ingredients and Total Program Cost

Once all of the ingredients which make up the program have been identified, the evaluator needs to put a value on those ingredients. Levin (1988) indicates that all ingredients have a cost, even when programs use volunteers or donated materials. Therefore, one should estimate the costs of volunteers or donated materials as if the organization actually paid for the goods or services. As part of the **sensitivity analysis**, variations in labor, as well as costs of materials, can be made. Doing so demonstrates how program costs differ when costs of labor or materials vary. When identifying personnel costs, one must make sure that fringe benefits are included. Fringe benefits include costs for health insurance, vacation, sick leave and other benefits, and often exceed 25% or more of the salary received by the employee.

Analyzing Costs

Once the ingredients and their associated costs are identified, total program costs can be estimated. For large programs, costs per unit or department can be considered as well. These program costs can be compared to benchmarks to see if the program is performing up to expectations. If not, adjustments can be made.

When examining the cost of education programs, one usually reports results in terms of the costs it takes to educate one person. When an evaluator formally examines the costs of a program, it is known as *cost-identification analysis*. When one identifies the lowest costs for different programs, the process is known as *cost-minimization analysis* (Eisenberg, 1989). So, after identifying the ingredients of a particular program, assigning costs to those ingredients, and determining total program cost, one might find out that a program costs $30 per student to complete. A program being implemented in another state, which has similar effects, but which costs just $20 per student, is one that ought to be reviewed carefully. The program administrator might take a look at the cheaper program, and if it is acceptable to the program stakeholders, implement the program at a greatly reduced cost. This example illustrates the principle of cost-minimization analysis.

Cost-Effectiveness Analysis

In 1996, the *Journal of the American Medical Association* published a series of three consensus statements concerning cost-effectiveness analysis (CEA) in health and medicine (Russell, Gold, Siegel, Daniels & Weinstein, 1996; Siegel, Weinstein, Russell & Gold,1996; Weinstein, Siegel, Gold & Kamlet, 1996). These three papers were the product of a U.S. Public Health Service group, the Panel on Cost-Effectiveness in Health and Medicine. The panel included experts representing cost-effectiveness analysis, clinical medicine, ethics, and health outcomes measurement. Its recommendations fell into the eight categories shown in Figure 15.1.

- The nature and limits of CEA and the reference case.
- Components belonging in the numerator and denominator of a cost-effectiveness (C/E) ratio.
- Measuring costs (numerator of the C/E ratio).
- Valuing health consequences (denominator of the C/E ratio).
- Estimating effectiveness of interventions.
- Time preference and discounting.
- Handling uncertainty.
- Reporting guidelines.

Figure 15.1 Recommendations for Conducting Cost-Effectiveness Analysis

Although the recommendations are described below in more detail, and are specifically for what is known as a reference case, the panelists argue that it should be the goal of all CEAs to follow the guidelines carefully. As the panel indicated: "In the interest of comparability, however, we urge that the reference case of assumptions and practices be included in every CEA that is designed, to permit broad comparisons across interventions, or that might be used for this purpose" (Weinstein, et al., 1996, p.1253).

The Nature and Limits of CEA and the Reference Case

Cost-effectiveness analysis can be defined as a "method for evaluating the health outcomes and resource costs of health interventions" (Russell, et al., 1996, p.1172). It provides a format for comparing various programs, their effects, as well as their associated costs. These comparisons can then be used to determine which program or intervention is best suited for the particular situation. CEA is, therefore, an administrative tool used to make rational decisions regarding the allocation of health resources.

There is increasing interest in the cost-effectiveness of programs in the fields of public health and medicine. For example, the U.S. Public Health Service convened the panel described above. The Centers for Disease Control and Prevention has placed more emphasis on training staff, and working with states regarding CEA. Agencies such as the National Institutes of Health and the Agency for Health Care Policy Research have begun to use CEA in their studies. There is growing acknowledgement of the importance of considering program costs as well as effects in the program evaluation.

One of the problems with CEA is that methods and criteria used to assess the costs and effects of different programs are not standardized. Different types of effects are measured, and, different costs are measured as well. What happens in these situations, then, is that it is nearly impossible to make fair or useful program comparisons. To address this issue, writers of the U.S. Public Health Service Consensus Statement recommend that a reference case be used in all CEAs, which enables program comparisons to be done more effectively.

A **reference case** "is defined by a standard set of methods and assumptions. It includes a set of standard results − the reference case results. While an investigator might also present results based on different methods and assumptions to serve other purposes of the analysis, the reference case serves as a point of comparison across studies" (Russell, et al., 1996, p.1173). The reference case is needed for three reasons:

- It sets standards for the ways costs and effects are measured and how they are valued, and serves as a benchmark to evaluate the quality of different studies, to determine if they are comparable to each other.
- It provides guidelines for reporting results, which makes it easier for those using the results to interpret the data, and to compare those results to ones obtained in other studies.
- Using reference cases encourages the development of a pool of studies which can be compared to each other.

A reference case can be thought of, then, as a standard type of CEA study which outlines the methods used to conduct the study, the assumptions of the study, and the effects of the study. The use of reference cases improves the comparability of results across programs.

As mentioned earlier in this chapter, the perspective of analysis is an important consideration in cost analytic studies. The writers of the consensus statement recommend that the "society's perspective" be used in the analysis. This perspective allows for a consideration of all program costs and all program effects, good and bad, for all stakeholders. An interesting example related to societal perspectives is that of the use of folic acid to reduce neural tube defects. Without question, folic acid reduces risk of neural tube defects, and, for this reason, many public health specialists have argued that we should add folic acid to different foods to ensure that women receive an adequate supply. However, "fortification puts older people at risk because it masks pernicious anemia, which if left untreated, can cause neurological problems" (Russell, et al., 1996, p.1174). A societal perspective of analysis would consider not only the positive effects of folic acid fortification for women, and their newborns, but also the negative effects for senior citizens.

Components Belonging in the Numerator and Denominator of a C/E Ratio

CEA results are usually expressed in terms of a ratio. The panel recommended that all costs for the program belong in the numerator of the ratio, while all health effects belong in the denominator. This formula yields a ratio which describes the amount of resources needed for a given program effect. Thus, an evaluator can make statements such as "for every dollar spent on this program, x number of people were not infected with the disease," or, "for every dollar spent on this program, **quality adjusted life years** (QALYs) in the target population improved 20%, which was 50% more effective than the reference case program."

Measuring Costs (Numerator of the C/E ratio)

The numerator of the C/E ratio measures the amount of resources used to implement the program. Resources are measured in monetary terms. Resource categories that should be included in the numerator are: costs of the health program or health care services, costs of patient time used to receive the treatment, costs related to providing the service (either paid or not paid), other costs, such as travel, child-care, and economic losses by employers and other employees while the program is taking place. As the panelists indicate: "A change in the use of a resource caused by a health intervention should be valued as its opportunity cost, which is the value of the resource if it were spent in its best available alternative use" (Weinstein, et al., 1996, p.1255).

Costs need to be measured in constant dollars. Therefore, if an evaluation is examining a program being implemented over several years, then the dollars need to be adjusted based on inflation or deflation. Health care costs often increase at rates higher than inflation, so these factors must be considered in the analysis. Of course, from a comparative perspective, one needs to ensure that the costs are measured similarly in the other programs being studied. Otherwise, inflation or deflation may have a major impact on the C/E ratio, and the comparison to other programs may be inappropriate.

The reference case will help analysts to identify which costs or resources must be placed in the numerator. Fair comparisons between programs regarding which costs are included in the analysis, along with the use of constant dollar values, will make the analysis cleaner and easier to interpret.

Valuing Health Consequences (Denominator of the C/E ratio)

There are a series of quality of life issues which need to be considered when conducting CEA. Evaluators are mistaken when they only consider whether someone lives or dies because of a specific intervention, or when they only consider whether the patients *do* or *do not* recover from an illness. For example, some studies show that two blood pressure medications can be equally effective in lowering blood pressure. However, one of the medicines has few side-effects, and the other renders a large proportion of male users impotent. Obviously, one must not only consider the direct effects of the medicine, but also consider indirect effects and quality of life issues.

To address these types of issues, the panel recommends that health consequences, which are put in the denominator of the C/E ratio, be measured in terms of quality adjusted life years (QALYs). In the past, effects have been measured in terms of number of years of life gained as a result of a particular procedure, the number of infections prevented, and so on. The panel argues that quality of life must also be considered when examining program effects, such as demonstrated in the blood pressure example above. There are many quality of life scales currently used, and they can be applied in a CEA study. In addition, the analyst must consider which perspective is being used when measuring QALYs. For the reference case, a societal perspective must be used. However, when evaluating individual treatment programs, the individual perspective is acceptable.

Estimating Effectiveness of Interventions

As mentioned earlier, the overall quality of CEA is directly related to the quality of the research design which examined the effects of the program. "The analyst should select outcome probabilities from the best-designed sources that are relevant to the question and population under study" (Weinstein, et al., 1996, p.1257). The data can come from randomized trials, observational studies, uncontrolled experiments, or descriptive studies. We recommend that the strongest design in terms of both internal and external validity (see Chapter 10) be used, especially for the reference case. Moreover, statistical modeling is an important aspect of estimation (see Chapter 14), which can help in the measurement of program effects and with sensitivity analyses described below.

Time Preference and Discounting

Different people value different health outcomes at different times. In addition, costs of programs increase or decrease due to inflation, interest rates, demand for goods and services, and other influences. From an economic perspective, although CEAs often use different rates to study inflation and discounting, the panel recommends a 3% discount rate for the reference case, and recommends that inflation be accounted for before discounting takes place.

Handling Uncertainty

Sensitivity analyses are conducted to explore different CEA results as a function of different assumptions for costs, as well as for effects. For example, if we believe that a new health education program will reduce the number of health problems in the target population by 10%, that would be a different effect than if we believe it will reduce the number of problems by 30%. If the same amounts of resources were used in the two programs, obviously, the program reducing the health problems by 30% would be more cost-effective. In Kahn's (1996) article on the cost-effectiveness of HIV prevention programs, he conducted a sensitivity analysis which adjusted for reduction in risk due to prevention. He varied the proportion of the population which would not be infected as a result of the program, as well as costs of the program (e.g., if the program cost half as much as originally assumed, twice as many people could be reached by the program, and twice as many infections could be prevented). Different assumptions created different results in Kahn's (1996) study.

Reporting Guidelines

Just as the panel recommended standards for the design and implementation of a CEA, it also made recommendations concerning the essential elements of a CEA report, especially the reference case. In general, the panel recommends more detail than less in the report, and asks the analyst not only to report results and recommendations, but also to provide technical appendices and addenda for the interested reader. Siegel, et al. (1996) give a detailed outline of the recommended components of the CEA report.

Cost-Benefit Analysis

Cost-benefit analysis (CBA) is a technique which estimates program benefits in dollar values (Posavac & Carey, 1980). There is considerable debate concerning the ethical issues related to assigning dollar values of health outcomes, and for these reasons, many health policy analysts prefer not to use CBA techniques, but rather, CEA strategies instead (Russell, et al., 1996). CBA *is* used, however, and it is one technique which allows for a comparison of various program types, not just programs focusing primarily on health. CBA is adaptable for many different types of programs, with many different goals and objectives, and a variety of situations. "CBA might be used to decide whether certain public resources should be allocated for construction of a dam, or for construction of a hospital" (Banta & Luce, 1983, p.147).

Ethics and Cost Analysis

A difficult aspect of cost analysis involves the ethical issues. As Russell, et al. (1996) suggest, when one makes choices, one makes ethical decisions. All cost analysis specialists suggest that CEA or other cost data should comprise only a portion of the information used to formulate decisions. Issues such as **distributive justice** (i.e., justice concerned with the apportionment of privileges, duties, and goods in consonance with the merits of the individual and in the best interest of society) go beyond simple costs. According to Kahn (1996): "Real-world HIV funding decisions reflect a constellation of criteria aside from cost-effectiveness, such as avoiding the stigmatization of socially marginalized groups, assuring equity and advocacy for prevention by spreading resources widely, and building on existing prevention infrastructure" (pp.1711-1712). Often, there are no simple answers to the complex questions and problems we seek to address. For example, should an intervention be implemented which helps a few very sick people, or should we implement an intervention that has benefits for a large number of people? Issues such as "fairness, feasibility, and values are not completely captured by the analysis and must be weighed against factors that are" (Russell, et al., 1996, p.1176).

Summary

In this chapter we have reviewed techniques which evaluators use to measure the costs and benefits of health programs: cost-identification analysis, cost-effectiveness analysis, and cost-benefit analysis. Special emphasis was placed on cost-effectiveness analysis. The recommendations for conducting such studies were based on the Panel on Cost-Effectiveness in Health and Medicine. The reference case was advanced as one method to make studies comparable with each other. Ethics, with respect to cost-analysis, was discussed, with the recommendation that cost data be only one component used when making resource allocations for programs.

Case Study

Rowland, J., Rivara, F., Salzberg, P., Soderberg, R., Maier, R., & Koepsell, T. (1996). Motorcycle helmet use and injury outcome and hospitalization costs from crashes in Washington State. *American Journal of Public Health*, *86*(1), 41-45.

Rowland and colleagues linked hospital record data to Washington State Patrol motorcycle crash records to study the effects of wearing helmets on injury reduction, as well as costs for medical treatment. Their data showed helmet use reduced the probability and severity of injuries, reduced chance of death, and reduced hospitalization costs. What were the limitations of this study? How would you use this study to lobby for mandatory helmet laws in your state? How would you design a similar study to measure the effects of helmet use among bicycle riders?

Student Questions/Activities

1. The local chief of police has just recommended to the city council an "up-grade" for the DARE program which is implemented in the school system. In addition to the purchase of more DARE materials, another "officer friendly" will be hired to work with the kids. This means that in your town you now have two DARE officers. You are opposed to this program, from a cost-analysis viewpoint, as well as from a health education perspective. Prepare a 1000-word presentation for City Hall, outlining the strengths and weaknesses of the DARE program, as well as your suggested alternative approach for dealing with the drug problem in your community. You may need to perform a literature search about DARE.

2.   You work as the coordinator of school health education in a large city, and have been asked to appear in front of the school board to discuss program effects and costs. Rumors of program cutbacks are rampant in the school system, as both the governor and the mayor have indicated that a reduction in funding in the schools is necessary, because of "excessive waste" in education programs. One of your school board members, a well-known person in business, asks: *Is health education cost-effective?* Respond.

3.   Select two programs which have similar goals (e.g., two programs focusing on helping people quit smoking). Using the ingredients approach, estimate the costs of the programs. On the basis of the cost data, as well as available effectiveness data, which program would you choose to implement? Will "setting" determine your answer, in part? If no data are available, what does this point tell you about the efficacy of decisions related to prevention programming?

Recommended Readings

Callahan, D. (1996). Controlling the costs of health care for the elderly - fair means and foul. *New England Journal of Medicine, 335*(10), 744-747.

Callahan comments on methods being proposed to control health care costs among the elderly. He poses some relevant questions: "What medical goals are appropriate for the elderly? Assuming we have a strong moral and social obligation to provide them with decent health care, is that obligation unlimited?" (p.745).

Hoffman, C., Rice, D., & Sung, H-Y. (1996). Persons with chronic conditions: Their prevalence and costs. *Journal of the American Medical Association, 276*(18), 1473-1479.

Hoffman and colleagues estimate the proportion of Americans with chronic conditions, as well as their related direct and indirect costs. Using 1990 data, they estimated that 90 million people had some type of chronic condition, and the costs of the chronic conditions were approximately $659 billion.

Kahn, J.G. (1996). The cost-effectiveness of HIV prevention targeting: How much more bang for the buck? *American Journal of Public Health, 86*(12), 1709-1712.

Using an epidemiologic model, target population scenarios, and cost and impact data, Kahn describes the benefits of targeting HIV prevention programs for high risk populations. Given the finite limits of HIV program funding, he concludes that ..."optimal prevention targeting represents a standard from which deviations should be carefully weighed" (p.1712).

References

Banta, H.D., & Luce, B.R. (1983). Assessing the cost-effectiveness of prevention. *Journal of Community Health, 9,* 145-165.

Eisenberg, J.M. (1989). Clinical economics: A guide to the economic analysis of clinical practices. *Journal of the American Medical Association, 262*(20), 2879-2886.

Ennett, S.T., Tobler, N.S., Ringwalt, C.L., & Flewelling, R.L. (1994). How effective is drug abuse resistance education? A meta-analysis of Project DARE outcome evaluations. *American Journal of Public Health, 84*(9), 1394-1401.

Gorman, D.M. (1995). The effectiveness of DARE and other drug use prevention programs. *American Journal of Public Health, 85*(6), 873.

Guba, E.G., & Lincoln, Y.S. (1989). *Fourth Generation Evaluation.* Newbury Park: Sage Publications.

Kahn, J.G. (1996). The cost-effectiveness of HIV prevention targeting: How much more bang for the buck? *American Journal of Public Health, 86*(12), 1709-1712.

Larson, K.D., Spoede, C.W., & Miller, P.B. (1994). *Fundamentals of Financial and Managerial Accounting.* Boston: Irwin.

Levin, H.M. (1988). Cost-effectiveness and educational policy. *Educational Evaluation and Policy Analysis, 10*(1), 51-69.

Posavac, E.J., & Carey, R.G. (1980). *Program Evaluation: Methods and Case Studies.* Englewood Cliffs, NJ: Prentice Hall.

Russell, L.B., Gold, M.R., Siegel, J.E., Daniels, N., Weinstein, M.C. (1996). The role of cost-effectiveness analysis in health and medicine. *Journal of the American Medical Association, 276*(14), 1172-1177.

Siegel, J.E., Weinstein, M.C., Russell, L.B., & Gold, M.R. (1996). Recommendations for reporting cost-effectiveness analyses. *Journal of the American Medical Association, 276*(16), 1339-1341.

Weinstein, M.C., Siegel, J.E., Gold, M.R., & Kamlet, M.S. (1996). Recommendations of the Panel on Cost-Effectiveness in Health and Medicine. *Journal of the American Medical Association, 276*(15), 1253-1258.

Chapter
16

Preparing the Evaluation Report

Chapter Objectives

After completing this chapter, you should be able to:

1. Identify the elements of content and style that are part of the preparation of an evaluation report.
2. Prepare an evaluation report that is useful to decision makers, planners, and other health education and promotion program stakeholders.
3. Provide several examples of ways to present evaluation results, and discuss the advantage of using certain graphic displays over others.
4. Identify the sections of evaluation reports that are of high priority to consumers, and therefore, command special effort and attention in preparation.
5. List and discuss several guidelines useful for the preparation of recommendations concerning a health education and promotion program.
6. Critique an evaluation report, pointing out strengths and weaknesses in style, balance, clarity, and objectivity.

Key Terms

executive summary
hard data
program context
soft data

Introduction

Designing and carrying out an evaluation project, as demonstrated in previous chapters, can be a complex task. In addition to other methodological concerns, measurement and analysis issues abound in evaluation. We hope that the descriptions, examples, and illustrations provided so far have illuminated and simplified the process to some extent. These issues aside, the final step in performing good evaluation is reporting the results, as well as the interpretation of those results, in a format that is useful, and which lends itself easily to understanding. An evaluation report is prepared in a satisfactory manner when it facilitates decision making by those stakeholders charged with such a task. Because of the nature of some evaluation research, reports stemming from such projects may be highly technical. However, they should not be unnecessarily esoteric. The readers of evaluations may (and probably will) be less interested in the sophistication of the sampling procedures and the statistical analyses than they will be in what the results mean for the future of their program, their company, or their job. However well written an evaluation report may be, it is impossible to guarantee that it will be read, understood, and enjoyed by all stakeholders. Having a clear view of the aims of the evaluation, and working closely with stakeholders on the front end of an evaluation, will assist the evaluator in producing a final report that is focused and *reader friendly*. As pointed out in Chapter 3, evaluations are more likely to be used if they address issues of importance to specific audiences. In this chapter, we will examine how one goes about displaying and reporting information that is useful to decision makers and other stakeholders.

Content of the Evaluation Report

While the design and general style of evaluation projects may have highly individualized characters (perhaps as unique as the personalities of the evaluators themselves), the documents detailing the results of evaluations tend to be fairly standard. It may be useful for you to look upon this section of the text as a sort of *checklist* of features. It is a reasonable assumption that you will be meeting the needs of 99 percent of report users if your document includes the components identified below. When in doubt about what to include, refer back to the original purpose of the evaluation and the specific questions to be addressed. If in doubt about how to organize the data in a manner that will be most useful to those people who will be making decisions based upon them, ask the person or persons who hired you. Avoid letting your ego get in the way, or making the assumption that you will somehow be held in less esteem if you ask for some guidance at this point. It is a good idea to have a plan for data presentation in mind, and to use the opportunity of a conference to affirm or modify the plan. It is the *experienced* evaluator who takes this particular step. Failing to affirm that the plan for presentation of data will be appropriate for the decisions to be made may culminate in:

- Producing a document that falls short of needs.
- Requiring a large scale rewriting of the report.
- Generating animosity between client and evaluator.

- Reducing the possibility of being asked to perform future evaluation tasks.
- Giving rise to other negative consequences.

What should most evaluation reports include? Typically, they should consist of: a front cover, a title page, acknowledgements, a table of contents, lists of figures, graphs, tables, exhibits, and other relevant displays, an executive summary, a background description of the program that was evaluated, including the aims of the program and other details, a description of the aims and methods relevant to the evaluation, the results, a discussion of the results, conclusions and recommendations about the program, and appendices (Fink, 1995; Salant & Dillman, 1994). In some reports, there may be a section that examines specific costs associated with the program (see Chapter 15). In the sections below, we shall take a look at each of these report components in some detail.

Front Matter

It might be argued that the reader's first impression of the professionalism of an evaluation document is its *front cover*. While this thought may conjure up the caution about not judging a book by its cover, it is nevertheless likely to be the first yardstick by which readers will evaluate the evaluator. A handsome cover will not compensate for a hastily prepared report, or an inadequate evaluation design, but it will get you off on the right foot. The cover should be of high quality or extra strength paper that will not easily fold or wrinkle. It should be of a quality that facilitates binding. Personnel at most office supply stores will be able to assist you in recognizing this type of paper. In addition to spiral bound or three-ring bound copies of the report, it may be useful to have at least one looseleaf copy from which additional reproductions can be made. Morris and Fitz-Gibbon (1978) offer the following suggestions for information to include on the cover:

- Title of the program and its location.
- Name of evaluator(s).
- Name(s) of the organization or the people to whom the evaluation report is to be submitted.
- Period of time covered by the report.
- Date of report submission.

The font type selected for the cover should be distinctive, and lettering on the front cover should be boldfaced. In this era of sophisticated word processing software, excellent computer hardware, and desktop publishing, there is no acceptable reason for a report to be prepared with anything less than a polished, professional appearance. Morris and Fitz-Gibbon (1978) say that the front cover "reflects [the author's] state of mind" (p.15).

The *title page* is the first page inside of the front cover. It ordinarily repeats the information on the front cover, and separates the cover from the rest of the document.

Rarely is one individual (i.e., the "evaluator") wholly responsible for all of the work that goes into an evaluation report. He or she gives way to data collectors, statistical package programmers, data preparers, typists, consultants, and other persons. The evaluator may be the person who oversees these activities, monitors them closely, and who has ultimate authority for the preparation of all interim and final report documents. Good work, monumental efforts, and even tedious, less skilled activities should not go unrecognized. Therefore, it is a good policy for the principal evaluator(s) to recognize the efforts of all persons who contribute to the report in an *acknowledgements* page. The list should provide names, and possibly, the tasks performed by each individual. The list needs not to be of unruly length, but it should include the names of at least those persons without whom the task may not have been completed. Acknowledging people not only helps their resumes, by having their contributions documented, but it contributes to their willingness to provide supportive services of a similar nature in the future.

As it is with textbooks and other publications, the *table of contents* is the reader's "road map" for locating key elements contained in the evaluation report. While it may seem abundantly obvious to have such an organizational structure, inexperienced report preparation personnel may overlook its inclusion. Each section of the report should be identified by title, and the page on which that section begins should be provided.

Figures, graphs, charts, diagrams, tables, exhibits, and other similar features of a report that present data or interpretations of data are known as *graphics*. Ordinarily, a report may contain many different types of graphic features. Integrated word processing programs, and special software programs provide persons preparing evaluation reports with tremendous versatility in generating graphics.

Each set of graphics (e.g., tables) should be listed on a separate page following the table of contents. Thus, a report might include a page with the heading "List of Tables." The title of each table should be provided, along with the page number in the document on which it can be located. Other page headings may be "List of Charts," "List of Figures," and so on. If a report contains relatively few visual portrayals of data, a single page headed by "List of Graphics" may suffice.

The Executive Summary

Perhaps the section of the report that will be most critical is the **executive summary**. This summary is an overview of the evaluation report. It explains what was evaluated, why the evaluation was performed, and what its major conclusions and recommendations are. The executive summary, and not the full report, is what *most people* who ever hear of the evaluation will read. It is written on behalf of people who have limited time to learn about the findings of the evaluation. In the case of evaluations of service programs done for state or federal officials, the executive summary may be what is consumed by legislators or legislative aides. Its content may provide the basis for the decision of recommending continued or discontinued funding for a program. The executive summary may be as brief as one page, and is usually two or two-and-one-half pages in length. Rarely will the summary be of greater length. It may be disappointing to hear that after all of the effort you pour into performing an evaluation, people will look at only a few pages. Believe it though, and keep it in mind as a gauge to weigh the dimensions that the executive summary can take on.

In addition to reporting what was evaluated, why it was evaluated, and what was found, other components of the executive summary may include an enumeration of the decisions that were to be made from the evaluation, the audience(s) for whom the report was intended, and any constraints under which the evaluation was done that may limit the applications of the findings. In the event that we have not sufficiently stressed the importance of the executive summary, we think that Morris and Fitz-Gibbon (1978) sum it up well: "Although the summary is placed first, it is the section that you *write* last!" (p.16).

Program Background and Evaluation Description

As pointed out in Chapter 3, programs do not exist in social or political vacuums. This section of the evaluation report provides an account of the **program context**. That is, it explains how and why the program was begun, and highlights what the program was intended to do. In addition to listing program objectives, the characteristics of program materials, activities, and administrative arrangements are delineated. It is critical to offer detail about what the program is *supposed* to look like, so that the section reporting results of what the program in fact *did* look like, can provide an appropriate comparison.

If the readers of the evaluation report are unfamiliar with the program, this section should provide as much detail as possible. Detail can be exchanged for brevity if the report is strictly for internal consumption, and the readers are fully aware of the purpose and scope of the program, and the historical events leading up to it.

It is wise to write this section of the evaluation report at the time that the evaluation plan is first being prepared. There are several reasons for preparing this part of the document then:

- Doing so will help the evaluator to understand the key elements of the program.
- It will provide direction to the evaluation.
- It will minimize the chance of bias raising its ugly head at the end of the evaluation. (It is easy to write program objectives retrospectively, and make them conform to program effects after the evaluative data have been analyzed thoroughly. However, this approach falls short of good science *and* good ethics!)
- It will offer the evaluator a framework for reporting data, and writing conclusions and recommendations.
- It will probably mean less work later on, such as when the remainder of the report is being prepared under the duress of deadlines. The time to concentrate efforts on the main part of the report will be appreciated.

Circulate a written draft of this background description among key program personnel for feedback with respect to accuracy. The evaluator *does* face somewhat of a dilemma, if the feedback received suggests there are discrepancies among program personnel concerning program elements and objectives. There should be some effort made for program personnel to arrive at a consensus of opinion concerning program aims (see Chapter 1).

The evaluation, itself, should be carefully described. According to Morris and Fitz-Gibbon (1978):

> The first part of this section describes and delimits the assignment that the evaluator has accepted. It explains *why* the evaluation was conducted, what it was intended to accomplish, and what it was *not* intended to accomplish. You should prepare the purposes of the evaluation immediately after accepting the job as evaluator (p.18).

In general, the content of this section of the report should address the purposes of the evaluation, and the evaluation design, including which measures will be used, when, how, and to whom they will be administered, and against which set of performance standards they will be compared.

Although most users of the evaluation are not likely to read this section, or at least, read it thoroughly, the people who want to know the nitty-gritty details of the evaluation (i.e., the "critics" and "skeptics") will scrutinize it closely. Individuals most likely to critique this section of the report will be those who hold viewpoints that differ from the posture of the report, or have the most to lose as a consequence of the evaluation's conclusions and recommendations. Study delimitations and limitations, constraints on time or money, instrumentation issues, data collection procedures, sampling methods, and other specific methodologic concerns about the rigor of the evaluation design should be addressed in utmost detail. One need not be apologetic for limitations that were beyond one's control. This section of the report is important for at least one other reason. It is important from the point of view of the evaluation connoisseur, or the student of evaluation who wishes to learn how others carry out evaluation assignments.

Presentation of Results

As in a basic or applied research paper, the results section presents the findings in factual, descriptive terms. You may hear investigators speak of results as being comprised of a combination of **hard data** and **soft data**. The former would be those findings that are relevant to the questions being investigated, and which have the properties of reliability and validity. The latter would be those commentaries, testimonials, casual observations, and other evidence of an anecdotal nature that tell evaluators about some of the characteristics of the program that may not have been measured directly. While decision makers are inclined to be more interested in hard data, soft data should not be disregarded. Soft data, because of its qualitative nature, may be extremely useful in providing insights about program strengths and weaknesses (see Chapter 11). Such anecdotal information also can help one develop the basis for making recommendations for what to evaluate in the next cycle of examination of the program's operation.

Before preparing the results section, the statistical analysis of all data should be completed. The specific analyses performed, ordinarily, will be a function of the specific questions that the evaluation is attempting to answer. While the evaluator has quite an arsenal of procedures that can be employed (see Chapter 14), the analytical scheme used should be only as complex as it needs to be. That is, if you are seeking answers to simple questions, use simple statistics that will be understood by readers; if you are addressing answers to complex issues, more sophisticated statistical procedures may not only be preferred, but actually required. The literature points out, however, that as the complexity of the analysis increases, the number of readers who can understand and interpret the analysis decreases (Emerson & Colditz, 1983; Rudolph, McDermott & Gold, 1985).

How the data are organized for presentation is a critical factor in reader comprehension. For quick perusal by readers, results of a survey questionnaire can be summarized directly on a facsimile of the instrument itself. Although these and other results can be presented clearly in a narrative format as well, a narration often is lengthy and tedious to read, and does not lend itself to rapid location of a particular point of interest. Therefore, a visual display of data often is preferred. Several options are possible.

Table 16.1 Florida Poison Information Center 1989 Poison Exposure Calls by Month

Month of Year 1989	Number of Calls
January	4603
February	4503
March	5078
April	5186
May	5290
June	5101
July	5271
August	5243
September	4799
October	4890
November	4685
December	4352
Unknown	6
Total:	59007

Tables provide ideal formats for displaying data. A large quantity of information can be scanned with ease. Tables lend themselves well to giving the reader a summary of descriptive statistical information such as frequencies and percentages. The title of each table should be descriptive and "stand alone." That is, a reader should be able to examine the title, and without benefit of further narrative, understand the nature of the data in the table. Nevertheless, few reports will contain "naked tables," but rather, will have ones with narrative descriptions that put the data in some appropriate context. A table should be referred to by number, and not simply as "the table shown below." Reference to a table is typically made prior to its actual appearance, though space considerations and "visual friendliness" will also determine placement within the report. The evaluator must keep in mind that tables, as well as other data displays, should be *reader friendly*. To illustrate the utility of graphic data presentation, the monthly call volume for a poison information center telephone hotline is illustrated in Table 16.1.

Figures are illustrations or diagrams that are particularly useful to readers in visualizing relational factors, or other aspects of a data set. A description of procedures, a set of graphed data, a sequence of steps, a series of diagnostic steps, or a decision tree are elements which lend themselves to portrayal as figures. Without further elaboration, though, a figure can be just about anything that its creator wishes it to be. While all figures should be clearly labeled, they may or may not stand alone without accompanying narrative.

Bar graphs are figures that are used commonly to portray data. They are among the easiest of all data displays to understand. Bar graphs are especially effective for illustrating levels of performance, degrees of achievement, or comparing the relative performances of individuals or organizations over time.

Figures 16.1a - 16.1c illustrate various bar graphs. Note that each graph is labeled (heading, horizontal (x) axis, vertical (y) axis) in such a way that it could stand alone with little or no narrative explanation. Figure 16.1a shows the level of performance of 25 individuals who were given a telephone survey consisting of 20 items related to poison knowledge. Notice how the strong performances, as well as the weak performances, on this inventory stand out clearly in a bar graph.

Figures 16.1b and 16.1c display a different set of data via two alternative formats. Figure 16.1b is a simple bar graph that approximates the month-by-month call volume at a poison control center. It reveals that call volume varies relatively little throughout the year. Figure 16.1c shows the same data with a more elaborate, three-dimensional graph, and an indication of the exact data being represented. Figure 16.1b is good because of its simplicity. Figure 16.1c is probably more attractive, if also somewhat more cluttered. Although we have shown bar graphs arranged vertically, they also may have the data represented horizontally.

Line graphs are valuable ways in which to display information graphically when the horizontal axis reports a measure that has a natural sequence, such as time. The data used for Figures 16.1b and 16.1c are displayed again in Figure 16.2a, as a line graph. When two or more groups are being compared over time, the line graph is helpful in visualizing trends and differences between groups. In Figure 16.2b, call volume data for two different years are superimposed on the same graph and compared. One can immediately see from these data that the months of June through August for 1989 produced more call volume. Using the same data in tabled form might not provide the reader with this insight as rapidly. Evaluators can experiment with data displays to determine which approach is most helpful, and as with so many other parts of the evaluation, can "pilot test" the report with colleagues and selected members of stakeholder groups.

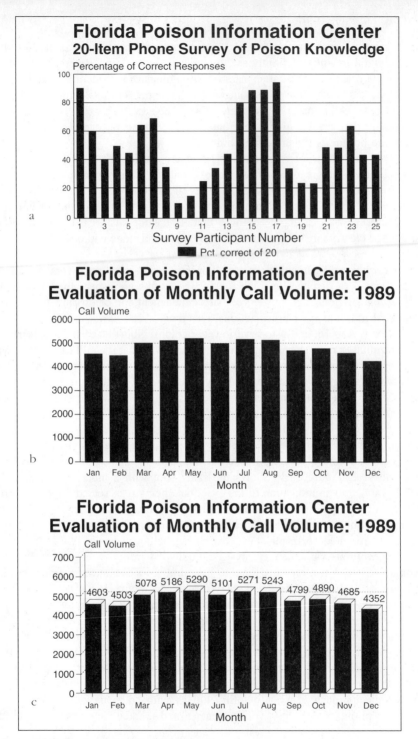

Figure 16.1a,b,c Examples of Bar Graphs

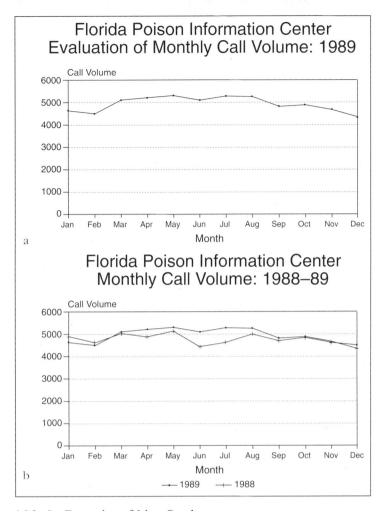

Figure 16.2a,b Examples of Line Graphs

Pie charts (also known as *circle* or *sector* charts) illustrate the division of a whole unit into its subunits or component parts. "They are frequently used to explain how a unit of government distributes its share of the tax dollar, how an individual spends his or her salary, or any other simple percentage distribution" (Best & Kahn, 1989, p.343). If properly labeled, pie charts require little additional explanation. Figures 16.3a and 16.3b are pie charts that display the monthly call volume of a poison control center for 1989. Notice that this information is identical to that provided in Table 16.1, Figure 16.1b, Figure 16.1c, and Figure 16.2a. The chart is shown as a "whole pie" in Figure 16.3a, and as a "cut pie" in Figure 16.3b. Raw frequencies, rather than percentages, are used in these illustrations. Even in the absence of actual percentages, inspection of the pie chart permits one to "visualize" that call volume varied little month-to-month for 1989.

Figure 16.3c displays data concerning another phase of this same poison control study: the age distribution of poisoning victims. In this illustration, the combination of identifying the age group, displaying the raw frequencies, and giving the rounded percentages, provides the reader with a relatively complete picture of this part of the data

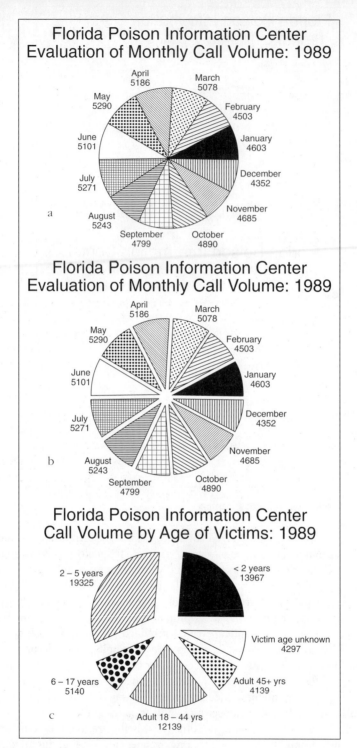

Figure 16.3a,b,c Examples of Pie Charts

set. The reader immediately sees that infants, toddlers, and pre-school children account for the majority of calls received by the poison center. (Consequently, one also draws the conclusion that preventive efforts and education programs for parents and children need to be designed with this age group in mind!) Would one draw the same conclusion as quickly if the data were in tabled form? Perhaps, but the question for the report writer to bear in mind is: "How can I best display my data to assist readers in interpreting them, and drawing relevant conclusions that will be helpful in program planning, future decision making, and other important tasks?"

Discussion, Conclusions, and Recommendations

Although this section appears toward the end of the report, it is one that attracts much reader attention. Next to the executive summary, this section is likely to be the part of the evaluation document most likely to be read or distributed. It is in this part of the report that the questions or hypotheses underlying the evaluation are addressed.

The keys to a well-written discussion section are *balance*, *clarity*, and *objectivity*. According to Windsor, Baranowski, Clark and Cutter (1984), writers make two common errors here: (1) drawing conclusions that go beyond what the data reveal; and, (2) reporting things for which there is no evidence at all. "Both are lethal errors to be avoided at all costs" (Windsor, et al., 1984, p.314). If evaluators and program managers have worked closely together, there may be a tendency by the evaluator to want to identify conclusions that will be pleasing and well received, regardless of their actual validity. There may be some pressure applied by key program players to report only selected findings, or to weight some results a great deal more than others. Good evaluators resist these political maneuvers, since objectivity becomes lost (see Chapter 3).

No matter how well a program operates, or how successfully it achieves or excedes its objectives, it is not without flaws or shortcomings. "The world rarely operates just as you expect, and an evaluation report that reads as if all went perfectly. is at best inaccurate, and at worst, dishonest" (Windsor, et al., 1984, p.314). Thus, a good evaluator will prepare a balanced report that cites both program strengths and weaknesses. Every question that was posed originally should be addressed as it relates to the purpose of the evaluation and the decisions emanating from it. If the data collected and analyzed fail to allow a decisive conclusion to be drawn, that fact should be pointed out.

The element of clarity should be of special concern when it comes to the presentation of recommendations. Although recommendations about health education and promotion efforts are likely to be program specific, certain generalizations can be made. Program topics typically addressed as recommendations are concerned with program content, delivery, personnel, budget, and scope. Therefore, items addressed in the recommendation section are likely to include:

■   Should the content of the health education and promotion program be revised? If so, then how or in what ways?

- Should there be modifications (increases or decreases) in the number or kinds of personnel associated with the program? Are certain personnel assigned improperly? How might changes be implemented effectively?
- Is the program overbudgeted in some areas, but underfunded in others? What reshuffling of appropriations is likely to produce the most efficient use of monetary resources?
- Should the program be expanded, maintained at its current level, curtailed, phased out, or eliminated? Why should this action be taken, and how should it be enacted?

The evaluator should bear in mind that recommendations need to be limited to the program under review, and not to the organization as a whole that supports the program. Thus, recommendations for revising a worksite health promotion program are legitimate concerns for the evaluator to ponder, but not recommendations about revising the priority of products or services turned out by the company that houses it. Ways to improve learning of health content in the classroom are fair game for an evaluator of a school health education program, but not the way that school districts make decisions about textbook purchases or class size.

Hendricks (1984) and Patton (1988) point out that the construction of *useful* recommendations is an art not well developed in the evaluation literature. This condition is perplexing if the recommendations constitute the critical products of an evaluation (Hendricks & Papagiannis, 1990). So, what qualities of a recommendation enhance its "user friendliness," or otherwise improve its utility? Some suggestions adapted from Hendricks and Papagiannis (1990) are offered below:

- Consider all *pertinent* issues to be "fair game," including both the preestablished ones, and those that arise during the course of the evaluation.
- Think about recommendations throughout the course of the evaluation, not just at the end of it. Possible recommendations should be recorded as soon as impressions are formed, and then reviewed for their relevance at the end of the evaluation.
- Draw recommendations from as wide a variety of sources as possible. This process may include the review of recommendations from other studies of similar programs, since they may have relevance to *this* program. The process may include garnering insights of any program personnel or clients.
- Work closely with program personnel throughout the evaluation process. Stakeholders should not be surprised by the nature of the recommendations with which they are eventually confronted. As data analysis "crystalizes," and likely recommendations begin to take shape, the evaluator should work actively with key decision makers (people who must approve and/or implement them) to build acceptance.
- Bear in mind the political, social, and organizational context of the program, so that realistic recommendations are ones primarily offered.

However, ethics and objectivity dictate that evaluators offer any recommendations they deem to be appropriate.

■ Recognize that recommendations can be *general*, (i.e., (corrective actions with respect to this program need to be taken), or *specific,* (problem "A" should be addressed by immediately enacting solution "X"). Furthermore, an evaluator can present a range of possible solutions, the merits and liabilities of which can be discussed at the organizational level.

■ Suggest the possible future implications of the recommendations, including the anticipated benefits to arise from enacting them.

■ Accompany each recommendation with a set of implementation strategies. Consider providing an implementation strategy that includes: (1) existing resources only; and, (2) future or anticipated resources.

■ Organize recommendations in meaningful ways to facilitate understanding. Examples of organizational approaches include: high priority versus lesser priority; short term versus long term; major versus minor; structural versus cosmetic; and so on.

Summary

The evaluation report is a developmental process that consists of much more than just the written preparation. The style and format of these documents is fairly standard, but can, and should be adapted to the needs of those who will be using the data and recommendations. Evaluation reports should have the quality of "reader friendliness." The way in which data are displayed is one technique for promoting this quality. The report writer has many options for the graphic presentation of results. The quality of a report is enhanced if it presents a clear, balanced, and objective review of the program's operation. Two of the most important sections of the report are the executive summary and the section that addresses conclusions and recommendations. Special care should be taken in preparing these aspects of the report. In making recommendations, the evaluator should consider developing a plan or strategy for guiding stakeholders in the implementation of changes suggested by the data.

Case Study

Office on Smoking and Health, Division of Adolescent and School Health, Centers for Disease Control and Prevention. (1998). Tobacco use among high school students – United States, 1997. *Morbidity & Mortality Weekly Report*, *47*(12), 229-233. (Also reprinted in *Journal of School Health*, Volume 68, Number 5, May, 1998, pp. 202-204.

Tobacco use by youth, as reported in the 1997 Youth Risk Behavior Survey, conducted by the Centers for Disease Control and Prevention, are broken out in this "executive summary." Prepare a 350-word written critique of this report, taking into account the elements that were identified in Chapter 16, concerning data dissemination in reports and the preparation of an executive summary. What recommendations would you make to the CDC for improving the usefulness and "reader friendliness" of similar reports in the future?

Student Questions/Activities

1. What does it mean when one says that an evaluation report has the property of "reader friendliness?"

2. Look again at the data presented in this chapter in Table 16.1 and Figures 16.1b, 16.1c, 16.2a, 16.3a, and 16.3b. Which graphic or set of graphics best presents these data? What is the basis for your judgment? Explain.

3. Write to a state or federal agency to see if you can obtain a copy of a recently completed evaluation of a health-related program. An aide in the office of the state legislator or congressional representative from your district may be able to assist you in identifying a report of this nature. Upon receipt, examine the report for its technical qualities. Compare its style and content to those suggested in this chapter.

4. Contact an agency for which an evaluation of a health education or related program was recently completed. Interview key personnel or other stakeholders concerning the extent to which recommendations were implemented. Ask about user satisfaction concerning the evaluation report. If implementation of specified recommendations was problematic, see if you can establish what some of the barriers to implementation were, and whether the evaluation document provided adequate guidance in this regard.

Recommended Readings

Fink, A. (Ed.). (1997). *The Survey Kit*. Thousand Oaks, CA: Sage.

This nine-volume work was composed by premiere survey research experts. The first volume is a survey researcher's handbook, and is followed by volumes addressing question development, carrying out self-administered and mailed surveys, conducting telephone and in-person interviews, designing surveys, sampling, measuring reliability and validity, analyzing data, and reporting results. This series can be useful to novices, as well as to more experienced survey researchers.

Patton, M.Q. (1997). *Utilization-Focused Evaluation*, 3rd edition. Thousand Oaks, CA: Sage

Among the many features of this book are descriptions of how to use evaluation and evaluation reports to change the culture of organizations, how evaluators can nurture results-oriented, reality-testing leadership in programs, and crafting effective reports. Readers should pay particular attention to Chapter 13 of the book, entitled, *Deciphering Data and Reporting Results: Analysis, Interpretations, Judgments, and Recommendations.*

Salant, P., & Dillman, D.A. (1994). *How To Conduct Your Own Survey.* New York: John Wiley.

This textbook is recommended because of its extensive examples and integration of survey construction and reporting on survey results. Hints for oral *and* written presentations are provided. Readers are especially directed to Chapter 10 of the book, entitled, *Reporting Survey Results.*

References

Best, J.W., & Kahn, J.V. (1989). *Research in Education*, 6th edition. Englewood Cliffs, NJ: Prentice Hall.

Emerson, J.D., & Colditz, G.A. (1983). Use of statistical analysis in the *New England Journal of Medicine. New England Journal of Medicine, 309,* 709-713.

Fink, A. (1995). *How To Report Surveys*. Thousand Oaks, CA: Sage.

Hendricks, M. (1984). Finis. *Evaluation News, 5*(4), 94-96.

Hendricks, M., & Papagiannis, M. (1990). Do's and dont's for offering effective recommendations. *Evaluation Practice, 11*(2), 121-125.

Morris, L.L., & Fitz-Gibbon, C.T. (1978). *How to Present an Evaluation Report*. Beverly Hills, CA: Sage Publications.

Patton, M.Q. (1988). The future and evaluation. *Evaluation Practice, 9*(4), 90-93.

Rudolph, A., McDermott, R.J., & Gold, R.S. (1985). Use of statistics in the *Journal of School Health* 1979-1983. *Journal of School Health, 55*(6), 230-233.

Salant, P., & Dillman, D.A. (1994). *How To Conduct Your Own Survey.* New York: John Wiley.

Windsor, R.A., Baranowski, T., Clark, N., & Cutter, G. (1984). *Evaluation of Health Promotion and Education Programs*. Palo Alto, CA: Mayfield Publishers.

Glossary of Key Terms

Academic Evaluation an evaluation whose purpose is, in part, driven by the requirement for faculty members to publish data-based studies in professional, peer-reviewed journals.

Accreditation Approach an evaluation model that examines program performance compared to a set of agreed upon standards or criteria, usually set by a professional body to which a program must be accountable.

Achievement Tests instruments which measure the degree to which an individual has mastered a body of knowledge or an assortment of skills.

Adversarial Approach an evaluation model that uses courtroom trial strategies to assess the value of a program, or its relative value compared to a competing program.

Alpha Test the initial test of a computer-based instruction program that ensures that the program is functioning adequately.

Analysis of Variance (ANOVA) a set of statistical procedures that examine variation among groups, especially when three or more groups are involved.

Anonymity a responsibility to protect the identify of human subjects under study from investigators, data collectors, and all other people.

APEX-PH an acronym for *a*ssessment *p*rotocol for *ex*cellence in *p*ublic *h*ealth; a strategy for prioritizing health problems, usually employed by local health departments.

Art Criticism Approach an evaluation model that considers the use of personal standards and criteria to assess how a "consumer" might judge the value of a program.

Attitudinal Inventories instruments that measure an individual's attitudes, values, beliefs, or opinions about individuals, objects, events, or constructs.

Authentic Measurement that used to assess skill mastery through techniques such as observations, games, and interviews; employed often by early childhood educators.

Autonomy (see Respect)

Behavior Rating Scales measures used by observers to judge the quality of a performance.

Behavioral Anchor the description of the behavior being rated on a scale or checklist.

Behavioral Data data that include the activity patterns of individuals, usually so that present performance can be compared to past performance following an intervention.

Behavioral Inventories instruments that measure behaviors of individuals, either through self-report or observation.

Benchmarks objectives used in the development and evaluation of programs, set by program planners, based on historical data or projected (and desirable) trends.

Beneficence the relative "good" that comes about as a result of an evaluation.

Beta Test the final testing of a computer-based instruction program that "fine tunes" the program, and prepares it for general dissemination.

Biomedical Instruments instruments that measure physiological functions of the body (e.g., blood pressure cuffs, height and weight scales, cholesterol meters, etc.).

Bogardus Social Distance Scale a scale used to estimate people's attitude or comfort level with social or geographic proximity to selected individuals, groups, or institutions.

Bogus Pipeline a technique used to increase validity of self-report measures, in which subjects believe they are undergoing a confirmatory physiological or biomedical test, when in fact, no such test is administered.

Budget Justification an investigator's defense of project costs, usually explaining such details as how personnel are to be used, why consultants are necessary, which materials are essential, how and why travel is to be performed, etc.

Central Location Intercept Interviews interviews which take place in central gathering locations, such as shopping malls, parking lots, and other similar spots, where potential respondents are "intercepted" to take part in a survey.

Chi-square Test a statistical test that compares the differences in frequencies or proportions by examining expected frequencies with observed frequencies.

CIPP Model a decision-oriented evaluation model that provides feedback about a program with respect to its *context*, *input*, *process*, and *product*.

Codebook whereas "coding" is the set of rules governing the translation of "raw data" to the formation of a data set, a codebook defines variables, describes their position in a data set, and assigns values to them.

Common Error Analysis a technique used in knowledge test development to design plausible foils for multiple-choice items.

Community Analysis a form of needs assessment that examines the traits and health problems of a community.

Compliance Evaluation an evaluation whose primary purpose is to demonstrate that a program meets or exceeds basic performance requirements or regulations, and is not violating laws or other principles of operation.

Confidence Interval the range of numerical values within which an investigator can be confident (usually 95% to 99%) that the population parameter lies.

Confidence Limits the upper and lower extremes of the confidence interval.

Confidentiality a responsibility to protect from disclosure the identity of human subjects being studied, under circumstances where identifying characteristics are known to investigators or data collectors.

Connoisseurship Approach (see Art Criticism Approach)

Construct Validity addresses the degree to which an instrument's score is a measure of the characteristic or construct of interest.

Constructed-response Items items that enable test takers to develop their own responses to questions (e.g., completion, short answer, essay).

Content Validity the extent to which a sample of items, tasks, or questions comprising an instrument are representative of some defined content domain or universe.

Continuous Quality Improvement a program management philosophy in which data form the cornerstone for ongoing improvement.

Correlation a set of statistical tests that describe the strength and direction of the relationship between two variables.

Cost-benefit Analysis a method of estimating the benefits of a program that usually applies a monetary value.

Cost-benefit Evaluation (see Cost-benefit Analysis)

Cost-effectiveness Analysis measures the cost of providing a service, as well as the outcomes obtained from the service, but without applying a monetary value.

Cost-identification Analysis a procedure that examines the costs associated with a program, sometimes called *cost-minimization analysis*, because it is used to identify the lowest cost possible for a particular program or treatment.

Cost-reimbursement Contract a contract between two parties in which the first party promises to reimburse the second party only for those expenses actually incurred, although a professional service fee may be paid in addition.

Cover Letter a letter that accompanies a survey that states the survey's purpose and encourages participation.

Criterion-referenced Tests those tests that have an absolute "pass" or "fail" score; an individual's score is compared to this pass/fail criterion, often referred to as a *cut score* or *passing score*.

Criterion-related Validity the degree to which an instrument's score is systematically related to one or more criteria; *predictive validity* and *concurrent validity* are two examples.

Critical Path Method a planning and evaluation strategy that plots all program tasks in a linear fashion, to project the most time efficient means of completing the project.

Cross-tabulation a statistical procedure that facilitates comparison of two nominal level or ordinal level variables.

Cultural Sensitivity the extent to which curriculum materials, instruments, individual items, and data collectors are free from faulty assumptions, and are responsive to the particular cultural traits of a group of people.

Cultural Tailoring the extent to which an intended audience participates in the identification, selection, preparation, and approval of curriculum materials, instruments, individual items, and data collectors.

Cumulative Scale a set of items that is ordered, based on difficulty or value-loading (e.g., a Guttman Scale).

Cut Score (see Criterion-referenced Tests)

Deception the purposeful or intentional withholding of, or misinforming about, details related to an investigation.

Dependent Variable a variable that is a consequence of, or dependent on, another (independent) variable.

Descriptive Data data that characterize a person's age, education, income, ethnicity, and other demographic information about an individual.

Descriptive Statistics statistical procedures used to organize and describe date sets, usually consisting of the mean, median, mode, and standard deviation.

Dichotomous Item an item that receives a score of "0" or "1" (or some other dichotomous score) depending on student/subject performance on an achievement test, where the individual is awarded 1 point for a correct response, but 0 points for an incorrect response.

Difficulty Index an item analysis procedure used to estimate the difficulty of an item (e.g., an index of .80 indicates that 80% of subjects answered an item correctly).

Direct Costs the actual costs of conducting a study or program, including personnel expenditures (salary, wages, employee benefits, consultants) and non-personnel expenditures (rent, office supplies and equipment, telephone and fax, postage, printing and photocopying, travel, etc.).

Discrepancy Evaluation an approach that examines the difference between program objectives and actual achievement, thereby guiding future management decisions.

Discriminant Analysis a multivariate statistical procedure that uses interval or ratio level data to classify or predict variables that are nominal (categorical) in nature.

Discrimination Index an item analysis procedure used to estimate the power of an item to differentiate between persons who score high and persons who score low on a scale or examination.

Distractors (see Foils)

Distributive Justice a perspective used in cost analysis that focuses on the way privileges, duties, and goods are distributed within society, in relation to the merits of the person and interests of society.

Drop-off Survey (see Home Delivery Interviews)

Equal Appearing Interval Scale a set of items designed to measure an individual's attitude toward the object of study, where each item has a scale value indicating a strength of attitude toward the object of study (e.g., a Thurstone scale).

Ethics principles dealing with the "rightness" or "wrongness" of a particular act or action.

Evaluability Assessment a systematic process for describing the key descriptive elements of a program, as well as its "readiness" to be evaluated.

Executive Summary an overview of an evaluation usually presented at the beginning of an evaluation report that highlights why a study was conducted, how it was conducted, the chief results, and recommendations.

Experimental Design (see True Experimental Design)

External Evaluator an evaluator who is not involved with, or a part of, the pro-gram being evaluated.

External Validity a property of investigations, studies, and research or evaluation designs that suggests the extent to which findings can be generalized from one group, setting, or time, to other groups, settings, and times.

Face Validity a trait an instrument is said to possess if, "on the face of things," it appears to measure what it is intended to measure, and appears to be appropriate for the audience for whom it is intended.

Factor Analysis a data reduction technique that studies patterns of occurrence among variables (i.e., underlying "factors") in large data sets.

Fidelity a term that describes the extent to which evaluators and clients are faithful, honest, and forthright with respect to a contract or agreement, and any related actual or implied promises.

Field Study (see Field Test)

Field Test a form of pilot testing that takes place in the setting where an evaluator will eventually implement the program or research project; field testing is often a second pilot test implemented "in the field" with a small group of subjects from the actual target population.

Fixed Price Contract a contract between two parties in which the first party promises to reimburse the second party a flat fee, usually tied to a schedule of producing certain "deliverables" (e.g., a midterm or final report).

Focus Group Interview a particular type of group interview, usually conducted with 8 to 12 subjects, where discussion is "focused" on a single issue, or a well-defined, limited number of issues; used in marketing research and in the formative stages of projects, such as in instrument design.

Foils the incorrect response options for a multiple-choice item; also known as *distractors*.

Forced-Choice Technique (see Paired Comparison Technique)

Formative Evaluation the monitoring activities that take place during the development and implementation phases of a program that provide feedback for consideration of program adjustments.

Frequency Distribution rank-ordered sets of raw scores.

Gantt Chart a planning and activity tool that involves the development of a matrix of program events and time periods to provide feedback on progress during the life of a project.

Generalizability the extent to which inferences based on a study of a particular sample can be made to other persons, places, settings, and times; (see External Validity)

Geographic Information Systems (GIS) a computer-based system that facilitates the data displays by geographic location.

Goal-free Approach an evaluation model established to reduce evaluator bias, by not revealing a program's prespecified intents, thereby permitting the identification of both desired program effects, as well as unintended "side effects."

Goal-oriented Approach an evaluation model that examines the articulation of program outcomes with a set of prespecified goals and objectives.

GOAMs an acronym for *g*oals, *o*bjectives, *a*ctivities, and *m*ilestones; a planning and evaluation tool for assessing tasks necessary to complete a project.

Graffiti a type of archival, qualitative data that describes certain phenomena, often political or social commentary, which can be used to corroborate data from other sources; an unobtrusive method for examining, reading, and interpreting people's casual, but purposeful writing and ideas on buildings, walls, etc.

Group Interviews interviews conducted simultaneously with more than one person to solicit multiple opinions, build consensus, and increase data collection efficiency; used extensively in marketing research.

Hard Data information of an objective nature obtained from valid, reliable sources that independent measures can confirm.

Hatchet Evaluation an evaluation whose intended purpose is to demonstrate the failures and weaknesses of a program or organization, thus discrediting it to the extent that funding or political support will evaporate or become greatly diminished.

Health-Risk Appraisals (HRAs) instruments that estimate an individual's health status at a particular point in time; HRAs purport to predict significant health events (e.g., probability of a heart attack) or future quality of life.

High-Stakes Tests examinations that have a major impact on an individual's life or career.

Home Delivery Interviews door-to-door surveys which enable an investigator to conduct interviews (or sometimes, written surveys) with specific individuals dwelling within a given household; permit surveys to be "dropped off" while the investigator waits for the survey to be completed, to return at a later time to collect the survey, or to leave a postage-paid, return envelope for the respondent to mail back.

Hypothesis a statement concerning the probable or expected relationship between a dependent variable and one or more independent variables.

Impact Evaluation the examination of the immediate effects of a program; a type of summative evaluation.

Incidence Rate the number of new occurrences of an event (e.g., a disease) over a specified period of time, usually in regard to a particular place and population.

Independent Variable a variable that is antecedent to, or determinant of, a dependent variable.

Indirect Costs costs that are not a part of direct costs, but which are usually estimated as a percentage of direct costs (e.g., utilities, security and protection, janitorial and housekeeping services, etc.).

Inferential Statistics a group of statistical procedures used to generalize results from a sample to a population.

Information Gathering Evaluation an evaluation whose primary purpose is to provide feedback of an ongoing and routine nature to a program manager.

Informed Consent a moral and ethical protocol in research and evaluation studies, that ensures that human subjects have been clearly and thoroughly informed of any potential risk to their physical or psychological well-being, prior to their participation.

Ingratiating Evaluation an evaluation whose deliberate purpose is to demonstrate the successes and strengths of a program, possibly without consideration of their actual validity, or in proportion to any program shortcomings, usually with the intent of securing continued funding, political support, and program survival.

Institutional Review Board (IRB) formal committees established by colleges and universities, government agencies, school districts, and other institutions to review ongoing and proposed research and evaluation projects for protecting the rights of human subjects.

Instrument Specifications the "blueprint" that describes exactly how an instrument is to be designed; common elements include purpose, target audience,

content domains, item types, and number of items.

Intact Group a cluster of people comprising a unit of study, usually selected when individual assignment to a group is not possible.

Internal Consistency Reliability a measure of the inter-correlation among items in a scale; the extent to which items are related to each other.

Internal Validity a property of investigations, studies, and research or evaluation designs that suggests the extent to which a cause-and-effect relationship can be implied from observed results following implementation of an intervention.

Inter-rater Reliability the level of agreement between two or more raters concerning the characteristics of a particular observation.

Interval Levels of Measurement measures that have the characteristic of "rank," but which also measure the distance between different points on a scale.

Interview Procedures face-to-face meetings between evaluators and subjects for the purpose of data collection.

Intra-rater Reliability the level of agreement or consistency for a single rater on repeated measures of the same observation.

Item Analysis a set of procedures employed by measurement specialists to appraise and increase the quality of instruments, usually with respect to instrument reliability.

Item Stem the part of a multiple-choice item that is the question or statement to which the examinee is to respond.

Justice the equitable treatment and representation of subgroups (usually those perceived to have less "power") within society.

Key Activity Chart a planning and

evaluation tool in which the main activities are identified, and sequenced and plotted on a schedule, to facilitate review of progress at a given point in time.

Least Publishable Unit the smallest unit of a research or evaluation study needed to prepare an article for professional publication; although not an uncommon practice, one that is generally viewed in a negative context.

Mean the arithmetical average in a set of scores.

Median the middle-most score in a set of scores.

Method Effect the impact of the particular method used in survey research on the type of data, quality of data, and utility of data that get reported.

Mini-pilot a form of pilot testing where the evaluator tests materials with a small group of subjects as they would be used in the actual study.

Mode the most commonly occurring score in a set of scores.

Multiple Regression a group of multivariate statistical procedures that combine several variables to predict some other variable.

Need something that is necessary or useful for the fulfillment of a purpose, and as such, must be judged and interpreted within the context of purposes, values, knowledge, and cause-effect relationships.

Needs Assessment the evaluation of *need*, including methods of determining things that are important for the fulfillment of defensible purposes.

Nominal Levels of Measurement measures that categorize individuals, objects, issues, or events into different groups (e.g., males vs. females, Republicans vs. Democrats, etc.).

Nonmalficence the actual or potential harm that could emanate from the result of performing research or evaluation.

Nonprobability Sample a means of selecting individuals from a population that is not based on probability theory.

Nonresponse Bias the error introduced by the failure of persons to respond to a survey, even though a probability sample was originally selected.

Norm-referenced Tests a type of test where an individual's score is compared to a group score.

Objectives-oriented Approach (see Goal-oriented Approach)

Observer Bias the conscious or unconscious activities of an observer that influences what is seen, recorded, measured, interpreted, reported, or judged to be important or relevant to the issue under investigation.

Observer Effect the alteration in behavior that occurs when people are aware of being observed, which in turn, threatens the validity of conclusions that may be drawn.

Odds Ratio a statistical procedure used to estimate risk or odds based on exposure to some event or condition.

Ordinal Levels of Measurement measures that rank-order individuals, objects, issues, or events.

Outcome Evaluation the examination of the long-term effects of a program; a type of summative evaluation.

Overhead Costs (see Indirect Costs)

Oversample a procedure employed to study a particular trait that occurs infrequently, and thus, requires selecting a sample of people possessing the trait that exceeds the proportion of such people in the overall population.

Paired Comparison Technique a method for assessing attitudes that asks subjects to select the more favorable choice from a series of paired statements.

Parallel Forms Reliability the degree

to which two or more parallel forms of the same test have equal means, standard deviations, and intercorrelations among items.

Passing Score (see Criterion-referenced tests)

PATCH Model an acronym for *p*lanned *a*pproach *t*o *c*ommunity *h*ealth; a strategy to involve individuals and groups within a community to plan, implement, and evaluate health programs in the community.

Perspective of Analysis the point of view one holds about a program's relative costs and benefits that is dependent on the nature of one's role as a stakeholder.

PERT an acronym for *P*rogram (or *P*erformance) *E*valuation *R*eview *T*echnique; a planning and evaluation tool for identifying and sequencing activities necessary to complete a project.

Pilot Study (see Pilot Test)

Pilot Test the "dress rehearsal" for a more expansive study whereby methods, materials, and all other procedures to be used are tested for feasibility, appropriateness, and so on.

Portfolio organization of various testing and measurement information about an individual, often a young child, that facilitates stakeholder understanding about learning achievement.

Posttest a test, observation, or measurement taken subsequent to the occurrence of a planned event, such as an intervention.

PRECEDE-PROCEED Model an acronym for *p*redisposing, *r*einforcing, *en*abling, *c*onstructs in *e*ducational/*e*nvironmental *d*iagnosis and *e*valuation (PRECEDE) and *p*olicy, *r*egulatory, and *o*rganizational *c*onstructs in *e*ducational and *e*nvironmental *d*evelopment (PROCEED); a conceptual and methodologic approach to needs assessment, program planning, and program evaluation.

Preferential Data data that report people's preferences, usually in regard to political or social issues.

Preliminary Review a preliminary, informal pilot test evaluators conduct using colleagues as subjects and critics.

Premise the "stem" of a matching test item.

Prepilot (see Mini-pilot)

Presurvey Letter a letter sent to potential respondents a few days prior to a telephone interview or mailed survey, to alert them to the forthcoming survey, obtain support, and motivate participation.

Pretest a test, observation, or measurement taken prior to the occurrence of a planned event, such as an intervention.

Prevalence Rate the number of existing cases (new and old) of a disease or condition at a given point in time, usually in regard to a specific place and population.

Probability Sample a means of selecting individuals from a population that seeks representativeness, and which is based on each individual having a known probability of being selected.

Process Evaluation the examination of the activities that take place while a program is being implemented; a type of formative evaluation.

Professional Review Approach (see Accreditation Approach)

Program Context the background description of a program that delineates its operating environment.

Program Evaluation the use of various procedures (both quantitative and qualitative) to determine the degree to which a program has been developed and implemented as planned, as well as to determine the degree to which the program has met its goals and objectives, and satisfied the needs of various program stakeholders.

Projective Testing   a procedure in which examinees must use their own beliefs and attitudes to respond to questions (e.g., Rorschach inkblot test).

Quality Adjusted Life Years (QALYs) a method used in cost-effectiveness analysis that measures not only the number of years of life gained as a result of following a particular protocol, but also the *quality* of those years gained.

Quality Assurance   the application of quality control procedures, as well as examination of critical processes, programs, projects, standards, materials, and outcomes as they relate to the program's overall goals and objectives.

Quality Control   a set of procedures used to assess the quality of a program and its materials; also used as a tool throughout a program's developmental phases.

Quasi-experimental Design   a design in which intervention and control (comparison) groups are used, but where random assignment of individuals to groups is not possible.

Quasi-legal Approach   (see Adversarial Approach)

Range   a measure of dispersion (spread) calculated by subtracting the lowest score in a distribution from the highest score.

Rater Reliability   the consistency with which an event is judged by two or more raters (or a single individual).

Ratio Scales   measures that rank individuals, objects, issues, or events, and which have a known distance between ranks, and which have a "0" value with absolute meaning.

Readability Level   the average grade level of reading achievement required to understand curriculum materials, or testing and measurement items.

Reference Case   a case that sets standards for the way that costs are measured and valued when results of studies are compared.

Regulatory Evaluation   (see Compliance Evaluation)

Reliability   the degree to which measures are free from errors; the extent to which an instrument's measurement is consistent, dependable, and stable.

Request for Proposal (RFP)   a funding agency's solicitation for proposals to conduct a specific research or evaluation task.

Respect   the consideration of the autonomy or freedom of persons, including nonautonomous persons such as minors, the mentally incompetent, prisoners, and other persons.

Response-selection Analysis   an item analysis procedure used to examine the patterns of responses on a forced-choice item, enabling evaluators to assess the plausibility of certain foils (for common-error analysis purposes), or the distribution of responses for a particular item.

Right of Privacy   a moral and ethical issue in research and evaluation studies that raises a question about the appropriateness of studying private (as opposed to public) activities of subjects without their knowledge or consent.

Sampling Error   the difference between a population parameter and a statistic measured in a sample.

Scheduled Interviews   in survey research, interviews that occur at a scheduled time in a person's home, school, worksite, or other agreed upon setting.

Selected-response items   the type of items that enable test takers to choose answers to questions from an array of options (e.g., multiple-choice, true-false, or matching items).

Selection Bias the error introduced to a study when the persons comprising a sample do not represent the true population parameters, or are not representative of the population to whom the investigator wants to make inferences.

Self-report a form of measurement in which subjects are asked directly to report some attitude, past behavior, current practice, or anticipated future activity, possibly without benefit of corroborating or validating evidence.

Semantic Differential Scale a type of a multiple-point scale with bipolar adjectival endpoints (e.g., hot/cold, bad/good, etc.) usually used to measure subtle facets of an attitude.

Sensitivity the ability of a test or procedure to identify persons with a particular trait (such as a disease) correctly.

Sensitivity Analysis a series of calculations based on the projected variations in program costs and outcomes that influence a study's conclusions; different program results are estimated based on different health outcomes and economic costs.

Social Desirability Response Bias the type of bias that arises from respondents' conscious or unconscious attempt to provide answers or responses in what they deem to be a desired or preferred manner or direction.

Soft Data information of a subjective or anecdotal nature that may provide insights about a program, but whose validity is uncertain given the casual means usually associated with its collection.

Specificity the ability of a test or procedure to identify persons *not* having a particular trait (such as a disease) correctly.

Stability Reliability (see Test-Retest Reliability)

Stakeholders persons on whom a program impacts, and for whom the program's evaluation affects.

Standard Deviation a measure of dispersion (spread) that describes the variability of scores around the mean.

Standard Error of Measurement a measurement statistic that estimates the standard deviation of the distribution of measurement error around a person's *true score*.

Statistical Significance an observed relationship between variables that exceeds the probability of chance.

Strategic Planning the process used by an organization to make decisions that help shape and guide what the organization is, what it does, why it does it, and who its constituent groups are.

Summated Rating Scale a set of items that are approximately equal in attitude value to which subjects respond with levels of agreement or disagreement (e.g., a Likert scale).

Summative Evaluation the evaluation of the end products of a program (see also *impact evaluation* and *outcome evaluation*).

SWOT Analysis a process used by an organization to examine its *s*trengths, *w*eaknesses, *o*pportunities and *t*hreats.

Systems Analysis an evaluation model that examines both program *effectiveness* and program *efficiency*.

t-**test** a procedure that compares the mean scores of two groups to determine if they are statistically different.

Table of Random Numbers a table often found as an appendix of a statistics book, that provides a list of random numbers, and that facilitates the selection of a simple random sample, and some other probability sampling procedures.

Tactical Planning a process conducted by an organization that defines a "best practice" for meeting the objectives set out in its strategic plan, i.e., implementation of the strategic plan.

Test-Retest Reliability the extent to which a test or other measure's results are similar when administered or assessed at two or more points in time.

Total Quality Management an approach to program management that considers the views of all stakeholders, and not merely a top-down view of.

Transactional Evaluation an evaluation model that examines the way a program is viewed by various stakeholders.

True Experimental Design a design that employs random assignment of individual subjects to intervention and control (comparison) groups.

Triangulation an effort to measure a particular phenomenon using multiple methods, or by taking multiple measures, sometimes mixing quantitative and qualitative techniques, thereby increasing validity.

Triangulation of Evidence (see Triangulation)

Untreated Control Group a group not receiving a given intervention or treatment, but which is "serving" as a comparison for a group that *is* receiving treatment, or otherwise, some special consideration.

Validity the appropriateness, meaningfulness, and usefulness of the specific inferences made from test scores or other types of measures; the extent to which something measures what it purports to measure.

Value Scale a measure of a person's preference for objects of study, such as people, ideas, institutions, behaviors, and things; sometimes called an *attitude rating scale*.

Whistle-blower a role of ethical or moral stance or posture, assumed by an evaluator or other stakeholder, when it is perceived that a program, one or more of its components, or the evaluation itself, compromises truth, principles, justice, respect for individual rights or safety, or other ethical concerns.

Word-of-Mouth Procedures (see Interview Procedures)

Name Index

Butts, J.M. 145,153

C

Cahill, J. 157,180
Callahan, D. 320
Campbell, D.T. 203-204,208,223
Cannell, C. 229,240
Caravella, T. 150,153
Carmine, E.G. 132,153
Carey, R.G. 43,55,318,321
Carlson, J.M. 308
Carr, P. 188-189,201
Casey, R.J. 277,289
Centers for Disease Control and
    Prevention 6,18,99,150,153,190-
    191,196,201,250,279,287,315,335
Center for Health Statistics 298-
    299,308
Chambers, L.C. 84
Chassin, M. 234,240
Chavez, D. 232,240
Chavez, E.L. 17
Chen, W.W. 29
Chronicle of Higher Education 88
Clark, N. 8,19,104,129,333,337
Clark, T.A. 6,19
Cleary, S.D. 17
Clifford, D.L. 32-33,54
Cochran, D. 145,153
Cochran, W.G. 285,288
Colditz, G.A. 232,240,328,337
Collins, J.L. 93-94,103,279,288
Cook, T.D. 208,223
Copeland, L.A. 304-305,308
Copple, C. 121,128
Corbin, J. 237,242
Corle, D.K. 83
Corry, J.M. 236,240
Coscarelli, W.C.C. 124,129
Costa, S.J., Jr. 35,54
Council for Education in Public Health
    25
Cousins, M. 222
Craig, R.C. 119,129
Crask, M.R. 258,262

Cronbach, L.J. 139,153
Cronin, F.J. 230,241
Cummings, K.M. 83
Cutter, G. 8,19,104,129,333,337

D

Daniel, L.G. 146,154
Daniels, N. 311,314,321
Darr, K. 73,85
Davis, C.A. 230,241
Davis, R.M. 150,153
Deeds, S.G. 189,201
De Grande, L. 236,241
deHaven-Smith, L. 197-198,201
Delbecq, A.L. 234-235,242
Dennison, D. 25,30
Department of Health and Human
    Services 48,182,184,201
Desmond, S.M. 131,153
Detert, R.A. 160,178,180
DeVellis, R. 154
Devore, J. 291,300,308
Dickersin, K. 51
DiClemente, C.C. 308
Dignan, M. 188-189,201
Dillman, D.A. 248,253-254,260,262,
    266,285,288-289,324,337
Doak, C.C. 254,262
Doak, L.G. 254,262
D'Onofrio, C.N. 50,55,161,180,254,263
Dovring, K. 232,240
Drolet, J.C. 232,242
Drug Enforcement Administration 107
Duyff, R.L. 117,127-128

E

Easterbrook, S. 179
Ebel, R.L. 95-96,103,107-109,128,
    133,139,153
Ebert, R. 24
Eheart, B.K. 122,128
Ehrle, B.J. 232,240
Eisenberg, J.M. 313
Eisenhower, D.D. 197
Eisner, E. 7,18,23,30

Hardin, P.C. 176,180
Harokopos, V. 277,289
Harrell, J.S. 180,308
Harris, K. 221
Harris, W.A. 102
Harrison, R.C. 134,154
Hastad, D.N. 120,128
Hatziandreu, E.J. 150,153
Health Education 232
Healthy People 2000 92-94,182-186,192
Henderson, M.E. 111,115,118,128
Hendricks, M. 334,337
Henriksen, L. 287
Henry, J. 209
Hernandez, S.R. 10,18
Hiatt, R.A. 55
Higgins, C.W. 152
Historical Perspectives on School Health 231
Hoey, J. 84
Hoffman, C. 320
Hogelin, G.C. 250,262
Holcomb, D.R. 230,241
Holsti, O.R. 232,240
Hooper, J. 143,154
Hopkins, K.D. 108,128
Horowitz, S.M. 152
House, E.R. 5,7-8,18,21-22,
24,26,30,36,39,45,48,54

I

Illinois Behavioral Risk Factor
Surveillance System 196
Illinois Criminal Justice Information
Authority 196
Illinois Department of Employment
Security 196
Illinois Department of Health 192,195-196,201
Illinois Department of Public Aid 196
Illinois Department of Transportation
196
Illinois Environmental Protection
Agency 196

Illinois Health Care Cost Containment
Council 196
Illinois State Board of Education 196
Illinois State Police 196
Institute of Medicine 183
IPLAN 192,195-196
Isaac, S. 142,154,216,218,223,257,
259,263

J

Jackson, C. 287
Jacobs, L.C. 44,53,214,223
James, D.C.S. 230,240
Jatulis, D. 307
Jenkins, C.N.H. 55,180
Jobe, J.B. 99,103
Johnson, B.G. 232,240
Johnson, G. 151
Johnson, J. 179
Johnson, R.A. 127
Johnson, R.R. 32-33,54
Johnston, L.D. 98,103
Joiner, C.L. 10,18
Joint Commission on Accreditation of
Healthcare Organizations 84
Joint Committee on Standards 48,54
Jones, R.A. 42,54
Jonghoon, K. 258,262
Journal of Educational Psychology 232
Journal of School Health 232
*Journal of the American Medical
Association* 314

K

Kachigan, S.K. 291,300,305,308
Kahn, J.G. 317-318,320-321
Kahn, J.V. 44,54,214,223,232,240,276,
285,288,331,337
Kahn, R. 229,240
Kalsbeek, W.D. 250,262
Kamlet, M.S. 314,321
Kann, L. 93-94,102-103,279,288
Kaufman, N.J. 59,85,206,223
Kaufman, R. 186-187,201
Keller, K.L. 230,232,240,242

W

Waksberg, J. 249,263
Wallen, N.E. 218,223,225-226,228,240
Waller, P.F. 304,308
Warren, C.W. 94,102-103,279,288
Weber, R.P. 232,242
*Webster's Third New International
    Dictionary* 185,201
Weiler, R.W. 101
Weinstein, M.C. 311,314,316-317,321
Weiss, C.H. 39-40,42,55
Werch, C.E. 150,154,308
Westhoff, W.W. 17,230,241,277,289
White, G.B. 53,55
Williams, B.I. 94,103,279,288
Wills, T.A. 17
Windsor, R.A. 8,19,28,95,104,115,
    118,129,134,154,333,337
Winkleby, M.A. 307
Wisconsin Department of Health and
    Social Services 186,201
Wodraska, J.R. 197-198,201
Wolf, R.L. 24,30
Wolfe, S.A. 145,153
Wood, N.D. 154
Woodby, L. 28
Wortham, S.C. 122,129
Worthen, B.R. 3,19,32,34,55,203,223
Wright, D.A. 307
Wright, S.R. 210,223
Wright, W.R. 230,240
Wulfeck, W.H. 108,128,143,147,
    153-154

X Y Z

Yaremko, R.M. 134,154
Young, D.R. 222
Zanna, M.P. 83
Zeller, R.A. 132,153
Zieky, M.J. 124-125,128

Subject Index

A

academic evaluation 41
accidental sample 266-267
accreditation approach to evaluation 25
achievement tests 94
adversarial approach to evaluation 24-25
age-adjusted rates 297-298
age-specific rates 298
Age of Accountability 3,5
Age of Efficiency & Testing 3-4
Age of Expansion 3-5
Age of Innocence 3-4
Age of Professionalism 3,5
Age of Reform 3-4
Agency for Health Care Policy Research 315
alpha level 300
ambiguity of direction of causal influence 208
American Assembly 197
American Association for Health Education 25,43
American Bar Association 88
American Cancer Society 6,163-165,192
American Educational Research Association 48,48,53,99,103,132, 142-146,153
American Evaluation Association 5,48,53
American Institute of Public Opinion 244
American Medical Association 182
American Psychological Association 48,53,103,131-132,153
American Public Health Association 182,191
analysis of variance (ANOVA) 300, 302-303
Angoff's strategy for cut score determination 101,125
anonymity 44

APEX-PH 181,191-192,199
archival data 236-237
art criticism approach to evaluation 23-24
Association for the Advancement of Health Education 43,53-54
attitudinal inventories 94
autonomy 45-46

B

bar graphs for presenting data 329-330
behavior rating scales 119-120
behavioral anchor 118
behavioral data (from surveys) 246-247
behavioral inventories 94-95
Behavioral Risk Factor Surveillance System (BRFSS) 190
benchmarks toward goal achievement 183
beneficence 45-46
bimodal distribution 294
biomedical instruments 94-95
bivariate statistics 300-305
Black Like Me 228
Bogardus social distance scale 114
bogus-pipeline 150
Bryson's model of strategic planning 193-194
budgets 64-70,177,198

C

case studies (use in qualitative evaluation) 232-233
ceiling effects 208
central location intercept interviews 173,248,268-269
Centers for Disease Control and Prevention 6,18,99,150, 153,190-191,196,201,250,279, 287,315,335

extreme case sample 269

F

face-to-face interviews 247-248
factor analysis 305-306
factorial designs 218-220
fidelity 45-46
field studies 159
film ethnography 233
fish bowl sample 276
fixed price reimbursement 69-70
floor effects 208
focus group interviews 173-174,230-231,249
foils 108
forced-choice technique (see paired-comparison)
formative evaluation 10-11,226
frequency distributions 292

G

Gantt chart 74-75
generalizability from samples 265,285-286
geographic information systems 306
goal-free approach to evaluation 26
goal-oriented evaluations 21-22
GOAMs 73
government data (use in validity studies) 150
grab sample 268-269
graffiti 237
group interviews 248-249
Guttman scales 113

H

haphazard sample 266-267
hard data 327
hatchet evaluation 40
Hawthorne effect 211
Health Belief Model 92
Health Education 232
health-risk appraisals (HRAs) 94-95
Healthier People in Wisconsin 186

Healthy People 2000 92-94,182-186,192
high stakes tests 89
historical analysis 231
Historical Perspectives on School Health 231
home delivery interviews 248
homogeneous sample 269
hypothesis 214,300

I

Illinois Behavioral Risk Factor Surveillance System 196
Illinois Criminal Justice Information Authority 196
Illinois Department of Employment Security 196
Illinois Department of Health 192,195-196,201
Illinois Department of Public Aid 196
Illinois Department of Transportation 196
Illinois Environmental Protection Agency 196
Illinois Health Care Cost Containment Council 196
Illinois State Board of Education 196
Illinois State Police 196
imitation by a control group (see diffusion)
incidence rate 297,299
independent variable 214,292
in-depth interviewing 229
indirect costs in a budget 64,69,313
indirect rate (institutional charges) 64,69
individual interviews 172-173
inferential statistics 291
information gathering evaluation 41-42
informed consent 44
Institute of Medicine 183
institutional review boards (IRBs) 44,48-49
instructional quality inventory (IQI) 143

instrument development   95-101
instrument specifications   96-97
instrument types   94-95
instrumentation and internal validity
    205-206
intact groups   217,267
interaction effects of selection biases
    and treatment   207,210
internal evaluators   32-33
interval levels of measurement   91,304-
    305
interviews   115-116,172-173,229-
    231,247-250
IPLAN   192,195-196
item analysis   147-149
item sampling   281
item stem   108

J

John Henry effect   209
Joint Commission on Accreditation of
    Healthcare Organizations   84
Joint Committee on Standards   48,54
Journal of Educational Psychology
    232
Journal of School Health   232
*Journal of the American Medical
    Association*   314
judgmental sample   269-270
justice   45-46
            distributive   318

K

Kendall's tau   304-305
Kessner Index   197
key activity chart   73-74
kinesics   233-234
KR-20 and KR-21 used for internal
    consistency   111

L

least publishable units (LPUs)   41
lie scales   150-151
Likert scales   111-112

line graphs for presenting data   329,331
logical error   147

M

mailed surveys and questionnaires   250-
    259
matching items   109
matrix sample   280-282
maximum score   291,296
mean   291-292
measurement in health education
            attitudes   111-117
            behavior   117-120
            children as subjects   121-122
            error measures   132-133,208
            health-related physical fitness
                tests   120
            knowledge   106-111
            levels of   89-92
            medical tests   122-124
            problems related to   87-89,208
            setting cut scores   124-126
            standard error of measurement
                133
measures of central tendency   292-295
measures of dispersion   295-297
median   292
method effect (in surveys)   260
minimum score   291,296
mini-pilot   158
mode   292-293
Monthly Nutrition Companion   117
multi-matrix sampling   281-282
multiple-choice items   108-109
multiple regression   305
multivariate statistics   305-306

N

National Aeronautics and Space
    Administration (NASA)   14
National Association of College and
    University Business Officers   194
National Association of County Health
    Officials   191,201

National Cancer Institute 162-163,171-172,175,178,180,268,289

National Center for Health Statistics 196

National Council on Accreditation of Teacher Education 25

National Council on Measurement in Education 103,132,153

National Commission for Protection of Human Subjects of Biomedical and Behavioral Research 43

National Commission on Health Education Credentialing, Inc. 6,18

National Heart, Lung, and Blood Institute 230,241

National Institutes of Health 14,315

National Institute on Drug Abuse 6,94,107

naturalistic observations 228

needs assessment and strategic planning
    benchmarks 183
    budget linkage to planning 198
    data sources 194-198
    definition and purposes of 185-187
    planning models for 187-194

New England Journal of Medicine 232

nominal group process 234-235

nominal levels of measurement 90-91,301

non-experimental quantitative evaluation designs 212-214

nonmalficence 45-46

nonprobability sampling methods
    grab samples 268-269
    homogeneous samples 269
    judgmental samples 269
    quota samples 270-271
    samples of convenience 266-267
    snowball samples 270
    volunteer samples 267-268

nonrandomized pretest-posttest control group design 217

nonresponse bias 283-284

normal distribution 294-295

norm-referenced tests 94

North Central Association of Colleges and Secondary Schools 4

O

observation 118-119,121,236-237

observed score 132

observer as participant 228

observer bias 228

observer effect 228

odds ratio 300-302

Office of Substance Abuse and Prevention 73,85

Office on Smoking and Health 308,335

one-group pretest-posttest design 213

one-shot case study 212

ordinal levels of measurement 91,301, 304

overhead costs in a budget 64

oversampling 272

P

p value (see probability level; alpha level)

paired comparison technique 114

Panel on Cost-Effectiveness in Health and Medicine 314,316-319

participant-observer studies 228

passing score (see cut score)

PATCH 181,190-192

Pearson's r 304-305

periodicity in systematic samples 277

PERT 73

physical traces (as evidence) 236-237

Phi Delta Kappa 5

pie charts for presenting data 331-333

pilot testing
    budget 177
    computer-based instructional materials 176-177
    curricula 171-174
    data analysis procedures 169-171

telephone interviews 249-250
theater testing 174
Thurstone scale 112
time-series designs 219-220
total quality management (TQM) 10
transactional approach to evaluation 22
triangulation of evidence 95,237
true-false items 108-109
true score 132
Tylerian Age 3-4

U

univariate statistics 292-295
unobtrusive techniques 236-237
untreated control group 47
United States Congress 43
U.S. Bureau of the Census 196
U.S. Centers for Disease Control and
    Prevention (see Centers for Disease
    Control and Prevention)
U.S. Department of Agriculture 196
U.S. Department of Health and Human
    Services (see Department of Health
    and Human Services)
U.S. General Accounting Office 196
U.S. Health Care Financing
    Administration 196
U.S. Postal Service 259
U.S. Public Health Service 314-315

V

validity
        concurrent 144-146
        construct 146,306
        content 142-144
        convergent 146
        criterion-related 144-145
        discriminant 146
        external 204
                threats to 210-211
        face 141-142
        internal 204
                threats to 204-210
        methods of enhancing validity
        146-151

predictive 144-145
procedures for attitudinal items
    116-117
procedures for knowledge tests
    111
situational 140
value scale 113
visual anthropology 233
vital statistics 297-299
volunteer sample 267-268

W

Western Electric Company 211
whistle-blowing 48
Wisconsin Department of Health and
    Social Services 186,201
Word-of-mouth procedures 115

X Y Z

Youth Risk Behavior Surveillance
    System (YRBSS) 6,93-94

About the Authors

Robert J. McDermott received his Ph.D. from the University of Wisconsin-Madison. From 1981 to 1986, he was a faculty member in the Department of Health Education, at Southern Illinois University, Carbondale. Dr. McDermott came to the University of South Florida College of Public Health in 1986, and has been Chair of the Department of Community and Family Health, since 1993. He received the 1997 *Award for Research* of the American School Health Association's Research Council. Also, in 1997, he was one of just 38 professionals identified through nominations of peers to be a founding member of the American Academy for Health Behavior. The American Association for Health Education (AAHE) named him its *AAHE Scholar* for 1999, and he is a past recipient of the American Alliance for Health, Physical Education, Recreation and Dance's *Mabel Lee Award* for early career achievements. Among his other activities, Dr. McDermott has been a member of the Centers for Disease Control and Prevention's invited working group on defining *Health Education in the 21st Century*, Visiting Professor at the University of Cologne (Germany) and at the University of Freiburg (Germany), and consultant to the Centers for Disease Control and Prevention's, Division of Adolescent and School Health, for collaboration with the Russian Federation.

Paul D. Sarvela received his Ph.D. from the University of Michigan. Before joining the faculty of the Department of Health Education and Recreation at Southern Illinois University (SIU), Carbondale, in 1986, he was a program evaluator for Ford Aerospace. Since 1993, Dr. Sarvela has been Director of the Southern Illinois University Center for Rural Health and Social Services Development, and has held a joint appointment in the SIU School of Medicine's Department of Family and Community Medicine. His primary expertise is in the area of needs assessment and strategic planning for communities. He was the principal investigator for the *Illinois Project for Local Assessment of Needs*, a model of community assessment for public health needs assessment and planning. He is a founding member of the American Academy for Health Behavior and a past recipient of the American Alliance for Health, Physical Education, Recreation and Dance's *Mabel Lee Award* for early career achievements. He received the 1996 *Quality Service Award* for his commitment to health care improvement in rural Illinois. He is also a former American Council on Education (ACE) Fellow. Dr. Sarvela has been a Visiting Professor at the University of Cologne (Germany), and also has lectured in Finland.